Adrenal Imaging

KU-726-209

McARDLE LIBRARY

0151 604 7223

CONTEMPORARY MEDICAL IMAGING

U. Joseph Schoepf, MD, SERIES EDITOR

Adrenal Imaging, edited by *Michael A. Blake, MB, BCh, and Giles W.L. Boland, MD, 2009*
CT of the Airways, edited by *Phillip M. Boiselle, MD, and David A. Lynch, MB, 2008*

Adrenal Imaging

Edited by

Michael A. Blake, MB, BCh

Massachusetts General Hospital, Department of Radiology,
Boston, MA, USA

and

Giles W.L. Boland, MD

Massachusetts General Hospital, Department of Radiology,
Boston, MA, USA

JET LIBRARY

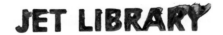 Humana Press

Editors
Michael A. Blake, MB, BCh
Massachusetts General Hospital
Dept. Radiology
55 Fruit St.
Boston, MA 02114
White Bldg.
USA
mblake2@partners.org

Giles W.L. Boland, MD
Massachusetts General Hospital
Dept. Radiology
55 Fruit St.
Boston, MA 02114
White Bldg.
USA
gboland@partners.org

Series Editor
U. Joseph Schoepf, MD
Department of Radiology
Medical University of South Carolina
Charleston, SC

ISBN: 978-1-934115-86-2   e-ISBN: 978-1-59745-560-2

DOI 10.1007/978-1-59745-560-2

Library of Congress Control Number: 2008940633

© Humana Press, a part of Springer Science+Business Media, LLC 2009
All rights reserved. This work may not be translated or copied in whole or in part without the written permission of the publisher (Humana Press, 999 Riverview Drive, Suite 208, Totowa, NJ 07512 USA), except for brief excerpts in connection with reviews or scholarly analysis. Use in connection with any form of information storage and retrieval, electronic adaptation, computer software, or by similar or dissimilar methodology now known or hereafter developed is forbidden.
The use in this publication of trade names, trademarks, service marks, and similar terms, even if they are not identified as such, is not to be taken as an expression of opinion as to whether or not they are subject to proprietary rights.
While the advice and information in this book are believed to be true and accurate at the date of going to press, neither the authors nor the editors nor the publisher can accept any legal responsibility for any errors or omissions that may be made. The publisher makes no warranty, express or implied, with respect to the material contained herein.

Printed on acid-free paper

9 8 7 6 5 4 3 2 1

springer.com

The small size of the adrenal gland belies its critical importance in medicine. Imaging of the adrenal gland has made tremendous strides in the last decade as new technologies continue to evolve. Consequently, we feel that it is an opportune time to distill, for the first time, the current state of knowledge available concerning imaging of the adrenal gland, into a single volume. In order for this text to offer widespread appeal and for completeness, we also considered it important to solicit current adrenal insights from medical disciplines other than imaging experts. These contributions are designed to be both independent (i.e. can be read on their own) and also be complementary to the remainder of the chapters. To allow this independence, specific information has been re-emphasized across different chapters according to the individual authors' different perspectives. We thus hope that the individual chapters and the complete text will serve as relevant and up-to-date references of adrenal gland imaging for both radiologists and non-radiologists (particularly oncologists, surgeons and endocrinologists), and will be helpful to physicians in practice and in training, and indeed to all interested in the adrenal glands.

We have tried to highlight the pertinent clinical and pathological information that underpins the accurate interpretation and use of adrenal imaging. Established adrenal imaging findings, algorithms and techniques in CT, MR, nuclear medicine, PET and PET/CT, as well as intervention and trauma, are reviewed. We chose to put the adrenal pathology chapter first as it provides a basis for the rest of the book serving as a comprehensive overview of the diseases that can effect the adrenal gland. We chose to place summary sections at the end of each of the other chapters, illuminating their key teaching points to enhance their retention.

We were also very fortunate to have been joined on this project by such a prestigious group of international contributors for whose support we are very grateful. Drs Ronald DeLellis and Sham Mangray give the overview of adrenal embryology and pathology in the first chapter. The pivotal adrenal role in endocrinology is highlighted by both Drs Subbulaxmi Trikudanathan and Robert Dluhy who cover adrenal cortical dysfunction, and also by Dr William Young who writes on adrenal medullary dysfunction. The important adrenal role in oncology from endocrinology, radiation oncology and radiology viewpoints is supplied by the collaboration of Drs Claire Higham, Peter Trainer, John Coen and Giles Boland. Adrenal surgeons Drs Antonia Stephen, Alex Haynes and Rich Hodin contribute a chapter from the adrenal surgeon's point of view. The imaging of adrenal hyperfunction and pheochromocytoma is then described by Drs Sahdev Anju and Rodney Reznek and Drs Eric Remer and Frank Millar respectively. The team of Drs Mel Korobkin, Mahmoud Al-Hawary and Isaac Francis demonstrate how to use CT to differentiate adrenal adenomas and metastases. Dr Phil Kenney gives an overview of adrenal MRI while Drs Jim Scott and Ted Palmer give their insight into adrenal nuclear medicine. Dr Johannes Roedl discusses with us the still emerging role of PET and PET/CT of the adrenals. Dr Brian Lucey shares his experience with adrenal intervention and trauma. To conclude the book, we look into the future with Dr Nagaraj Holalkere, who highlights new developments in adrenal imaging.

We are very grateful to our world-renowned adrenal experts whose contributions have made this a practical, well-illustrated, and authoritative text. We are most thankful to Springer and Humana for giving us this opportunity and for all their support and, in particular, to Yana Mermel and Paul Dolgert.

Boston, USA   Michael A. Blake
                                                                Giles W.L. Boland

Contents

Contributors

Mahmoud M. Al-Hawary, MD, Department of Radiology, University of Michigan Hospitals, Ann Arbor, Michigan

Michael A. Blake, MB, BCh, BAO, MRCPI, BSc, FRCR, FFR (RCSI), Division of Abdominal Imaging and Intervention, Department of Radiology, Massachusetts General Hospital, Boston, MA

Giles W.L. Boland, MD, Division of Abdominal Imaging and Intervention, Department of Radiology, Massachusetts General Hospital, Boston, MA

John J. Coen, MD, Department of Radiation Oncology, Massachusetts General Hospital Boston, MA

Ronald A. DeLellis, MD, Department of Pathology, Rhode Island Hospital and The Miriam Hospital, The Warren Alpert Medical School of Brown University, Providence, R.I.

Robert G. Dluhy, MD, Endocrine-Hypertension Division, Brigham and Women's Hospital, Boston, MA

Isaac R. Francis, MD, Department of Radiology, University of Michigan Hospitals, Ann Arbor, Michigan

Alex B. Haynes, MD, Division of General Surgery, Massachusetts General Hospital, Boston, MA

Claire E. Higham, DPhil, Department of Endocrinology, Christie Hospital, Manchester, UK

Richard A. Hodin, MD, Division of General Surgery, Massachusetts General Hospital, Boston, MA

Nagaraj Setty Holalkere, MD, DNB, Department of Radiology, Boston Medical Centre, Boston, MA

Philip J. Kenney, MD, Department of Diagnostic Radiology, University of Alabama at Birmingham, Birmingham, AL

Melvyn Korobkin, MD, Department of Radiology, University of Michigan Hospitals, Ann Arbor, Michigan

Brian C. Lucey, MB, BCh, BAO, MRCPI, FFR (RCSI), Department of Radiology, VA Healthcare System, West Roxbury, MA

Shamlal Mangray, MB, BS, Department of Pathology, Rhode Island Hospital and The Miriam Hospital, The Warren Alpert Medical School of Brown University, Providence, R.I.

Frank H. Miller, MD, Department of Radiology, Northwestern University Feinberg School of Medicine, Chicago, IL

Edwin L. Palmer III, MD, Division of Nuclear Medicine, Department of Radiology, Massachusetts General Hospital, Boston, Massachusetts

Erick M. Remer, MD, Section of Abdominal Imaging, Division of Diagnostic Radiology, Cleveland Clinic, Cleveland, OH

Rodney H. Reznek FRANZCR (Hon), FRCP, FRCR, Cancer Imaging, Institute of Cancer, St Bartholomew's Hospital, West Smithfield, London, UK

Johannes B. Roedl, MD, Department of Radiology, Massachusetts General Hospital, Boston, MA

Anju Sahdev, MB, BS, MRCP, FRCR, Department of Diagnostic Imaging, St Bartholomew's Hospital, West Smithfield, London, UK

James A. Scott, MD, Division of Nuclear Medicine, Department of Radiology, Massachusetts General Hospital, Boston, Massachusetts

Antonia E. Stephen, MD, Division of Surgical Oncology, Massachusetts General Hospital Cancer Center, Boston, MA

Peter J. Trainer, MD, FRCP, Department of Endocrinology, Christie Hospital, Manchester, UK

Subbulaxmi Trikudanathan, MD, Department of Medicine, St Elizabeth's Medical Center, Boston, Massachusetts

William F. Young Jr, MD, Division of Endocrinology, Diabetes, Metabolism, Nutrition and Internal Medicine, Mayo Clinic Rochester, Rochester, MN

Adrenal Embryology and Pathology

1

Shamlal Mangray and Ronald A. DeLellis

Contents

S. Mangray (✉)
Attending Pathologist, Rhode Island Hospital
and The Miriam Hospital, The Warren Alpert Medical
School of Brown University, Providence, R.I. 02903
E-mail: SMangray@Lifespan.org

Introduction

The adrenal glands are composite endocrine organs consisting of the steroid hormone producing cortex and the catecholamine synthesizing medulla. Each of these compartments can give rise to a variety of proliferative lesions that can be visualized by computed tomography (CT), magnetic resonance imaging (MRI) or positron emission tomography (PET). The increased use of these modalities has demonstrated the presence of varying sized mass lesions in up to 5% of individuals subjected to CT studies for reasons unrelated to adrenal dysfunction [1]. Most of these incidentally discovered lesions (incidentalomas) are asymptomatic and the vast majority are of cortical origin.

The specific goals of this chapter are to provide an overview of the anatomy and development of the adrenal glands together with a review of the pathological features of a variety of adrenal abnormalities presenting as mass lesions with or without endocrine hyperfunction. In addition, this chapter will review adrenal abnormalities associated with hypofunctional states.

Embryology and Developmental Disorders of the Adrenal Glands

The adrenal glands have a dual embryological origin with the cortex being derived from the celomic mesoderm of the urogenital ridge and the medulla arising

M.A. Blake, G. Boland (eds.), *Adrenal Imaging*, DOI 10.1007/978-1-59745-560-2_1,
© 2009 Humana Press, a part of Springer Science+Business Media, LLC

from the neural crest [2]. In the 5th week of gestation (9-mm embryo stage), mesothelial cells from the posterior abdominal wall, between the root of the bowel mesentery and developing mesonephros/gonad (urogenital ridge), proliferate and form the primitive cortex of the adrenal gland [3]. In the 6th week, a second wave of mesothelial cells surrounds the primitive cortex. By 8 weeks, the cortical cells separate from the mesothelium and become surrounded by a fibrous capsule. In the fetus, the cortex is divisible into a broad inner zone composed of large eosinophilic cells (provisional zone or fetal cortex) and an outer zone that is destined to become the adult (definitive) cortex. The major secretory product of the fetal cortex is dehydroepiandrosterone sulfate, reflecting its importance in the development of the genital system during gestation, whereas the cells of the adult cortex produce cortisol, aldosterone and sex steroids.

The combined weight of the glands at birth is approximately 10 g, with 75% of the cortical volume represented by fetal cortex. At this time the adrenal glands are 10–20 times larger than adult glands relative to body weight and approximately one third the size of the neonatal kidney. Shortly thereafter, a series of involutional changes occurs associated with an approximate 50% reduction in the gland weight [3, 4]. Much of the fetal cortex involutes while the permanent cortex proliferates toward the center of the gland. As a result, the fetal cortex accounts for 20% of cortical volume by the 12th postgestational week.

The intra- and extra-adrenal paraganglia and the sympathetic nervous system are intimately associated during embryonic development and arise from the neural crest. The cortical anlage is invaded on its medial aspect by primitive sympathetic cells and nerve fibers that originate from the contiguous prevertebral and paravertebral sympathetic tissue in the 14-mm embryo (about 7 weeks of gestation). Some primitive sympathetic cells, however, may penetrate the anlage without associated nerve fibers [5, 6]. The primitive sympathetic cells are first apparent as nodular aggregates in the cortex, where they may form rosettes or pseudorosettes. Chromaffin cells (mature medullary cells) are identifiable among the primitive sympathetic cells between the 27- and 33-mm stages and gradually increase in number. The nodules of primitive sympathetic cells peak in number and size between 17 and 20 weeks and

then decline. Groups of primitive cells may, however, persist until birth and may also be apparent in early infancy (see section on neuroblastoma). In the fetus, the extraadrenal chromaffin cells account for most of the chromaffin tissue and are most prominent in the organ of Zuckerkandl in the region proximal to the aortic bifurcation, where they are identifiable grossly [7]. There is a progressive involution of the extraadrenal chromaffin cells while the medullary chromaffin cells reach maximum volume at birth.

The eventual shape of the adrenal glands is affected by the development of the kidneys and gonads. The gonadal component of the urogenital ridge is located medial to the mesonephros. The gonads descend caudally, the mesonephros becomes largely involuted and the kidneys are derived predominantly from the metanephros of the pelvis migrating cephalad to lie eventually inferolateral to the adrenal glands [2, 3]. The ultimate pyramidal or crescent shape of the adrenal glands is dependent on the normal development and migration of the kidneys as is demonstrated by the flattened appearance of the adrenal glands in cases of renal agenesis.

The most common congenital anomaly of the adrenal is *heterotopia* [8]. Although the term "heterotopia" is commonly used for this condition, a more accurate description is *accessory* adrenal tissue since in most cases orthotopic adrenal gland is also present. Most accessory adrenals consist exclusively of cortical tissue, but a few examples, particularly those in the region of the celiac ganglion, may also contain medulla [7]. Accessory adrenal cortex is most frequently found in the retroperitoneal space along the course of the urogenital ridges. In addition, accessory adrenal tissue may also be discovered incidentally just beneath the renal capsule in the upper pole, at the hilar regions of the ovaries and testes, and along the course of the spermatic cord. The studies of MacLennan [9] have shown that adrenal cortical tissue is present in approximately 1% of inguinal hernia sacs from children undergoing inguinal herniorrhaphy. Rare sites of accessory adrenal tissue include pancreas, spleen, liver, mesentery, lung and brain. Accessory adrenals may undergo hyperplasia in response to increased levels of ACTH and may serve as the site of origin of cortical neoplasms [7, 10]. True heterotopic adrenals may be fused with the liver or kidney and are typically surrounded by a common connective tissue capsule [11, 12].

Adrenal *union (fusion)* and adhesion are rare anomalies that are distinguished respectively by the presence (adrenal union) or absence (adhesion) of a connective tissue capsule. Fusion is occasionally associated with midline congenital defects, including spinal dysraphism, indeterminate visceral situs, and the Cornelia de Lange syndrome [7]. Fusion of the adrenals can occur in patients with bilateral renal agenesis.

Aplasia of the adrenals has been reported in association with anencephaly; however, in most instances, the adrenals are markedly hypoplastic rather than completely absent. In approximately 10% of patients with unilateral renal agenesis, the ipsilateral adrenal is also absent. Several types of adrenal hypoplasia have been reported. Affected infants typically show signs and symptoms of adrenal insufficiency. In so-called primary hypoplasia, the adult cortex is markedly hypoplastic, but the fetal zone is retained and often demonstrates cytomegalic features [12]. This disorder has an X-linked pattern of inheritance and is associated with mutations or deletions of the DAX-1 gene (Xp21) [13, 14]. The miniature adult type of hypoplasia may appear sporadically or as an inherited abnormality with an autosomal recessive pattern of inheritance. The adrenals have a normal architecture despite their small size.

Gross and Microscopic Anatomy of the Adrenal Glands

In the normal adult, each gland weighs between 4 and 5 g, although greater weights have been recorded in hospitalized patients dying after prolonged illnesses presumably due to prolonged stimulation by endogenous ACTH [7]. Adrenals from patients treated with prolonged corticosteroid administration, on the other hand, are atrophic. Each normal adrenal measures approximately $5 \times 3 \times 1$ cm. The right gland has a roughly pyramidal shape, while the left gland has a crescent shape (Fig. 1.1). The glands have a tripartite structure that consists of head (medial), body (middle), and tail (lateral) portions [7]. The central vein emerges from the ventral aspect of the gland at the junction of the head and body (Fig. 1.1B). Within the gland itself, the muscle bundles of the central vein are eccentric and are oriented toward the medulla.

In the fresh state, the outer cortex is bright yellow, while the inner cortical zone is brown to tan. The cortex measures approximately 1 mm in thickness in adults and comprises approximately 90% of the total glandular weight. It consists of the glomerulosa, fasciculata, and reticularis zones [6]. The glomerulosa comprises up to 15% of the cortical volume and is composed of relatively small lipid-poor cells (Fig. 1.2A), which synthesize mineralocorticoids. Since this layer is often incomplete, the fasciculata may abut the capsule of the gland directly. The fasciculata is composed of columns of lipid-rich cells, which synthesize both glucocorticoids and sex steroids. This zone occupies 70%–80% of the cortical volume. Stimulation of the adrenal by adrenocorticotropic hormone (ACTH) leads to depletion of lipid stores from the fasciculata [12]. The remainder of the cortex is composed of the reticularis, which is capable of synthesis of both glucocorticoids and sex steroids. These cells are characterized by eosinophilic cytoplasm, scanty lipid vacuoles, and prominent deposits of lipochrome pigment, which are responsible for the brown color of the reticularis. Adrenal cortical cells demonstrate positive immunohistochemical staining with antibodies to the intermediate filament proteins vimentin and cytokeratin, and the steroid cell markers inhibin and calretinin. In addition, cortical cells are positive with the monoclonal antibody, A103 (*melan-A*).

On microscopic examination cortical extrusions are found frequently in association with the adrenal glands of adults. They are characterized by the presence of nodular groups of cortical cells that extend into the peri-adrenal fat. Typically, they are attached to the adjacent cortex by a small pedicle and are surrounded by a fibrous capsule; however, they may be completely separated from the gland in some instances.

In the adult, the adrenal medulla occupies 8%–10% of the gland volume and has an average weight of 0.44 g [7]. The major portion of the medulla lies within the head of the gland (*medial*), while the body of the gland contains medullary cells within its crest and usually within one alar region [7]. The average corticomedullary ratio is 5:1 in the head of the gland and 14.7:1 in the body. The tail (*lateral*) of the adrenal does not normally contain medullary tissue. An understanding of the normal distribution of the medulla is essential for the recognition of the early phase of adrenal medullary hyperplasia.

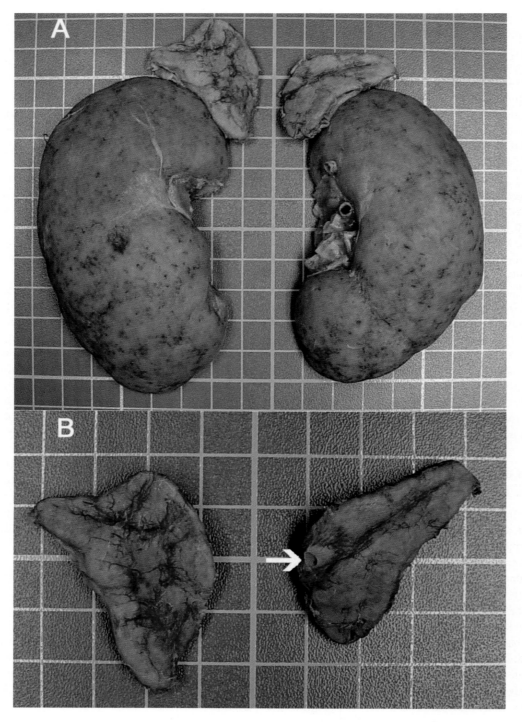

Fig. 1.1 Normal relationship of adrenals to kidneys (autopsy specimen). The adrenal glands are located superiorly and medially to the kidneys (A). Close up view of the adrenal glands with the head located medially and tail located laterally (B). The adrenal central vein is easily seen in the left gland (*arrow*)

Fig. 1.2 Microscopic section demonstrating the layers of the adrenal cortex. The *zona glomerulosa* (ZG) is present just beneath the capsule, the clear cell containing *zona fasciculata* (ZF) occupies an intermediate position and the *zona reticularis* (ZR) is present in the lowest portion of the figure (A). The medulla (B) is composed of large cells with basophilic cytoplasm and large nuclei that demonstrate variation in size and shape. Sustentacular cells have spindle shaped nuclei (*arrows*). A few cells from the *zona reticularis* are present in the lowest portion of the field

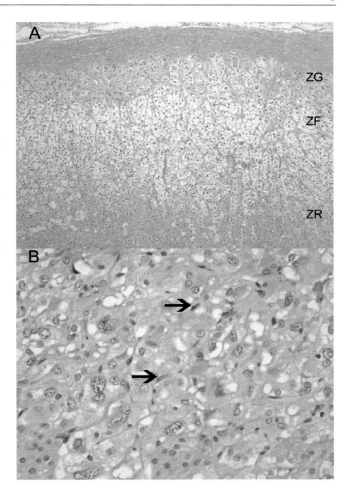

Medullary cells are typically arranged in small nests and cords that are separated by a rich capillary network (Fig. 1.2B). A few ganglion cells are present within the medulla either as single cells or small cell clusters. Sustentacular *or supporting* cells are present at the peripheries of the medullary cords and nests and are also evident around the ganglion cells. In current pathology practice, immunohistochemical stains can be used to demonstrate the component cells of the adrenal medulla. The most commonly utilized antibodies are the neuroendocrine markers chromogranin and synaptophysin that stain the cytoplasm of the medullary cells while the S-100 protein antibody stains the sustentacular cells.

The medulla contains both norepinephrine and epinephrine in addition to their biosynthetic intermediaries. The major catecholamine product of the medulla is epinephrine, which affects the activities of a wide variety of cells and tissues following its interactions with specific receptors. The extra-adrenal sympathetic paraganglia are identical morphologically and histochemically to the adrenal medulla.

Hyperplastic Disorders

Cortical Hyperplasia

Hyperplasia of the adrenal cortex, which represents an increased cortical mass resulting from stimulation of the cortex by ACTH derived from the pituitary or from a variety of extrapituitary sources, can be associated with a wide variety of clinical syndromes. Cortical hyperplasia can also selectively involve the zona glomerulosa in patients with idiopathic hyperaldosteronism.

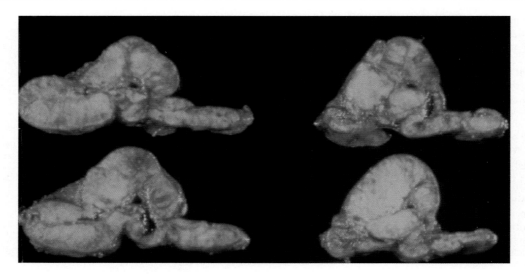

Fig. 1.3 Diffuse and nodular hyperplasia of the cortex

Pituitary/Hypothalamic-based Hyperplasia (Cushing's Disease)

Hyperplasia may be the result of stimulation of the adrenal glands by ACTH-producing pituitary adenomas or of hypothalamic stimulation of the pituitary ACTH cells by corticotropin releasing hormone (CRH) [15–17]. Basophilic pituitary adenomas were originally observed in association with hypercortisolism by Harvey Cushing in 1932, and this association has been termed Cushing's disease or ACTH-dependent Cushing's syndrome. Many pituitary tumors associated with Cushing's syndrome are microadenomas, measuring less than 1 cm.

Cortical hyperplasia in patients with ACTH-dependent Cushing's syndrome can be either diffuse or nodular, and combinations of diffuse and nodular hyperplasia are common. In diffuse hyperplasia, gland weights may be increased only slightly [12]. In more advanced cases, the combined average weight varies between 12 and 24 g. The glands have rounded contours rather than the sharp outlines typical of normal glands. The inner portion of the cortex is widened and often appears pale brown or tan. The outer layers of the cortex are typically yellow. On microscopy, the inner brown zone corresponds to lipid-depleted cells of the fasciculata, whereas the cells of the outer cortex are more characteristically vacuolated [18]. The glomerulosa in adults with Cushing's disease is often difficult to identify, but in children the glomerulosa may also appear slightly hyperplastic [19].

In some cases, the cortex may appear nodular with individual nodules measuring less than 0.5 cm or 1.0 cm in diameter, depending on relatively arbitrary criteria used by different authors [7]. This type of change has been referred to as diffuse and micronodular hyperplasia. If the nodules exceed 1 cm in diameter, the hyperplasia is defined as diffuse and macronodular.

In diffuse and nodular (micro- or macro-) hyperplasia, multiple cortical nodules are superimposed upon a diffusely hyperplastic cortex (Fig. 1.3). Formation of nodules is often asymmetric, and while one adrenal may show diffuse and nodular cortical hyperplasia, the contralateral adrenal may appear diffusely hyperplastic. The nodules are often composed of admixtures of clear- and compact-type cells. In contrast to the atrophic cortex adjacent to a functioning adenoma, the cortex between or adjacent to the nodules in nodular hyperplasia is diffusely hyperplastic.

Cortical Hyperplasia Associated with Ectopic Production of Adrenocorticotropic Hormone or Corticotropin-releasing Hormone

Hyperplasia can be found in association with a variety of neoplasms producing ACTH or CRH [17]. In most series, bronchial carcinoids and small-cell carcinomas account for the majority of cases. Other tumors associated with the ectopic ACTH syndrome include pancreatic endocrine neoplasms, medullary thyroid carcinoma, thymic carcinoids, and pheochromocytomas. In patients with the ectopic ACTH syndrome associated with bronchogenic small-cell carcinoma or other tumors, the adrenals are usually larger (average combined weight of 20–30 g) than those seen in association with diffuse hyperplasia stemming from pituitary ACTH overproduction. The cortex is diffusely hyperplastic and appears tan-brown throughout its width. On microscopy, there is evidence of diffuse hyperplasia of the fasciculata cells, which are characterized by a compact or lipid-depleted appearance [20]. Both bronchial carcinoids and small cell bronchogenic carcinomas may also produce CRH ectopically. Exceptionally, secretion of both ACTH and CRH from a single tumor has been documented [21].

Cortical Hyperplasia Associated with Hyperaldosteronism

Primary hyperaldosteronism is characterized by the excessive secretion of aldosterone from the adrenal glands and is associated with suppression of plasma renin activity with resultant hypokalemia and hypertension. At least six subtypes of primary hyperaldosteronism have been recognized, including aldosterone-producing adenoma, idiopathic hyperaldosteronism, primary adrenal hyperplasia, aldosterone-producing adrenal cortical carcinoma, aldosterone-producing ovarian tumor, and familial hyperaldosteronism (FH) [17]. FH is subdivided into two groups: FH-I (glucocorticoid-remediable hyperaldosteronism) and FH-II (aldosterone-producing adenoma and idiopathic hyperaldosteronism). FH-I is linked to a defect in a hybrid gene at chromosome 8q24 while FH-II has been linked to chromosome 7p22 [22].

Primary hyperaldosteronism is most often associated with adrenal cortical adenomas; however, in approximately 40% of cases the only apparent adrenal abnormality is hyperplasia of the cortex with or without the formation of micronodules [7, 12, 23]. Less commonly macronodular glands are present with nodules ranging from 0.25 to 1.0 cm, and in rare instances up to 3.0 cm [17]. Generally, biochemical abnormalities in patients with hyperplasia are less severe than in those with adenomas. On histologic examination, hyperplasia of the glomerulosa is characterized by thickening of this cell layer, with tongue-like projections of the glomerulosa extending toward the fasciculata. Micronodules, when present, are usually composed of clear fasciculata-type cells [10] and are thought to be a consequence of the associated hypertension. In about 10% of cases, it may not be possible to distinguish such a micronodule from a true adenoma associated with aldosterone production.

Macronodular Hyperplasia (Massive Macronodular Adrenal Cortical Disease)

In macronodular hyperplasia with marked adrenal enlargement, the adrenals together may weigh up to 200 g, and individual nodules may measure up to 4.0 cm in diameter [13, 17]. Because of the very large size of the glands and confluence of adjacent nodules, the resected adrenals may be mistaken for neoplasms. Macronodular hyperplasia is ACTH independent, and this entity can (rarely) involve a single gland [12]. The cortex between the nodules is often atrophic, as might be expected in an ACTH independent process. This entity, which has also been referred to as massive macronodular adrenal cortical disease (MMAD), has a bimodal age distribution. A small proportion of patients may present during the first year of life and this form of the disease may be associated with the McCune-Albright syndrome. Most of the patients present clinically in the fifth decade with a male to female ratio of 1:1. Rare examples of familial MMAD have also been reported. This disorder has been associated with aberrant expression and regulation of various G-protein coupled receptors [24].

Primary Pigmented Nodular Adrenocortical Disease—Microadenomatous Hyperplasia of the Adrenal

Primary pigmented nodular adrenocortical disease (PPNAD), a rare disorder, is characterized by the presence of multiple pigmented nodules of cortical cells with intervening atrophic cortical tissue usually seen in association with features of ACTH-independent Cushing's syndrome [17, 25]. The glands may be either smaller than normal or enlarged. Individual nodules, which can vary in color from gray to black, typically measure from 1 to 3 mm in diameter, although larger nodules measuring up to 3 cm in diameter may also be evident [7]. The nodules are composed of large, granular eosinophilic cells that often contain enlarged

Table 1.1 Inherited tumor syndromes associated with adrenal neoplasms

Tumor Type/Syndrome	Extra-Adrenal Features	Gene(s)
Adrenocortical tumors and neuroblastic tumors		
Beckwith-Wiedemann	Exomphalos, macroglossia, pancreatic islet cell hyperplasia, gigantism/hemihypertrophy, Wilms tumor, hepatoblastoma, pancreaticoblastoma	*CDKN1/NSD1, KCNQ1, KCNQ1OT1 (domain 2); IGF2 and H19 (domain 1)*
Adrenocortical tumors		
Li-Fraumeni syndrome (cortical carcinoma)	Other neoplasms/cancers	*TP53*
Carney complex (PPNAD)	Lentigines and other pigmented skin lesions, myxomas, LCCST of testis, pituitary adenoma	*PRKAR1A*
MEN 1 (Wermer's syndrome) (cortical adenoma)	Endocrine lesions of parathyroid, pituitary, pancreas, GI tract; skin lesions	*MEN1*
Pheochromocytomas		
Von Hippel-Lindau disease	Retinal and cranial hemangioblastoma, RCC, cysts of multiple organs, pancreatic endocrine tumors, ELST of ear	*VHL*
Pheochromocytoma-paraganglioma	Paraganglioma of abdomen, thorax, head and neck	*SDHD, SDHC, SDHB*
MEN 2A (Sipple syndrome)	1° hyperparathyroidism (hyperplasia), MTC	*RET*
MEN 2B	Mucosal neuromas, ganglioneuromatosis of intestine, marfanoid habitus, MTC, corneal nerve lesions	*RET*
Neurofibromatosis type 1	Café au lait macules, neurofibromas or plexiform neurofibroma, optic glioma, axillary or inguinal freckling, Lisch nodules, osseous lesions	*NF1*

MEN multiple endocrine neoplasia; RCC renal cell carcinoma, MTC medullary thyroid carcinoma; GI gastrointestinal; ELST endolymphatic sac tumors; LCCST large cell calcifying Sertoli cell tumor; PPNAD primary pigmented nodular adrenocortical disease

hyperchromatic nuclei with prominent nucleoli. Because of the atypical nuclear features, this entity has also been referred to as micronodular dysplasia. The cells are generally filled with lipochrome pigment, which is responsible for their dark color on gross examination.

The origin of PPNAD is unknown, although some studies suggested an autoimmune etiology [26]. PPNAD arises sporadically or in a familial form that can be associated with Carney's complex (CNC), which includes cardiac myxomas, spotty pigmentation, neurofibromatosis, testicular Leydig or Sertoli cell tumors, mammary myxoid fibroadenomas, and cerebral hemangiomas [17, 27] (Table 1.1). CNC may occur sporadically or may be inherited as an autosomal dominant trait. The responsible genes have been mapped by linkage analysis to loci at 2p16 and 17q22-24. Other loci have also been implicated in the development of this syndrome. The gene encoding the protein kinase A (PKA) type Iα regulatory subunit PRKAR1A has been mapped to 17q22-24 and

LOH studies from patients with CNC have revealed mutations in this gene in approximately 50% of affected individuals. No mutations were found on 2p16. Studies of sporadic and isolated cases of CNC have also revealed inactivating mutations of PRKAR1A. The wild type alleles could be inactivated by somatic mutations consistent with the hypothesis that the gene belongs to the tumor suppression class [28, 29].

Other Types of Adrenal Hyperplasia

The entity of congenital adrenal hyperplasia is discussed in the section on metabolic disorders while the subject of adrenal medullary hyperplasia is discussed in the context of familial pheochromocytoma.

Adrenal Neoplasms

Most adrenal neoplasms occur as sporadic or nonsyndromic tumors; however, some may be associated with heritable disorders. Inherited syndromes with an increased predisposition to developing adrenal cortical or medullary tumors include Beckwith-Wiedemann syndrome, Li-Fraumeni syndrome, Carney complex, multiple endocrine neoplasia (MEN) types 1, 2A and 2B, familial pheochromocytoma-paraganglioma, neurofibromatosis type 1 and von Hippel-Lindau disease (Table 1.1). While the manifestations of most syndromes more commonly occur later in life, characteristic features of macroglossia, prenatal and postnatal overgrowth (gigantism/hemihyperplasia), abdominal wall defects (exomphalos) and pancreatic islet cell hyperplasia leading to hypoglycemia permit early recognition of Beckwith-Wiedemann syndrome. The adrenal glands are typically hyperplastic and contain numerous cytomegalic cells [13, 17]. Hemorrhagic adrenal cortical macrocysts may also be found [30]. Patients with Beckwith-Wiedemann syndrome are predisposed to the development of malignant tumors such as Wilms tumor, adrenocortical carcinoma, neuroblastoma, hepatoblastoma and pancreaticoblastoma [7, 30]. Benign adrenal cortical adenomas and ganglioneuromas have also been reported [30]. An autosomal dominant inheritance is well established in Beckwith-Wiedemann syndrome, but approximately 85% of cases are actually sporadic. The molecular basis of this syndrome is complex and involves downregulation of imprinted genes within the chromosome 11p15 region (IGF2 and H19 at domain 1; CDKN1C, KCNQ1 and KCNQ1OT1 at domain 2) [30]. Unlike Beckwith-Wiedemann syndrome, which predisposes to both cortical and medullary tumors, the other syndromes give rise to either cortical or medullary tumors. Of note, the manifestations of MEN 2B, which include oral, ocular and gastrointestinal ganglioneuromatosis associated with a Marfanoid habitus, may also be present at birth or early infancy.

Cortical Adenomas

Cortical adenomas are a functionally heterogeneous group of benign neoplasms that can arise from any of the cortical layers [7, 31]. These tumors can be associated with the overproduction of glucocorticoids (Cushing's syndrome), androgenic or estrogenic steroids (adrenogenital syndrome), or mineralocorticoids (Conn's syndrome). Mixed syndromes can develop, and cortical adenomas without apparent functional activity are common.

Nonfunctional Cortical Adenomas and Cortical Nodules

Cortical nodules are common findings in patients without clinical or biochemical evidence of steroid hormone hypersecretion [7]. Autopsy studies have revealed cortical nodules in approximately 25% of individuals. These nodules are also commonly detected with abdominal computed tomography (CT) and magnetic resonance imaging (MRI) scans and have been grouped among the lesions classified as "incidentalomas". Although cortical nodules are commonly multicentric and bilateral, single nodules measuring up to 2–3 cm in diameter may be evident. Smaller nodules are often nonencapsulated, whereas larger single nodules may be surrounded by a fibrous capsule. The nodules are bright yellow with foci of brownish discoloration and are composed of fasciculata-type cells predominantly. Occasionally, foci of myelolipomatous change or ossification may be evident within the nodules. In contrast to functional adenomas associated with glucocorticoid production, the cortex adjacent to nonfunctional nodules is not atrophic.

Cortical nodules are most frequently encountered in the adrenals of elderly individuals or in patients with essential hypertension or diabetes mellitus. The studies of Dobbie have suggested that nodules represent foci of compensatory cortical hyperplasia that have developed in response to focal atrophy of the cortex induced by narrowing of adrenal capsular arterioles [32]. Non-functional cortical nodules may be particularly prominent in patients with aldosterone-secreting adenomas, presumably as a result of the associated hypertension. Cortical nodularity may also be evident in the zona reticularis. Nodules arising in this zone often appear brown to black owing to the presence of lipofuscin pigment. Incidental pigmented nodules may be found in up to one-third of normal adult adrenal glands.

Cushing's Syndrome

Tumors associated with Cushing's syndrome are typically unilateral and present as sharply circumscribed or encapsulated masses that weigh less than 50 g and measure 3–4 cm in average diameter. Tumors weighing more than 100 g should be approached carefully to exclude malignancy [7, 10, 13]. On cross section, adenomas vary from

Fig. 1.4 Gross photograph of a cortisol producing adenoma (2.5 cm) with focal hemorrhage (A). The neoplasm is yellow, similar to the adjacent non-neoplastic cortex (*arrow*) which appears mildly atrophic. The microscopic section shows that the tumor cells resemble those of the normal zona fasciculata (B). There is no evidence of cellular atypia, mitotic activity or necrosis

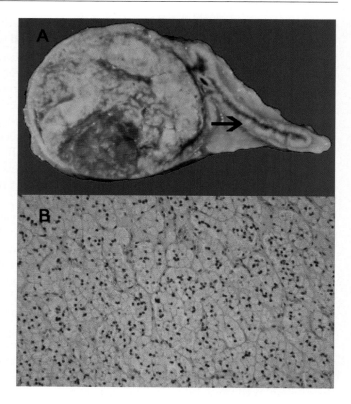

yellow to brown, and occasional examples of heavily pigmented (black) adenomas have been reported (Figs. 1.4A and 1.5). Necrosis is rare in the absence of prior arteriographic or venographic study, but cystic change is relatively common in larger tumors.

Adenomas are most often composed of small nests, cords, or alveolar arrangements of vacuolated clear cells that most closely resemble those of the normal fasciculata (Fig. 1.4B). Generally, adenoma cells are somewhat larger than normal cortical cells, have a low nuclear/cytoplasmic ratio and only rare mitotic figures. Black adenomas may be composed exclusively of lipochrome-rich compact cells [12]. Foci of myelolipomatous change or calcification may be seen, particularly in larger adenomas [10]. The cortex adjacent to functional adenomas and in the contralateral adrenal is typically atrophic, with cortical cells that have a clear or vacuolated cytoplasm. The atrophy, however, does not involve the glomerulosa [23].

Clonality studies using chromosome inactivation analysis have shown that some adenomas are clonal while others are polyclonal. Monoclonal adenomas are larger than polyclonal lesions and more

frequently show nuclear pleomorphism [33]. Such heterogeneity may reflect different pathophysiological mechanisms or different stages of a common multi-step process.

Conn's Syndrome

Initial studies suggested that cortical adenomas were responsible for Conn's syndrome in up to 90% of cases; however, more recent studies indicate that adenomas are present in a considerably smaller proportion of cases. Most adenomas associated with hyperaldosteronism measure less than 2.0 cm in diameter and are round to ovoid in configuration [34]. Most commonly they are unilateral, although bilateral tumors have been reported. They are characteristically bright yellow and are sharply demarcated from the adjacent cortex, most often by a pseudocapsule. The tumor cells are generally arranged in small nests and cords. They can resemble cells of the glomerulosa, fasciculata, or reticularis or combine the features of both glomerulosa and fasciculata cells (hybrid cells) [10, 34]. Rarely, black adenomas have been associated with Conn's syndrome [12]. In patients treated with

Fig. 1.5 Gross photograph of an aldersteronoma (3 cm) which is tan yellow in color (A) and non-functional black adenoma (2.5 cm) (B)

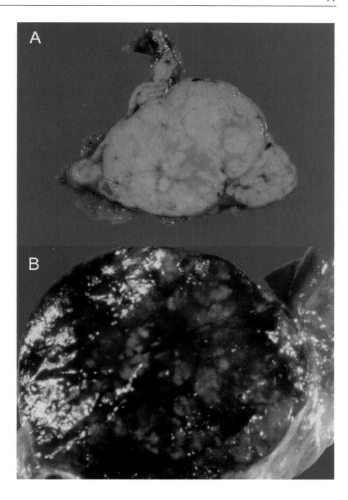

spironolactone, some cells within the adenoma may contain lamellated eosinophilic inclusions (spironolactone bodies). The fasciculata adjacent to aldosterone-secreting adenomas is typically normal, but hyperplasia of the zona glomerulosa may be present [34].

Adrenogenital Syndromes (Sex Steroid Overproduction)

Benign cortical tumors may be associated with syndromes of virilization or feminization, but the presence of a pure adrenogenital syndrome, particularly feminization, should raise the possibility of malignancy. Some authors, in fact, consider all feminizing cortical neoplasms to be potentially malignant. Virilizing adenomas are generally larger than those found in the context of pure Cushing's syndrome, and a few adenomas associated with adrenogenital syndromes have been reported to weigh up to 500 g [7, 10]. Similar to those tumors associated with glucocorticoid overproduction, virilizing adenomas are sharply circumscribed or encapsulated; however, they tend to be red-brown rather than yellow on cross section [10]. Smaller tumors have an alveolar pattern of growth, whereas larger tumors tend to have a more solid or diffuse growth pattern. Although most tumor cells have a low nuclear/cytoplasmic ratio, single cells and small cell groups may exhibit nuclear enlargement and hyperchromasia. The cytoplasm is usually eosinophilic and granular. Sex steroid-producing adenomas are not associated with atrophy of the adjacent cortex or the contralateral adrenal.

Oncocytic Adenoma (Oncocytoma)

Tumors with oncocytic features (oncocytomas) rarely develop as primary adrenal cortical neoplasms and may be functional or non-functional. They tend to be large neoplasms with average weights of 130–300 grams. Most have behaved as benign neoplasms, although some may be malignant, as discussed in a subsequent section. Typically, oncocytomas are dark brown in color, similar to oncocytomas at other sites. They have abundant granular eosinophilic cytoplasm, which corresponds to the presence of numerous mitochondria. Sasano and co-workers described three adrenal cortical oncocytomas that were unassociated with clinical syndromes of steroid excess and that lacked steroid hormone synthetic enzymes, as determined by immunohistochemical analysis [35].

Cortical Carcinoma

Adrenocortical carcinomas (ACC) are rare tumors with an incidence of about one to two cases per million population. They account for 0.05–0.2% of all malignancies. There is a bimodal age distribution, with a small peak in the first two decades and a larger peak in the fifth to seventh decades [12, 22]. ACCs have been reported in approximately 1% of patients with the Li Fraumeni syndrome and most affected individuals have demonstrated mutations in p53 at chromosome locus 17p13. Cortical carcinomas, in fact, may be the only manifestation of this disorder in childhood [36]. The frequency of these tumors is also increased in patients with the Beckwith-Wiedemann syndrome and some patients with congenital adrenal hyperplasia may develop cortical malignancies.

ACCs develop somewhat more commonly in women, although some studies have demonstrated a slight male predominance. Most patients have initial signs of abdominal pain, and up to 30% may have a palpable abdominal mass. The tumors may be associated with Cushing's syndrome or evidence of sex steroid overproduction, and mixed syndromes occur more often than with cortical adenomas. Rarely, mineralocorticoid production may be present in patients with cortical carcinomas. A significant proportion of cortical carcinomas (up to 75% in some series) may be unassociated with syndromes of hormone overproduction [37]. In some instances, patients may show signs of hypoglycemia due the production of insulin like growth factors by the tumor or hypercalcemia due to the production of parathyroid hormone or parathyroid hormone-like peptide.

As a rule, ACCs are large tumors weighing more than 100 g in adults; most often, tumor weight is in excess of 750 g [38–41]. Rarely, however, tumors weighing less than 50 g will metastasize, while a small proportion of tumors weighing more than 1000 g may not [7]. Benign tumors associated with adrenogenital syndromes, however, can weigh considerably more than 100 g. Tumor weight is also a useful predictor of malignancy in children; tumors weighing more than 500 g in a series of 23 cases reported by Cagle et al. [42] were malignant, whereas only a single tumor weighing less than 500 g pursued a malignant course despite the presence of histologic features that would fulfil criteria for malignancy in adults (see below).

On gross examination, most ACCs have a coarsely nodular appearance with individual nodules varying from pink to yellow-tan, depending on their lipid content. Carcinomas associated with feminization or virilization tend to be red-brown in color, while those associated with Cushing's syndrome are more often yellow-tan. Foci of necrosis, hemorrhage, and calcification are common, particularly in large tumors (Fig. 1.6A). The larger tumors often invade contiguous structures, including the kidney and liver. Histologically, they may have alveolar, trabecular, or solid patterns of growth, and admixtures of these patterns are common [7, 10, 13]. Foci of myxoid change, pseudoglandular patterns, and spindle-cell growth may be prominent in some tumors [43]. Depending on their lipid content, the cytoplasm may vary from vacuolated to eosinophilic. Some tumors may have eosinophilic globular inclusions resembling those seen in pheochromocytomas. There may be considerable variation in the appearance of the nuclei. In some instances, they may appear relatively small and uniform (Fig. 1.6A), while in others they may exhibit pronounced atypia manifested by pleomorphism, coarse chromatin granularity, and multiple prominent nucleoli (Fig. 1.7). Mitotic activity, including atypical forms, is often prominent. Nuclear pseudoinclusions, representing invaginations of the cytoplasm into the nucleus, may be particularly striking in some cortical carcinomas. Some adrenal cortical carcinomas may be composed of oncocytic cells [44]. While some of these tumors may be associated with Cushing's syndrome, others may be non-functional.

Fig. 1.6 Gross photograph of a large adrenal cortical carcinoma with extensive necrosis (A). A microscopic section shows neoplastic cells with cellular atypia and necrosis (lower portion of field) (B)

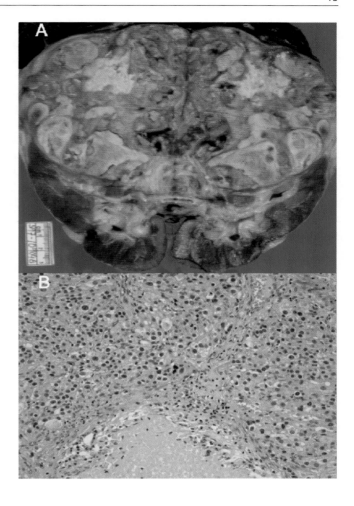

Fig. 1.7 Microscopic section of an adrenal cortical carcinoma demonstrating nuclear pleomorphism and an atypical mitotic figure (*arrow*)

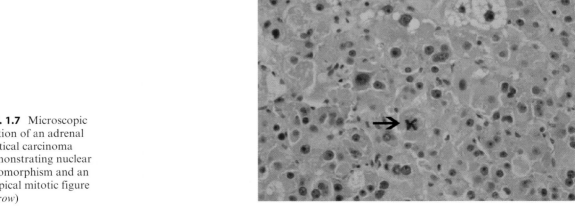

The most generally accepted criteria for the distinction of benign and malignant tumors include: high nuclear grade; more than five mitoses per 50 high power fields (HPF); atypical mitoses; diffuse patterns of growth; necrosis (Fig. 1.6B); invasion of venous, sinusoidal, or capsular structures; and clear cells comprising less than 25% of the tumor [38]. In a series of 43 cases, Weiss [38] found that tumors with fewer than two of these features never metastasized, whereas those with more than four almost invariably recurred or metastasized. Subsequently, Weiss et al. lowered the threshold for malignancy from four to three parameters [45]. Some groups have determined the tumor proliferating fraction (TPF) using the marker MIB-1 as well as p53 expression in an attempt to discriminate benign from malignant adrenal cortical tumors. In general, the majority of adenomas have a TPF less than 4% and are p53 negative while carcinomas generally have a TPF greater than 4% and are p53 positive in about half of the cases [46].

In the pediatric population, benign cortical tumors are significantly more likely to have mitotic activity, necrosis, broad fibrous bands, and nuclear pleomorphism than adenomas in adults [42]. Recently it has been suggested that the same criteria be used for malignancy in patients older than 3.5 years [22]. One approach used by some experts in pediatric pathology has been to label tumors having features fulfilling the criteria of malignancy in adults as "atypical adenomas".

There are no generally accepted criteria for the grading of cortical carcinomas. In an analysis of 42 carcinomas, the only parameter that had a strong statistical association with patient outcome was mitotic rate [45]. Tumors with more than 20 mitoses per 50 high power fields were associated with a mean survival of 14 months while tumors with fewer than 20 mitoses had a mean survival of 58 months.

ACCs must be distinguished from a variety of secondary tumors involving the adrenal, including renal cell carcinoma, hepatocellular carcinoma, metastatic carcinoma, and liposarcoma. Immunohistochemistry may be of particular value in discriminating cortical carcinomas from these tumor types [6], as summarized in Fig. 1.17.

The monoclonal antibody A103, which reacts with Melan-A, an antigen recognized by cytotoxic T cells and expressed in melanocytes, has also been used for the identification of adrenocortical and other steroid tumors [12, 47]. With the exception of melanoma, the only tumors that are reactive with A103 are adrenocortical adenomas and carcinomas, testicular Leydig cell tumors, and ovarian Sertoli-Leydig cell tumors. Antibodies to inhibin A also provide, an additional useful approach for the identification of steroid producing cells. Renshaw and Granter have demonstrated that inhibin A and A103 are both useful for the identification of adrenal cortical neoplasms and that A103 is marginally more specific and inhibin A slightly more sensitive [48]. Calretinin is also expressed in adrenal cortical neoplasms and is a useful adjunct in cases where stains for inhibin A are negative. Jorda and co-workers demonstrated that 24 of 33 (73%) cortical neoplasms were positive for inhibin A; however, when calretinin was added, the numbers of tumors staining positively for the two markers alone or in combination increased to 94% (31/33 cases) [49]. Synaptophysin is also expressed in a significant proportion of cortical tumors, but chromogranin is absent, in contrast to pheochromocytoma which are typically positive for both of these markers.

Didolkar and co-workers [37] have studied the natural history of a large series of patients with adrenal cortical carcinoma. The mean duration of symptoms in patients with or without hormonal manifestations was 6 months. Fifty-two percent had distant metastases at the time of diagnosis, 41% had locally advanced disease, and 7% had tumor confined to the adrenal. The overall median survival was 14 months, and the 5-year survival rate was 24%. The median survival of patients with functional tumors was somewhat longer than that of those patients with nonfunctional tumors. In order, the most common sites of metastasis were the lung, retroperitoneal lymph nodes, liver, and bone.

In a recent analysis of the Surveillance, Epidemiology and End Results (SEER) database between 1988 and 2002, Paton et al. identified 602 ACCs [50]. Three percent of tumors were less than 5 cm and localized (stage I), 36% were greater than 5 cm and localized (stage II) and 20.3% invaded adjacent structures (stage III). There were distant metastases (stage IV) in 31.4% of cases and stage was unknown in 8.8%. While 5-year survival was better in localized disease (62%) compared to 7% in advanced disease, tumor stage and survival did not improve over the 15-year study period. They concluded, that despite improvements in sensitivity of radiographic imaging modalities, ACC was not diagnosed at an earlier stage and there was no trend towards improved survival.

Neuroblastic Tumors

Neuroblastic tumors (NTs) are embryonic neoplasms of the sympathetic nervous system, and are the most common solid neoplasms in childhood other than central nervous system tumors. They account for approximately 15% of all neoplasms in children 4 years and younger (mean age of 21 months) [12]. The current classification system in use is International Neuroblastoma Pathology Committee (INPC) classification system [51, 52]. In this system, NTs are divided into four major categories (Table 1.2): neuroblastoma (Schwannian stroma-poor NT); the composite tumor ganglioneuroblastoma, nodular (composite Schwannian stroma-rich/stroma-dominant and stroma poor NT), ganglioneuroblastoma, intermixed (Schwannian stroma-rich NT) and ganglioneuroma (Schwannian stroma-dominant NT). The epidemiologic and clinical characteristics of NTs are largely related to neuroblastoma (NB), which account for the majority of these neoplasms.

Most cases of *neuroblastoma (Schwannian stroma-poor NT)* occur sporadically, although isolated cases of familial neuroblastomas (NBs) have been recorded

Table 1.2 International Neuroblastoma Pathology Committee (INPC) classification of neuroblastic tumors (NT)

Terminology and Grade
Neuroblastoma (Schwannian stroma-poor NT)
Undifferentiated
Poorly-differentiated
Differentiating
Ganglioneuroblastoma, nodular (Composite Schwannian stroma-poor and Schwannian stroma-rich/stroma-dominant NT)
Ganglioneuroblastoma intermixed (Schwannian stroma-rich NT)
Ganglioneuroma (Schwannian stroma-dominant NT)
Maturing
Mature

[53]. The tumors may be found in association with the Beckwith-Wiedemann syndrome, von Recklinghausen's disease, Hirschsprung's disease, opsoclonus/ myoclonus, heterochromia iridis, watery diarrhea, or Cushing's syndrome [7]. Rare examples of NB have been reported in adults [12].

NB most commonly develop in relationship to the sympathetic nervous system and most often appear as abdominal masses. The ratio of adrenal to extraadrenal primary sites is approximately 1.5–2:1. The remaining tumors may develop within the head and neck region, mediastinum, or pelvic area. In approximately 10% of cases, it is not possible to establish the primary site of origin with certainty.

Increased levels of catecholamines and their metabolites are found in most patients with NBs; however, hypertension is present only rarely in affected patients. Rare cases of neuroblastoma have been associated with cardiogenic shock [12]. Mass screening with analysis of urinary catecholamines in infants has been successful in detecting occult cases of NB both in Japan and other countries [54]. However, recent studies have suggested that little or no survival advantage has been gained by detecting occult cases in infants [55–57].

The concept of in-situ neuroblastomas was initially proposed by Beckwith and Perrin in 1963 [58] for neuroblastomatous foci confined to the adrenals of newborns. At the microscopic level, these lesions are composed of clusters of immature neuroblasts with frequent foci of cystic change. The incidence rate varies from 0.4 to 2.5% in different autopsy series, much higher than the incidence of clinically apparent neuroblastoma (Schwannian stroma-poor NT). It is thought that a substantial number undergo spontaneous regression, degeneration or maturation. Bolande has suggested that neuroblastic nodules measuring more than 2000 μm in diameter represent latent NB [59] while those of smaller diameter are thought to be an integral part of adrenal morphogenesis.

NTs vary in size from those measuring less than 1 cm in diameter to those that may fill the abdomen or thorax. The gross appearance ranges from soft and white to gray-pink in NB [7, 10] to a yellow tan appearance and firmer consistency in ganglioneuroma (Fig. 1.8). With increasing size, NBs tend to

Fig. 1.8 Gross photograph
of neuroblastoma demon-
strating a hemorrhagic cut
surface with white stippling
on the right indicating the
presence of calcification
(*arrow*) (A). A low power
photomicrograph demon-
strates a "small blue cell
tumor" with a lobular
growth pattern
(neuroblastoma) (B)

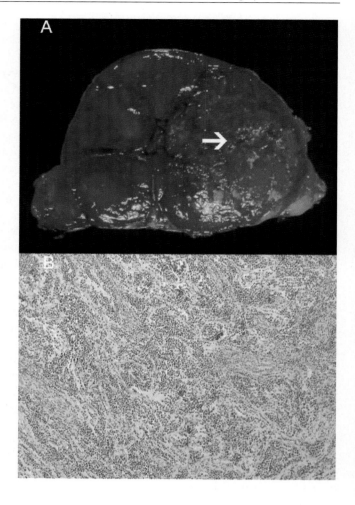

undergo hemorrhage, necrosis, cyst formation, and
calcification; however cyst formation and hemorrhage may also be evident in small tumors. Adrenal
primaries tend to grow toward the midline and can
extend to the contralateral adrenal. Large, right-
sided tumors can invade the liver directly, whereas
large, left-sided tumors can invade the pancreatic
parenchyma.

NBs are composed of sheets of small cells with
hyperchromatic nuclei and scanty cytoplasm with a
lobular appearance owing to the presence of thin
fibrovascular septa between groups of tumor cells
(Fig. 1.8B). Most contain a finely fibrillary matrix
(neuropil) between the tumor cells. At the ultrastructural level, this material corresponds to masses
of unmyelinated axons [12]. Homer Wright pseudorosettes, composed of one or two layers of neuroblasts surrounding a central space filled with

neuritic processes, are found in about 30% of
cases [10] (Fig. 1.9). Grading of NBs is based on
the presence of neuropil and the proportion of cells
differentiating towards mature ganglion cells.

The most commonly employed immunohistochemical markers in the diagnosis of NB are synaptophysin
and chromogranin. The latter marker is more
specific for a diagnosis of NB as synaptophysin is
positive in adrenocortical tumors as well. These
markers are used to differentiate NBs from other
small round cell tumors such as Ewing sarcoma/
primitive neuroectodermal (EWS/PNET) family of
tumors, lymphoma, rhabdomyosarcoma and desmo-
plastic small round cell tumor (DSRCT), along with
the use of other immunohistochemical markers and
specific molecular genetic translocations associated
with the latter lesions. Increased levels of catecholamines and their metabolites support a diagnosis of NB.

Fig. 1.9 High power photomicrograph of neuroblastoma shows eosinophilic fibrillary neuropil centrally among neuroblasts (Homer-Wright pseudorosette)

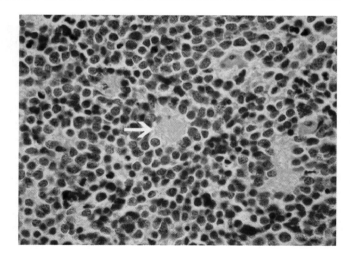

NBs can metastasize widely through both lymphatic and vascular routes [10]. The most common sites include bone marrow (78%), bone (69%), lymph nodes (42%) and liver (20%) while pulmonary and brain metastases are uncommon. Less commonly lung (3%), skin (2%) and testes (2%) may also be involved. Spontaneous regression is well documented.

Ganglioneuroblastoma, nodular (composite Schwannian stroma-rich/stroma-dominant and stroma-poor neuroblastic tumor) is characterized by a gross appearance in which commonly hemorrhagic neuroblastoma nodules (Fig. 1.10A inset) are present in a background that may resemble the gross appearance of ganglioneuroblastoma, intermixed or the glistening tan-pink whorled cut surface of ganglioneuroma (GN) (Fig. 1.10A). Microscopically, there is usually an abrupt demarcation of the neuroblastic (stroma-poor) component from the stroma-rich (ganglioneuroblastoma, intermixed) or stroma-dominant component (GN) (Fig. 1.10B). These nodules, therefore, have pushing borders and may even have a fibrous pseudocapsule.

The proportion of both components may vary in ganglioneuroblastoma, nodular (GNB, nodular). The stroma-rich/stroma-dominant component is often located at the periphery of the tumor, but it can appear as thin or broad septa between contiguous nodules. In rare cases the neuroblastic component may dominate the tumor with the stroma-rich/stroma-dominant component being in the periphery.

Cases in which ganglioneuroblastoma, intermixed (GNB, intermixed) or GN is found in the sections from the primary site, but NB is found in sections from a metastatic site, are classified as GNB, nodular.

Ganglioneuroblastoma, intermixed (Schwannian stroma-rich NT) can have the same gross appearance as NB or GN depending on the extent of differentiation. It is characterized by the random intermingling of neuroblastic nests and ganglion cells within the stroma-rich (ganglioneuromatous) component.

The most mature NT is *ganglioneuroma (Schwannian stroma-dominant NT)*. Less than 30% of these tumors occur in the adrenal glands and they are most commonly asymptomatic [12]. The remainder develop in the posterior compartment of the mediastinum, retroperitoneum and other sites. Rarely, they are associated with hypertension, watery diarrhea, and hypokalemia or masculinization [12]. Adrenal GNs are generally smaller than those in the mediastinum or retroperitoneum. They are sharply circumscribed but do not have a true capsule. On cross section they are gray to tan, and their consistency differs from soft and gelatinous to firm and whorled with an appearance similar to that of a leiomyoma (Fig. 1.10A). Microscopically, GN contains varying numbers of mature ganglion cells and Schwann cells together with variable amounts of collagen (Figs. 1.10B and 1.14). A few multinucleated ganglion cells may also be evident. The Schwann cells and collagen are often arranged in interlacing

Fig. 1.10 Gross photograph demonstrates the
typical appearance of a
ganglioneuroma with a
gelatinous and fibrous cut
surface (A). The overall size
of the tumor was 12 cm;
however, a 1-cm white and
focally hemorrhagic nodule
of neuroblastoma (*arrow
and inset*) was found;
accordingly this tumor was
classified as a ganglioneuroblastoma, nodular. On
microscopic section, the
boundary between
neuroblastoma (NB)
and ganglioneuroma (GN)
is sharply demarcated

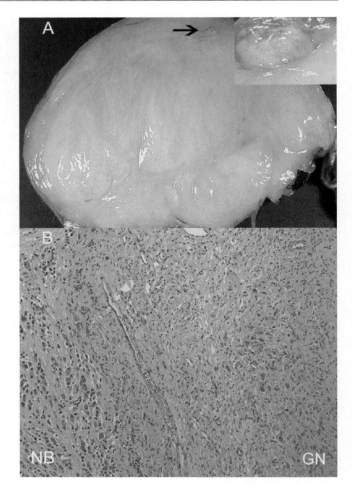

bundles. Ganglion cells may be distributed
diffusely throughout the tumor or arranged in small
clusters. Distinction from GNB, intermixed is based on
the Schwannian stroma constituting much more than
50% of the tumor and absence of nests of neuroblasts.

The *prognosis* of NTs is dependent upon a number
of variables, including age, histopathologic features,
stage, biochemical, genetic and biologic parameters

(Table 1.3). NBs are separated into favorable and
unfavorable histology groups based on the patient's
age at diagnosis, grade of tumor and the mitosis
karyorrhexis index (MKI) [60]. The MKI is derived
by counting cells at high power and determining the
percentage of cells undergoing mitosis and karyorrhexis. MKI is expressed as low ($<2\%$), intermediate (2–4%) or high ($>4\%$).

Table 1.3 Prognostic factors for neuroblastic tumors

Prognostic Factor	Favorable	Adverse
Age	<1 year	>1 year
Stage	Stage 1, 2A, 2B and 4S (localized disease)	Stage 3 and 4 (advanced disease)
Histopathology	Favorable histology	Unfavorable histology
Biochemical markers	Low serum ferritin	High serum ferritin
Genetic and biologic markers	Hyperdiploid and triploid tumors	Diploid and tetraploid tumors
	MYCN non-amplified	MYCN amplification
	Lack of chromosome 1p loss or 17q gain	Chromosome 1p loss or 17q gain
	High TRK-A/C expression	Low TRK-A/C expression

Pheochromocytoma

Pheochromocytomas (intra-adrenal paragangliomas) are uncommon tumors that have been reported in 0.005%–0.1% of unselected autopsies [12]. Their average annual incidence is eight per million person-years in the United States, and they are responsible for less than 0.1% of cases of hypertension. Approximately 70% of pheochromocytomas arise in the adrenal glands, but tumors of identical morphology and function may also appear in a wide variety of extraadrenal sites from the sympathetic paraganglia. While the extraadrenal tumors have also been termed "extra-adrenal pheochromocytomas" by some authors, the preferred terminology for such neoplasms is extra-adrenal paraganglioma [22].

In most series, the majority of pheochromocytomas are sporadic (non-familial). Although previous studies indicated that approximately 10% were familial, more recent studies indicate that a considerably higher proportion have a genetic basis. This distinction is of particular importance since most familial tumors are bilateral and multicentric while most sporadic tumors are unilateral. Several different genes have been implicated in the development of familial pheochromocytomas and paragangliomas: the *VHL* (von Hippel Lindau) gene which is responsible for the VHL syndrome, the *RET* gene which causes the MEN 2 syndromes, the neurofibromatosis (NF)-1 gene which is responsible for von Recklinghausen's disease and the genes encoding the B and D subunits of succinate dehydrogenase (SDH) which are associated with the development of familial paragangliomas and pheochromocytomas. Neumann and coworkers demonstrated that 66 of 271 patients (24%) with apparent sporadic pheochromocytomas had germline mutations in one of these genes with 45% involving the VHL gene, 19.6% the RET gene and 16.6% and 18.2% involving the SDHD and SDHB genes respectively [61].

The clinical manifestations in patients with pheochromocytomas are protean but are generally dominated by signs and symptoms of catecholamine hypersecretion or the complications of hypertension. Common symptoms include headache, diaphoresis, palpitations, anxiety, chest pain, and weight loss. In most series, hypertension, which may be sustained or paroxysmal, is the most common sign at presentation. A few patients with pheochromocytomas are normotensive, and a few may even be hypotensive. Most pheochromocytomas produce a combination of norepinephrine and epinephrine, with a predominance of norepinephrine. Tumors producing epinephrine exclusively may be associated with hypotension. The clinical diagnosis depends on the presence of increased urinary and plasma levels of catecholamines and their metabolites.

In patients with nonfamilial forms of pheochromocytoma, the right adrenal is somewhat more commonly involved than the left. Most nonfamilial tumors are unilateral, sharply circumscribed, solid masses with fibrous pseudocapsules. Most tumors from surgical series measure 3–5 cm in diameter, with tumor weights ranging from 70 to 150 g [10]. Size and weight variations may be considerable and even very small tumors can be associated with serious symptoms. The tumors vary in color from gray-white to pink-tan, with foci of congestion (Fig. 1.11A). Larger tumors can contain central areas of fibrosis. Occasionally, very large pheochromocytomas undergo cystic degeneration, and they may be difficult to distinguish from nonneoplastic adrenal cysts (see section on adrenal cysts).

Familial pheochromocytomas are typically bilateral and multicentric and the adjacent medulla is often hyperplastic [12, 62, 63]. Large tumor masses in patients with familial pheochromocytomas most likely develop as a result of the confluence of multiple small tumor nodules developing in a background of diffuse medullary hyperplasia (Figs. 1.11B and 1.12). Molecular studies of microdissected nodules in patients with MEN 2A associated adrenal medullary hyperplasia have shown that this disorder is a multifocal monoclonal proliferation. The same X-chromosome is inactivated in individual nodules from the same patient suggesting an early clonal expansion of adrenal medullary precursors in these patients. Rarely, adrenal medullary hyperplasia may occur in patients without a known hereditary syndrome.

The tumors are composed of intermediate to large polygonal cells that may be arranged in alveolar, trabecular, or solid patterns. Most pheochromocytomas exhibit admixtures of these growth patterns. In tumors with alveolar arrangements, the groups of

Fig. 1.11 Gross photograph
of pheochromocytoma (A).
The characteristic tan cut
surface of this tumor
contrasts with the yellow
rim of adjacent cortex.
Gross photograph of
diffuse and nodular (*arrow*)
medullary hyperplasia from
a patient with type 2A MEN

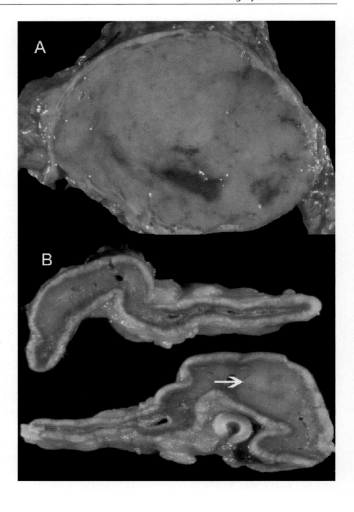

tumor cells are surrounded by a capillary-rich frame-work that results in a characteristic "Zellballen" appearance (Fig. 1.13A). Pheochromocytoma with oncocytic features has been described [64]. Although most pheochromocytomas are composed of inter-mediate to large-sized polygonal cells, some tumors may be composed of spindle cells or relatively small cells resembling pheochromoblasts. Moreover, very large cells resembling ganglion cells may also be evident in some cases. In addition to chromaffin cells, pheochromocytomas also contain a population of sustentacular cells, which are difficult to recognize in hematoxylin and eosin–stained preparations; how-ever, they can be demonstrated selectively with anti-bodies to S-100 protein (Fig. 1.13B). Typically, the sustentacular cells are present at the peripheries of the cell nests. The nuclei of pheochromocytoma cells are round to ovoid, with coarsely clumped chromatin

and a single prominent nucleolus. Nuclear pleo-morphism and hyperchromasia may be particularly prominent in some pheochromocytomas, but this finding does not correlate with malignant behavior. Benign pheochromocytomas can occasionally con-tain mitotic figures.

Large tumors frequently display areas of hemor-rhage and necrosis. The stroma may have areas of myxoid change with foci of lymphocytic infiltration. Amyloid deposits have been identified in up to 70% of pheochromocytomas in some series, while other series have reported the presence of amyloid in a significantly smaller proportion of cases [65]. Foci of capsular and venous invasion may also be evident, but these features do not correlate with malignant behavior. Brown fat has been reported in the retro-peritoneum surrounding pheochromocytomas; this change, however, is not specific [12].

Fig. 1.12 An adrenalectomy specimen from a patient with multiple endocrine neoplasia shows multiple nodules on the external aspect (A). The medulla between the two nodules is diffusely hyperplastic (arrow) (B)

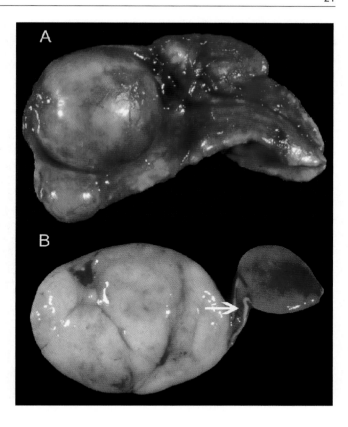

Pheochromocytomas usually show negative results on tests for cytokeratins in the majority of cases, but stain positively for vimentin and neurofilament proteins. They exhibit positivity for chromogranin proteins and synaptophysin, but synaptophysin is also present in a large proportion of adrenal cortical carcinomas. S-100 protein is restricted to the sustentacular cells and is particularly evident in those areas with a "Zellballen" pattern (Fig. 1.13B). Pheochromocytomas may also contain a large array of regulatory peptide products, including leu- and met-enkephalin, endorphins, ACTH, somatostatin, and calcitonin [66, 67]. The overproduction of these substances may give rise, in rare cases, to syndromes of hormone excess, including Cushing's syndrome.

Pheochromocytomas are rare in childhood, and they are more likely to be bilateral and multicentric than in adults [68]. Approximately 90% of affected children have sustained hypertension, and polydipsia, polyuria, and convulsions are considerably more common than in adults. In addition, the rate of metachronous or synchronous extra-adrenal paragangliomas is considerably higher in children than in adults [12]. The high rate of bilaterality and multicentricity suggests that many of these cases may represent unrecognized examples of familial pheochromocytomas.

Composite pheochromocytomas or compound tumors of the adrenal medulla are complex neoplasms containing pheochromocytoma together with foci of neuroblastoma, ganglioneuroblastoma, ganglioneuroma, or malignant peripheral nerve sheath tumor [7]. Composite pheochromocytomas are rare tumors that comprise less than 3% of sympathoadrenal pheochromocytomas. Rarely, they may be associated with neurofibromatosis type I [69]. The predominant component of the tumor is usually the pheochromocytoma while the most common second component is ganglioneuroma (Fig. 1.14). Interestingly, normal and neoplastic chromaffin cells are capable of differentiation into ganglion cells under the influence of nerve growth factor [70]. It has been suggested that the sustentacular cells of pheochromocytomas could serve as the progenitors of the malignant peripheral nerve

Fig. 1.13 This microscopic
section of a pheochromcy-
toma highlights the
"Zellballen" pattern (A).
A stain for S-100 protein
highlights the sustentacular
cells (B)

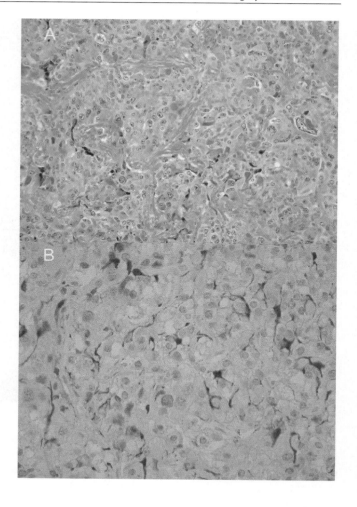

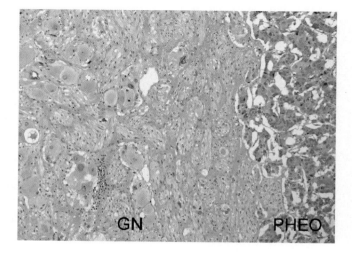

Fig. 1.14 Microscopic
section of a composite
tumor composed of pheo-
chromocytoma (PHEO)
and ganglioneuroma (GN).
Large mature single
ganglion cells and in nests
surrounded by the spindle
cell Schwannian stroma are
present on the left

sheath component of some composite pheochromocytomas. Many of the reported composite tumors have been associated with signs and symptoms typical of pheochromocytomas, and some have been found in the context of the Verner-Morrison syndrome of watery diarrhea and hypokalemia. A unique case of composite pheochromocytoma consisting of typical pheochromocytoma and neuroendocrine carcinoma has been reported [71].

The diagnosis of *malignancy* in pheochromocytomas is particularly difficult. Differences in criteria have resulted in considerable variation in the reported rates of malignant pheochromocytomas, which have ranged from 2.4% to 14%. With the exception of the presence of distant metastases, there are no absolute criteria that distinguish benign from malignant pheochromocytomas reliably. In a study of adrenal and extra-adrenal sympathoadrenal paragangliomas, Linnoila and co-workers noted that malignant tumors occurred more commonly in males, were of larger size with coarse nodularity and necrosis, had extensive local and vascular invasion and were less likely to have cytoplasmic hyaline globules than their benign counterparts [72]. In this study, four parameters were most predictive of malignancy: extraadrenal location, coarse nodularity of the primary tumor, confluent tumor necrosis, and absence of cytoplasmic hyaline globules. Although most malignant tumors had two or three of these features, most benign tumors had only one or none.

Although there is some suggestion that tumor weight correlates with malignant behavior, Thompson was unable to demonstrate a statistically significant difference between benign and malignant pheochromocytomas in the series from the AFIP [73]. A system for the assessment of malignancy of pheochromocytomas has been developed by Thompson (PASS, Pheochromocytomas of the Adrenal Gland Scaled Score). In this system, each of the following features was assigned a value of 1: vascular invasion, capsular invasion, profound nuclear pleomorphism and hyperchromasia. Features assigned a value of 2 included: periadrenal adipose tissue invasion, large tumor nests or diffuse growth pattern, focal or confluent necrosis, high cellularity, tumor cells spindling, cellular monotony, mitotic figures in excess of 3 per 10 high power fields and atypical mitoses. Among 50 tumors that were classified as histologically malignant and assigned a PASS ≥ 4, 33 patients developed metastases while 17 did not. Patients with tumors with a PASS < 3 remained free of metastases with a mean follow-up of 14.1 years.

Other parameters that have been assessed for determining benign and malignant pheochromocytomas include the proliferative fraction as assessed with the monoclonal antibody MIB-1 and the number of S-100 positive sustentacular cells. However, neither of these approaches has provided conclusive parameters of malignancy.

Malignant pheochromocytomas are generally slowly growing neoplasms with five-year survival rates in the range of 40%–50%. The most common sites of metastatic spread include lymph nodes, bone, and liver. In assessing lymph node metastases, all efforts should be directed to distinguishing concurrent extraadrenal paragangliomas that compress adjacent lymph nodes from true nodal metastases.

Other Adrenal Mass Lesions

The advent of high-resolution abdominal imaging techniques, including CT, MRI and PET has markedly increased the rate of discovery of nonfunctional adrenal mass lesions [1, 12]. As a group, these lesions have been referred to as "incidentalomas", and the differential diagnosis includes primary and metastatic tumors, cysts, myelolipomas, a variety of other entities, lymphoid hyperplasia, and periadrenal lesions. Nonfunctional cortical adenomas as well as cortical nodules, which are also frequently detected by this approach, are discussed in other sections.

Metastatic Malignancies and Malignant Lymphoma

Adrenal metastases have been reported in almost 30% of patients with metastatic tumors of diverse sites of origin [10], with bilateral involvement in almost 50% of cases. The high frequency of adrenal metastases is most likely related to the rich sinusoidal blood supply of the glands. In most series, from the US and Western Europe, primary tumors of the lung and breast account for 60% of the cases, followed by primary tumors of the gastrointestinal tract, kidney, skin (melanoma), and thyroid gland. Adrenal cortical carcinomas may also occasionally metastasize to the contralateral adrenal. Patients

Fig. 1.15 Adrenal gland involved by metastatic renal cell carcinoma (2 cm). The tumor is white and has lobular contours

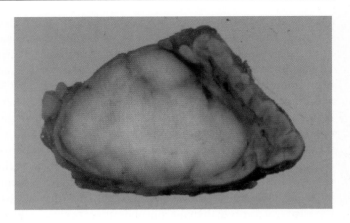

with metastatic carcinoma involving one or both adrenals may be seen initially for diagnosis of an intra-adrenal mass, and in such cases the primary tumor may not be evident until the time of autopsy. Overt adrenal insufficiency is rare in patients with adrenal metastasis; however, mild degrees of adrenal insufficiency may be evident in affected patients [74]. Clinically significant adrenal hemorrhage secondary to adrenal metastases is rare [12].

On gross examination, adrenal metastases may appear as multiple or single firm masses that replace all or part of the gland (Fig. 1.15). Larger metastases frequently exhibit foci of necrosis and hemorrhage, and may therefore simulate primary adrenal cortical carcinomas. Their microscopic appearances differ according to their sites of origin. While most such lesions are recognizable as metastases, some may be impossible to distinguish from adrenal primary tumors. The differential diagnosis of metastatic carcinoma is discussed in the section on "Needle Biopsy of Adrenal Masses" and is summarized in Fig. 1.17.

Secondary involvement of the adrenals may occur in up to 25% of patients with disseminated malignant lymphoma studied at autopsy [7]. Both Hodgkin's and non-Hodgkin's lymphomas have been reported, with a somewhat higher frequency for non-Hodgkin's lymphomas. Rarely, however, is the lymphomatous involvement associated with adrenal insufficiency. This complication occurs primarily in patients with high-grade tumors [75].

Adrenal involvement can be unilateral or bilateral, and tumors can range in size from those of microscopic dimensions to those that replace the adrenal and adjacent structures. The gross appearance can be identical to that of primary cortical or metastatic carcinomas. The histologic characteristics vary according to the type of lymphoma. The differential diagnosis includes metastatic carcinoma, primary adrenal cortical carcinoma, metastatic amelanotic melanoma, and pheochromocytoma. Malignant lymphomas can be distinguished from other tumor types on the basis of positive staining for leukocyte common antigen and other markers of lymphoid differentiation. Very rare examples of primary lymphomas of the adrenal glands have also been reported [76, 77]. Virtually all of the primary adrenal lymphomas have been of the non-Hodgkin's large-cell type, including the large-cell angiotropic variant [78].

Cysts and Pseudocysts

Although adrenal cysts are uncommon, their rate of detection as a result of CT and MRI scanning has increased dramatically. Most adrenal cysts are unilateral, with a predominance in women. They have been divided into four major categories, including epithelial cysts (retention cysts, embryonal cysts, and cystic neoplasms), parasitic cysts (predominantly echinococcal), endothelial cysts, and pseudocysts [7, 12, 17]. Mesothelium-lined cysts have also been reported.

The term pseudocyst describes a lesion that lacks recognizable endothelial or epithelial cells. In the series of eight pseudocysts reported by Medeiros and co-workers [79], seven of the patients were women with a median age of 41 years. Pseudocysts range in size from 1.8 to 10 cm, but lesions of considerably larger size have been reported. The cyst contents are usually hemorrhagic fibrinous material. The wall is composed of dense fibrous tissue with areas of calcification and foci of chronic inflammation. Most adrenal pseudocysts probably develop as lymphangioendothelial cysts that undergo episodes of hemorrhage, fibrosis, and hemosiderin deposition with the ultimate disappearance of the endothelial lining [80]. This conclusion is based on the occasional presence of residual lining cells that are positive for factor VIII-related antigen. Occasionally, abundant elastic tissue may be present within the cyst wall, further suggesting a vascular origin.

As noted previously, any adrenal neoplasm may undergo cystic change. In rare instances, this may involve the neoplasm almost entirely so that on imaging studies they simulate a cyst or pseudocyst, but on pathologic examination residual mural tumor nodules are found. Erickson et al. reported 2 adrenal cortical carcinomas, 2 adrenal cortical adenomas and 2 pheochromocytomas associated with 6 of 32 pseudocysts from the archives of the Mayo Clinic over a 25-year period [81]. An additional case of pheochromocytoma was associated with an endothelial cyst.

Myelolipoma

The myelolipoma is an uncommon, benign, tumor-like lesion of the adrenal composed of mature adipose tissue admixed with hematopoietic cells. Most myelolipomas appear as unilateral adrenal masses; however, similar lesions may develop in extraadrenal sites in the retroperitoneum. The mean age at diagnosis is approximately 50 years, and most patients are asymptomatic. The typical myelolipoma is a nonencapsulated lesion that is bright yellow with foci of red-brown discoloration (Fig. 1.16A) [7]. These tumors vary considerably in size, from those that are of microscopic dimensions

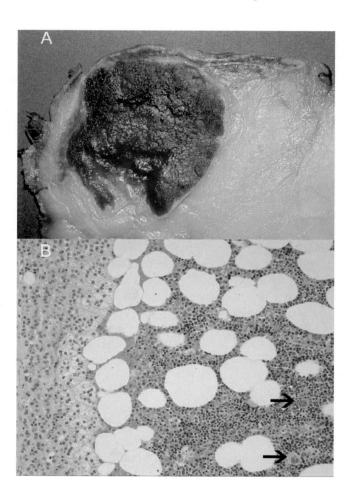

Fig. 1.16 Gross photograph of myelolipoma (5 cm) demonstrates a focally red cut surface surrounded by yellow cortical tissue and extra-adrenal fat (A). The microscopic section shows adrenal cortex on the left while hemopoietic and adipose tissue is present on the right (B). The large multinucleated cells are megakaryocytes (*arrows*)

to those that fill the abdomen. At the microscopic level, they are composed of mature adipose tissue with scattered islands of hematopoietic cells [7, 12] (Fig. 1.16B). Areas of necrosis, hemorrhage, cyst formation, and calcification may also be evident, particularly in larger tumors. Foci of myelolipomatous change may be found in a variety of otherwise normal and neoplastic adrenal tissue [10]. As a result, it is debatable as to whether these lesions are neoplastic or not. However, Bishop et al. demonstrated nonrandom X-chromosome inactivation in the hematopoietic elements and fat in 8 of 11 myelolipomas from female patients suggesting a clonal origin of these tumors [82].

Connective Tissue Tumors

A variety of mesenchymal tumors may arise within the adrenal, including hemangiomas, lipomas, leiomyomas, osteomas, neurofibromas, and neurilemomas [7, 10]. Among the benign tumors, cavernous hemangiomas are the most common and are detected as incidental findings at surgery or autopsy. Most hemangiomas are solitary lesions involving a single adrenal. These lesions should be distinguished from adrenal cortical adenomas with degenerative changes and secondary vascular proliferation. The gross and histologic features of adrenal neurofibromas and neurilemomas are similar to those of tumors found at other sites. Leiomyomas are rare and most likely originate from vascular smooth muscle cells. Prevot and co-workers have reported a single case of a solitary fibrous tumor of the adrenal [83]. The lesion was well circumscribed but not encapsulated and infiltrated the adrenal and surrounding adipose tissue. On microscopic examination, it was composed of spindle cells that were arranged in small, interlacing fascicles separated by bundles of collagen with focal collections of lymphocytes.

Angiosarcomas arising within the adrenal gland are extremely rare. In a series of nine angiosarcomas reported by Wenig et al. [84], the tumors ranged in size from 6 to 10 cm and were composed of spindle-shaped and/or epithelioid cells. A vascular origin was confirmed by the finding of factor VIII-related antigen and CD34 immunoreactivity. Epithelioid angiosarcomas may show focal keratin immunoreactivity, as reported for epithelioid angiosarcomas

at other sites. Rarely, extensive hemorrhagic infarction of an adrenal adenoma with the formation of pseudovascular spaces lined by large, atypical fibroblasts may mimic a primary adrenal angiosarcoma [85]. Leiomyosarcomas and malignant peripheral nerve sheath tumors may infrequently develop as primary adrenal gland malignancies [86, 87]. Some cases of leiomyosarcoma have occurred in patients with acquired immune deficiency syndrome [87, 88].

Other Tumors

A variety of other neoplasms including malignant melanoma, carcinosarcoma and dysembryonic neoplasms have been reported as adrenal primaries, but are exceptionally rare. The relatively few reported cases of mixed corticomedullary tumors in all likelihood represent examples of collision tumors. Adenomatoid tumors of mesothelial origin have also been reported as adrenal primaries, but are uncommon. Rarely, ovarian thecal metaplasia may result in gross enlargement of the adrenal glands.

Needle Biopsy of Adrenal Masses

Adrenal biopsy is typically performed when adrenal lesions cannot be accurately characterized with CT, MR imaging, or PET in order to establish a definitive diagnosis. However, the pathologic work-up of adrenal masses on core needle or fine needle aspiration biopsies is a challenging process. Foremost, is determination of whether or not the biopsy is lesional or not. Indeed, in the case of benign adrenal cortical nodules or tumors, the lesion may recapitulate the histology of the adrenal cortex precluding a definite diagnosis of neoplasm on needle biopsy. As noted in a previous section, the diagnosis of adrenocortical carcinoma can be difficult on resection specimens. Because of variability in a neoplasm, the area sampled may only permit a diagnosis of, "consistent with adrenal cortical neoplasm," to be rendered. Clearly in functional tumors, differentiation from metastatic tumor or primary tumor from adjacent structures is aided by biochemical studies when available. However, since the majority of cases that are encountered on needle biopsies are non-functional tumors, an immunohistochemical approach is employed because of morphologic overlap.

Metastatic carcinomas are positive for cytokeratins while cortical tumors may be positive or negative (Fig. 1.17). Most melanomas and sarcomas are negative for cytokeratins. However, some sarcomas can have positive staining (e.g. synovial sarcoma), but a spindle cell morphology usually aids in making the distinction. Thyroid transcription factor 1 (TTF-1) is commonly positive in metastatic lung and thyroid carcinomas, but negative in primaries of breast, gastrointestinal tract, liver and kidney. Thyroglobulin (THY) is used to differentiate lung (THY negative) from thyroid carcinoma (THY positive). Other commonly used antibodies include gross cystic disease fluid 15 (GCDFP-15) for breast; CDX2 (protein product of a homeobox gene involved in intestinal development) for gastrointestinal primaries; polyclonal carcinoembryonic antigen (pCEA) and HepPar-1 (a protein of unknown function in liver cells) for hepatocellular carcinoma

(HCC); and CD10 (a zinc metallopeptidase expressed in early lymphoid progenitors and normal germinal center cells of lymph nodes) and renal cell carcinoma antigen (RCC), both of which may be expressed in renal cell carcinoma. CD45 (a membrane protein tyrosine phosphatase found on all leukocytes) is positive in, and is used to screen for lymphoreticular and hematopoietic neoplasms. Additional lineage specific markers are used for further classification into T-cell or B-cell lymphoma. As mentioned previously, melan A detected by A103 is positive both in melanoma and in adrenal cortical tumors, but the use of additional melanoma markers (e.g. HMB-45, a monoclonal antibody to glycoproteinaceous antigenic group of melanocytes, or S-100 potein) and steroid associated antibodies for adrenal cortical tumors assist in making the distinction [47]. It must be emphasized that the algorithmic approach, summarized in Fig. 1.17, is

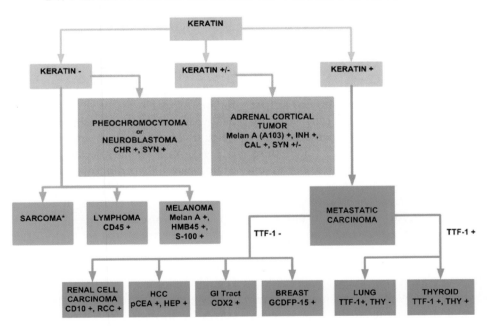

Fig. 1.17 A simplified algorithm showing the immunohistochemical work-up of an adrenal mass on needle biopsy. * Some sarcomas are keratin positive (e.g. synovial sarcoma, epithelioid sarcoma)
Abbreviations; A103- Melan A; CAL- Calretinin; CHR- Chromogranin; CD45- Leukocyte common antigen; GCDFP- Gross cystic disease fluid protein; GI- Gastrointestinal; HCC- Hepatocellular carcinoma; HEP- Hepatocyte-1 (HepPar-1); INH –Inhibin; pCEA- Polyclonal carcinoembryonic antigen; RCC- Renal cell carcinoma antigen; SYN- Synaptophysin; THY- Thyroglobulin; TTF- Thyroid transcription factor

a simplification, since sensitivity and specificity of the different immunohistochemical markers vary, so that despite adequate material on a biopsy, one neoplasm can only be favored over another, without a definitive diagnosis in some cases.

Metabolic Disorders
Storage Diseases

Adrenoleukodystrophy (Addison-Schilder's disease) is a rare, X-linked recessive disorder characterized by progressive demyelination of the central and peripheral nervous systems and by adrenal cortical insufficiency [12, 17]. The disorder is caused by mutations of the gene on chromosome Xq28 encoding an ATP-binding transporter ALDP-adrenoleukodystrophy protein (ALDP) that is localized in the peroxisomal membrane. A variety of mutations resulting in the defective oxidation of very long fatty acids have been identified [89]. The adrenal glands in this disorder are grossly atrophic with weights ranging from 1 to 2 g or less, with ballooning and striation of the cells of the inner zona fasciculata and zona reticularis. Groups of ballooned cells form nodules which may undergo degenerative changes with the formation of large cortical vacuoles. An adult variant of this disorder with an onset in the second or third decades is known as adrenomyeloneuropathy, a condition that can be associated with unexplained adrenal insufficiency in the absence of neurologic manifestations at first clinical presentation [17]. Cortical cells typically appear ballooned and contain linear lamellar inclusions at the ultrastructural level [12, 17]. A third form of the disease has been reported in women who are carriers of the abnormal gene.

Wolman's disease (primary familial xanthomatosis) is a rare lipid storage disorder caused by an autosomal recessive deficiency of lysosomal acid lipase [12, 17]. The disease is characterized by the accumulation of triglycerides and cholesterol esters in a variety of tissues including the liver, spleen and adrenal glands. Most affected individuals die by the age of 6 months. Typically, the adrenal glands are markedly enlarged even though they often retain their normal configurations and glands often demonstrate multiple foci of calcification in association with necrosis and fibrosis [12]. Other storage diseases (e.g. Niemann-Pick disease) may result in adrenal enlargement and hypofunction.

Congenital Adrenal Hyperplasia

The syndromes of congenital adrenal hyperplasia (congenital adrenogenital syndromes) result from a series of autosomal recessive enzymatic defects in the biosynthesis of adrenal steroids. The most common deficiency affects the enzyme 21-hydroxylase ($P\text{-}450_{c21}$) and is responsible for approximately 95% of cases of congenital adrenal hyperplasia [90]. The worldwide incidence of classic 21-hydroxylase deficiency is 1 in 14,500 births, with a heterozygote frequency of approximately 1 in 60. Affected individuals have evidence of cortisol deficiency, aldosterone deficiency with salt wasting, and excess adrenal androgen production with evidence of virilization. Excess adrenal androgen production is a consequence of the accumulation of 17-hydroxypregnenolone, which is subsequently metabolized to androgenic steroids. Non-classic 21-hydroxylase deficiency has a frequency of one in 100 in certain parts of the United States and is one of the most common autosomal recessive disorders. Affected individuals have mild degrees of cortisol deficiency, normal aldosterone production, and excess production of adrenal androgens. This form of 21-hydroxylase deficiency is most often diagnosed in childhood or early adulthood. A small proportion of individuals with 21-hydroxylase deficiency may have no apparent symptoms.

Deficiency of 11β-hydroxylase ($P450_{c11}$) accounts for approximately 5% of all cases of congenital adrenal hyperplasia and is associated with increased production of androgens and deoxycorticosterone [12, 91]. As a result, affected individuals typically exhibit signs of hyperandrogenism and hypertension. Deficiency of 17α-hydroxylase is responsible for approximately 1% of cases. External genitalia are female in both sexes. Increased levels of deoxycorticosterone are responsible for the hypertension seen in these patients.

Adrenal hyperplasia in the congenital adrenogenital syndromes results from inadequate production of glucocorticoids, leading to stimulation of the cortex by increased pituitary ACTH production. The adrenals become markedly enlarged, with a characteristic cerebriform appearance; they are brown to tan in color [7]. On microscopy, cortical cells are lipid depleted. In individuals with deficiency of 20,22-desmolase ($P\text{-}450_{scc}$), the adrenals are pale yellow and are characterized on microscopic examination by vacuolated cells, occasionally with formation of cholesterol clefts and an accompanying giant-cell reaction. These disorders are usually treated by replacement of the deficient steroid hormone and surgical correction of ambiguous genitalia.

Adrenal cortical adenomas and carcinomas may develop, though rarely, in the setting of congenital adrenal hyperplasia [12, 92]. Testicular tumors can also arise in affected patients. These lesions are not autonomous neoplasms, since they are dependent on the presence of elevated levels of ACTH. They are commonly bilateral and are most typically located in the hilar regions of the testes. The cell of origin is unknown, but the component cells of these lesions contain abundant amounts of eosinophilic cytoplasm, but lack crystalloids of Reinke as are seen in Leydig cell tumors. The diagnosis of congenital adrenal hyperplasia may only become apparent after examination of such testicular tumors in 18% of the cases [93].

Hypofunctional States

Cortical hypofunction may occur as the result of a primary disorder of the adrenal cortex or as a secondary change due to a disorder of the pituitary–hypothalamic axis.

Primary Hypofunction

Primary hypofunction may result from autoimmune adrenalitis, type I and type II polyglandular autoimmune syndrome, infections including bacterial, fungal and viral, amyloid deposition and hemorrhage.

Autoimmune Adrenalitis

Inflammation of the adrenal glands occurs as a result of autoimmune mechanisms in approximately 75% of cases of cortical hypofunction. In idiopathic (autoimmune) Addison's disease, the glands are markedly atrophic, and the residual cortical tissue is infiltrated by chronic inflammatory cells, including lymphocytes and plasma cells. All layers of the cortex are involved, but the medulla is unaffected. Typically, the capsule of the gland is fibrotic. Both humoral and cell-mediated immune mechanisms have been implicated in the development of autoimmune adrenal hypofunction. Autoantibodies to cortical cells are present in 50% of patients and in more than 70% of women with newly diagnosed disease. The major targets for autoantibody reactivity are the adrenal cytochrome p-450 enzymes [94]. Affected patients can also have antibodies to gonadal, gastric parietal, and thyroid follicular cells.

Adrenal cortical hypofunction may be associated with hypofunction of other endocrine glands [95]. The type I polyglandular autoimmune syndrome is associated with mucocutaneous candidiasis, hypoparathyroidism, adrenal insufficiency, autoimmune thyroiditis, and diabetes mellitus. Alopecia may also be present. This form of the disease has also been termed autoimmune polyendocrinopathy-candidiasis-ectodermal dystrophy (APECED). Mutations in the APECED or autoimmune regulatory gene (21q22.3) have been implicated in the development of this syndrome [96, 97]. The type II polyglandular autoimmune syndrome is characterized by adrenal insufficiency, autoimmune thyroiditis, and insulin-dependent diabetes mellitus. The type I syndrome is inherited as an autosomal recessive trait, while the pattern of inheritance of the type II syndrome is usually dominant.

Infectious Disorders

Infectious disorders, including tuberculosis and fungal diseases (histoplasmosis, North and South American blastomycosis, coccidiomycosis, cryptococcosis), can affect both the cortical and medullary regions of the adrenal glands. Although tuberculosis is now a rare cause of adrenal insufficiency in the United States and Western Europe, it is a common cause in parts of the world where tuberculosis is endemic. In contrast to the shrunken appearance of the adrenals in idiopathic Addison's disease, the glands in mycobacterial infection are typically enlarged and are replaced by caseous material. Infection with *Mycobacterium avium intracellulare*, on the other hand, is typically associated with the presence of confluent masses of histiocytes containing the acid-fast organisms.

Cytomegalovirus (CMV) has been identified in the adrenals of a large proportion of patients dying of the acquired immunodeficiency syndrome [98]. Adrenal cortical necrosis associated with CMV infection can be severe enough to result in acute adrenal insufficiency in some instances. Both herpes simplex and varicella zoster may also involve the adrenals and may lead to adrenal cortical insufficiency when they are associated with extensive cortical necrosis.

Amyloidosis

Rarely, amyloid deposition can result in cortical hypofunction [12, 17]. Typically, adrenal involvement is associated with extensive systemic amyloid disease of the AA type. The adrenal glands may have a normal shape and size or may be massively enlarged. In severe cases, the glands are pale tan to yellow. Microscopically, amyloid deposits affect the fasciculata and reticularis zones and are typically present between the cortical cells and capillary endothelium. The cortical cells ultimately become atrophic as a result of the progressive deposition of intercellular amyloid. In patients with AL disease, the amyloid deposits are usually perivascular in distribution.

Adrenal Hemorrhage

Adrenal hemorrhage may develop in a segmental fashion or may involve the entire adrenal [99]. This syndrome may be seen in association with sepsis and shock due to meningococcal infection or infection with other bacteria, including *Haemophilus influenzae* and *Streptococcus pneumoniae* (Waterhouse-Friderichsen syndrome). Typically, the glands are enlarged and hemorrhagic, with necrosis of both cortical and medullary tissue. Adrenal hemorrhage in the Waterhouse-Friderichsen syndrome is regarded as the consequence rather than the cause of shock. Anticoagulant therapy may also be associated with adrenal hemorrhage.

Corticomedullary necrosis of a milder degree has been reported in association with hypotension and shock [100]. In patients with segmental lesions, examination of the capsular vessels and sinusoids will reveal evidence of thrombus formation. Affected cortical areas show a pattern of ischemic necrosis that ultimately heals by the process of fibrosis.

Secondary Hypofunction

Adrenal cortical atrophy may be found in association with lesions primarily affecting the adenohypophysis or hypothalamus, leading to diminished secretion of ACTH [12, 17]. The administration of exogenous corticosteroids will effect similar changes as a result of suppression of ACTH. The adrenals in secondary hypofunctional states are considerably smaller than normal, although the overall configurations of the glands are retained. Typically, the cortex is bright yellow owing to lipid accumulation in the cortical cells, the capsule is fibrotic, and the medulla is unaffected. The zona glomerulosa is usually of normal thickness in these cases.

References

1. Young WF (2007) The incidentally discovered adrenal mass. N Engl J Med 356:601–610
2. Barwick TD, Malhotra A, Webb JA et al. (2005) Embryology of the adrenal glands and its relevance to diagnostic imaging. Clin Radiol 60:953–959
3. Sadler TW (2006) Langman's medical embryology, 10th edn. Philadelphia. Lippincott Williams & Wilkins, pp314–315
4. Beck K, Tygstrup I, Nerup J (1969) The involution of the fetal adrenal cortex: a light microscopic study. Acta Pathol Microbiol Scand 76:391–400
5. Coupland RE (1980) The development and fate of catecholamine secreting endocrine cells. In: Parvez H, Parez S (eds) Biogenic amines in development. Elsevier/North Holland, Amsterdam, pp 3–28
6. Mills SE (ed) Sternberg's histology for pathologists, 3rd edn. Lippincott Williams & Wilkins, Philadelphia, pp 1167–1188 and 1211–1233
7. Lack EE (1997) Tumors of the adrenal gland and extra-adrenal paraganglia. Armed Forces Institute of Pathology, Washington, D.C.
8. Gutowski T, Gray GF (1979) Ectopic adrenal in inguinal hernia sacs. J Urol 121:353–354
9. MacLennan A (1919) On the presence of adrenal rests in hernial sac walls. Surg Gynecol Obstet 29:387
10. Page DL, DeLellis RA, Hough AJ (1985) Tumors of the adrenal. In: Atlas of tumor pathology, 2nd series, fascicle 23. Armed Forces Institute of Pathology, Washington, D.C.
11. Dolan MF, Janouski NA (1968) Adrenohepatic union. Arch Pathol 86:22
12. DeLellis RA, Mangray S (2004) The adrenal glands. In: Mills SE (ed) Sternberg's diagnostic surgical pathology. Lippincott Williams & Wilkins, Philadelphia, pp 621–667
13. Lack EE (1990) Pathology of the adrenal glands. Churchill Livingstone, New York
14. Burris TP, Guo W, McCabe ER (1996) The gene responsible for congenital adrenal hypoplasia DAX-1, encodes a nuclear hormone receptor that defines a new class within the superfamily. Recent Prog Hormone Res 54:241
15. Burch C (1985) Cushing's disease: a review. Arch Intern Med 145:1106–1111

16. Upton GV, Amatruda TT (1971) Evidence for the presence of tumor peptide with corticotropin-releasing factor like activity in the ectopic ACTH syndrome. N Engl J Med 285:419–424

17. Lloyd RV, Douglas BR, Young WF (2002) Atlas of nontumor pathology: endocrine diseases. American Registry of Pathology & Armed Forces Institute of Pathology (AFIP), Washington, D.C., pp 171–257

18. Reibord H, Fisher ER (1968) Electron microscopic study of adrenal cortical hyperplasia in Cushing's syndrome. Arch Pathol 86:419–426

19. Neville AM, Symington T (1972) Bilateral adrenal cortical hyperplasia in children with Cushing's syndrome. J Pathol 107:95–106

20. Neville AM, Symington T (1967) The pathology of the adrenal in Cushing's syndrome. J Pathol Bacteriol 93:19–35

21. Zarate A, Kovacs K, Flores M et al. (1986) ACTH and CRF-producing bronchial Carcinoid associated with Cushing's syndrome. Clin Endocrinol Oxf 24:523

22. DeLellis RA, Lloyd RV, Heitz PU, Eng C (2004) World Health Organization classification of tumors. Pathology & genetics. Tumors of endocrine organs. IARC Press, Lyons, pp 135–174, 209–262

23. Conn JW, Knopf RF, Nesbit RM (1964) Clinical characteristic of primary aldosteronism from an analysis of 145 cases. Am J Surg 107:159

24. Bourdeau I, Stratakis CA (2002) Cyclic AMP dependent signaling aberrations in macronodular adrenal disease. Ann NY Acad Sci 968:240–255

25. Meador CK, Bowdoin B, Owen WC, Farmer TA (1967) Primary adrenocortical nodular dysplasia: a rare cause of Cushing's syndrome. J Clin Endocrinol Metab 27:1255–1263

26. Wulffraat NM, Drexhage HA, Wiersinga WM et al. (1988) Immunoglobulins of patients with Cushing's syndrome due to pigmented adrenocortical micronodular dysplasia simulate in vitro steroidogenesis. J Clin Endocrinol Metab 66:601

27. Carney JA, Young WF (1992) Primary pigmented nodular adrenal cortical disease and its associated conditions. Endocrinologist 2:6–21

28. Groussin L, Jullian E, Perlemoine K et al. (2002) Mutations of the PRKAR1A gene in Cushing's syndrome due to sporadic primary pigmented nodular adrenal cortical disease. J Clin Endocrinol Metab 87:4324–4329

29. Stratakis CA (2002) Mutations of the gene encoding the protein kinase A Type Iα regulatory subunit (PRKAR1A) in patients with the "complex of spotty skin pigmentation, myxomas, endocrine overactivity and Schwannomas" (Carney Complex) Ann NY Acad Sci 968:3–21

30. Cohen MM (2005) Beckwith-Wiedemann syndrome: historical, clinicopathological, and etiogenetic perspectives. Pediatr Dev Pathol 8:287–304

31. Bertagna C, Orth DN (1981) Clinical and laboratory findings and results of therapy in 58 patients with adrenocortical tumors admitted to a single medical center (1951–1978). Am J Med 71:855–875

32. Dobbie JM (1969) Adrenal cortical nodular hyperplasia: the aging adrenal. J Pathol 99:1–18

33. Gicquel C, Leblond-Francillard M, Bertagna X et al. (1994) Clonal analysis of human adrenal cortical carcinomas and secreting adenomas. Clin Endocrinol (Oxf) 40:465–477

34. Neville AM, Symington T (1966) Pathology of primary aldosteronism. Cancer 19:1854–1868

35. Sasano H, Szuki T, Sano T, Kameya T, Sasano N, Nagwa H (1991) Adrenocortical oncocytoma: a true nonfunctioning adrenal cortical tumor. Am J Surg Pathol 15:949–956

36. Sameshima Y, Tsunematsu Y, Watanabe S et al. (1992) Detection of novel germline p53 mutations in diverse cancer prone families identified by selecting patients with childhood adrenocortical carcinoma. J Natl Cancer Inst 84:703–710

37. Didolkar MD, Bescher RA, Elias EG, Moore RH (1981) Natural history of adrenal cortical carcinoma: a clinicopathologic study of 42 patients. Cancer 47:2153–2161

38. Weiss LM (1984) Comparative histological study of 43 metastasizing and nonmetastasizing adrenocortical tumors. Am J Surg Pathol 8:163–169

39. Hutter AM, Kayhoe DE (1966) Adrenal cortical carcinoma: clinical features of 138 patients. Am J Med 41:572–592

40. Hough AJ, Hollifield JW, Page DL, Hartmann WH (1979) Prognostic factors in adrenal cortical tumors: a mathematical analysis of clinical and morphologic data. Am J Clin Pathol 72:390–399

41. Hajjar RA, Hickey RC, Samaan NA (1979) Adrenal cortical carcinoma: a study of 32 patients. Cancer 35:549–554

42. Cagle PT, Hough A, Pysher J et al. (1986) Comparison of adrenal cortical tumors in children and adults. Cancer 57:2235–2237

43. Brown FM, Gaffey TA, Wold LE, Lloyd RV (2000) Myxoid neoplasms of the adrenalcortex: a rare histologic variant. Am J Surg Pathol 24:396–401

44. Hoang MP, Ayala AG, Albores-Saavedra J (2002) Oncocytic adrenal cortical carcinoma: a morphologic, immunohistochemical and ultrastructural study of four cases. Mod Pathol 15:973–978

45. Weiss LM, Medeiros LJ, Vickery AL Jr (1989) Pathologic features of prognostic significance in adrenocortical carcinoma. Am J Surg Pathol 13(3):202–206

46. Vargas MP, Vargas HI, Kleiner DE, Merino MJ (1997) Adrenocortical neoplasms: role of prognostic markers MIB-1, p53, and RB. Am J Surg Pathol 21:556–562

47. DeLellis RA, Shin SJ (2006) Immunohistology of endocrine tumors. In: Diagnostic immunohistochemistry. Dabbs DJ (ed) Churchill Livingstone, Philadelphia, pp 261–300

48. Renshaw AA, Granter SR (1998) A comparison of A103 and inhibin reactivity in adrenal cortical tumors: distinction from hepatocellular carcinoma and renal tumors. Mod Pathol 11:1160–1164

49. Jorda M, De MB, Nadji M (2002) Calretinin and inhibin A are useful in separating adrenal cortical neoplasms from pheochromocytomas. Appl Immunohistochem Mol Morph 10:67–70

50. Paton BL, Novitsky YW, Zerey M et al. (2006) Outcomes of adrenal cortical carcinoma in the United States. Surgery 140(6):914–920

51. Shimada H, Ambros IM, Dehner LP et al. (1999) Terminology and morphologic criteria of neuroblastic tumors. Recommendations by the International Neuroblastoma Pathology Committee. Cancer 86:349–363

52. Shimada H, Ambros IM, Dehner LP et al. (1999) The international neuroblastoma pathology classification (the Shimada system). Cancer 86:364–372

53. Hardy PC, Nesbit ME Jr (1973) Familial neuroblastoma: report of a kindred with a high incidence of familial tumors. J Pediatr 80:74–77

54. Sawada T (1992) Past and future of neuroblastoma screening in Japan. Am J Pediatr Hematol Onco 14:320–326

55. Woods WG, Gao RN, Shuster JJ et al. (2002) Screening of infants and mortality due to Neuroblastoma. N Engl J Med 346:1041–1046

56. Schilling FH, Spix C, Berthold F et al. (2002) Neuroblastoma screening at one year of age. N Engl J Med 346:1047–1053

57. Yamato K, Ohta S, Ito E et al. (2002) Marginal decrease in mortality and marked increase in incidence as a result of neuroblastoma screening at 6 months of age:cohort study in seven prefectures in Japan. J Clin Oncol 20:1209–1214

58. Beckwith JB, Perrin EV (1963) In situ neuroblastomas: a contribution to the natural history of neural crest tumors. Am J Pathol 43:1089–1104

59. Bolande RP (1979) Developmental pathology. Am J Pathol 94:623–683

60. Shimada H, Umehara S, Monobe Y et al. (2001) International neuroblastoma pathology classification for prognostic evaluation of patients with peripheral neuroblastic tumors. A report from the Children's Cancer Group. Cancer 92:2451–2461

61. Neumann HPH, Bausch B, McWhinney S et al. (2001) Germ-line mutations in non syndromic pheochromocytoma. New Engl J Med 346:1459–1466

62. DeLellis RA, Dayal Y, Tischler AS, Lee AK, Wolfe HJ (1986) Multiple endocrine neoplasia (MEN) syndromes: cellular origins and inter-relationships. Int Rev Exp Pathol 28:163–215

63. Carney JA, Sizemore GW, Sheps SG (1976) Adrenal medullary disease in multiple endocrine neoplasia, type 2. Am J Clin Pathol 66:279–290

64. Li M, Wenig BM (2000) Adrenal oncocytic pheochromocytoma. Am J Surg Pathol 24:1552–1557

65. Steinhoff MN, Wells SA, DeSchryver-Kelskemeti K (1992) Stromal amyloid in pheochromocytomas. Hum Pathol 23:33–36

66. Hassoun J, Monges G, Giraud P et al. (1984) Immunohistochemical study of pheochromocytomas: an investigation of methionine enkephalin, vasoactive intestinal peptide, somatostatin corticotropin, β-endorphin and calcitonin in 16 tumors. Am J Pathol 114:56–63

67. DeLellis RA, Tischler AS, Lee AK et al. (1983) Leu-enkephalin-like immunoreactivity in proliferative lesions of the human adrenal medulla and extra-adrenal paraganglia. Am J Surg Pathol 7:29–37

68. Stackpole RH, Melicow MM, Uson AC (1953) Pheochromocytoma in children. J Pediatr 63:315–330

69. Kimura N, Watanabe T, Fukase M et al. (2002) Neurofibromin and NF1 gene analysis in composite pheochromocytoma and tumors associated with von Recklinghausen's disease. Mod Pathol 15:183–188

70. Tischler AS, DeLellis RA, Biales B et al. (1980) Nerve growth factor induced neurite outgrowth from normal human chromaffin cell. Lab Invest 43:399–409

71. Juarez D, Brown RW, Ostrowski M et al. (1999) Pheochromocytoma associated with neuroendocrine carcinoma. A new type of composite pheochromocytoma. Arch Pathol Lab Med 123:1274–1279

72. Linnoila RI, Keiser HR, Steinberg SM, Lack EE (1990) Histopathology of benign versus malignant sympathoadrenal paragangliomas: clinicopathologic study of 120 cases including unusual histological features. Hum Pathol 21:1168–1180

73. Thompson LDR (2002) Pheochromocytoma of the adrenal gland scaled score (PASS) to separate benign form malignant neoplasms. A clinicopathologic and immunophenotypic study of 100 cases. Am J Surg Pathol 26:551–556

74. Redman BG, Pazdur R, Zingas AP, Loredo R (1987) Prospective evaluation of adrenal insufficiency in patients with adrenal metastasis. Cancer 60:103–107

75. Gamelin E, Beldent V, Rousselet M-C et al. (1992) Non-Hodgkin's lymphoma presenting with primary adrenal insufficiency: a disease with an underestimated frequency? Cancer 69:2333–2336

76. Choi GH, Durishin M, Garbudawala ST, Richard J (1990) Non-Hodgkin's lymphoma of the adrenal gland. Arch Pathol Lab Med 114:883–885

77. Schnitzer B, Smid D, Lloyd RV (1986) Primary T-cell lymphoma of the adrenal glands with adrenal insufficiency. Hum Pathol 17:634–636

78. Chu P, Costa J, Lackman MF (1996) Angiotropic large cell lymphoma presenting as primary adrenal insufficiency. Hum Pathol 27:209–211

79. Medeiros LJ, Levandrowski KB, Vickery AL (1989) Adrenal pseudocyst: a clinical and pathological study of eight cases. Hum Pathol 20:660–665

80. Incze JS, Lui PS, Merriam JC, Austen G, Widrich WC, Gerzof SG (1979) Morphology and pathogenesis of adrenal cysts. Am J Pathol 95:423–432

81. Erickson LA, Lloyd RV, Hartman R, Thompson G (2004) Cystic adrenal neoplasms. Cancer 101:1537–1544

82. Bishop E, Eble JN, Cheng L et al. (2006) Adrenal myelolipomas show nonrandom X-chromosome inactivation in hematopoietic elements and fat: support for a clonal origin of myelolipomas. Am J Surg Pathol 30:838–843

83. Prevot S, Penna CT, Imbert J-C et al. (1996) Solitary fibrous tumor of the adrenal gland. Mod Pathol 9:1170–1174

84. Wenig B, Abbondanzo SL, Heffess C (1994) Epithelioid angiosarcoma of the adrenal glands. A clinicopathologic study of nine cases with discussion of implications of finding "epithelial-specific" markers. Am J Surg Pathol 18(1):62–73

85. Granger JK, Hoan H-Y, Collins C (1991) Massive hemorrhagic functional adrenal adenoma histologically mimicking angiosarcoma: report of a case with immunohistochemical study. Am J Surg Pathol 15:699–704

86. Lack EE, Graham CW, Azumi N et al. (1991) Primary leiomyosarcoma of adrenal gland: case report with immunohistochemical and ultrastructural study. Am J Surg Pathol 15:899–905

87. Zetler PJ, Filipanko JD, Bilbey JH, Schmidt N (1995) Primary adrenal leiomyosarcoma in a man with acquired immunodeficiency syndrome (AIDS): further evidence for an increase in smooth muscle tumors related to Epstein Barr virus infection in AIDS. Arch Pathol Lab Med 119:1164–1167

88. Linos D, Kiriakopoulos AC, Tsakayannis DE et al. (2004) Laparoscopic excision of bilateral primary leiomyosarcomas in a 14-year-old girl with acquired immunodeficiency syndrome (AIDS). Surgery 136:1098–1100

89. Cartier N, Lopez J, Moullier P et al. (1995) Retroviral-mediated gene transfer connects very long chain fatty acid metabolism in adrenoleukodystrophy fibroblasts. Proc Natl Acad Sci USA 92:1674

90. White PC, New MI, Dupont D (1987) Congenital adrenal hyperplasia. N Engl J Med 316:1519–1524, 1580–1586

91. Hughes I (2002) Congenital adrenal hyperplasia: phenotype and genotypes. J Pediatr Endocrinol Metab 15(suppl 15):1529–1340

92. Jaursch-Hancke C, Allollio B, Meltzer U, Bidlingmaier F, Winkelmann W (1988) Adrenal cortical carcinoma in patients with untreated congenital adrenal hyperplasia. Acta Endocrinol 117:146–147

93. Rutgers JL, Young RH, Scully RE (1988) The testicular tumor of the adrenogenital syndrome: a report of 6 cases and review of the literature on testicular masses in patients with adrenocortical disorders. Am J Surg Pathol 12:503–513

94. Weetman AP (1995) Autoimmunity to steroid producing cells and familial polyendocrinopathy. Ballieres Clin Endocrinol Metab 9:157–174

95. Neufeld M, MacLaren NK, Blizzard RM (1981) Two types of autoimmune Addison's disease associated with different polyglandular autoimmune syndromes. Medicine 60:355–362

96. Wang CY, Davoodi-Semiromi A, Huang W et al. (1998) Characterization of mutations in patients with autoimmune polyglandular syndrome type I (APSI). Hum Genet 103:681–685

97. Ahonen P (1985) Autoimmune polyendocrinopathy-candidosis ectodermal dystrophy (APECED): autosomal recessive inheritance. Clin Genet 27:535–542

98. Grinspoon SK, Bilezikian JP (1992) HIV disease and the endocrine system. N Engl J Med 327:1360–1365

99. Friderichsen C (1955) Waterhouse-Friderichsen syndrome. Acta Endocrinol 18:482–492

100. Kuhajda FP, Hutchins GM (1979) Adrenal corticomedullary junction necrosis: a morphological marker for hypotension. Am Heart J 98:294–297

Adrenocortical Dysfunction

2

Subbulaxmi Trikudanathan and Robert G. Dluhy

Contents

S. Trikudanathan (✉)
Department of Medicine, St Elizabeth's Medical Center,
736 Cambridge Street, Boston, Massachusetts 02135
E-mail: Subbulaxmi.Trikudanathan@caritaschristi.org

M.A. Blake, G. Boland (eds.), *Adrenal Imaging*, DOI 10.1007/978-1-59745-560-2_2,
© 2009 Humana Press, a part of Springer Science+Business Media, LLC

Normal Physiology and Regulation of Adrenocortical Function

The adrenal cortex secretes three classes of steroid hormones: glucocorticoids, mineralocorticoids and androgens. A five-ring nucleus forms the backbone of adrenal steroids with 19(androgen) or 21(glucocorticoid, mineralocorticoid) carbon atoms. The mineralocorticoid aldosterone, secreted in the outer zona glomerulosa plays a pivotal role in the maintenance of blood pressure, vascular volume and potassium homeostasis. The central zona fasciculata consists of large lipid-laden cells, which produce cortisol. Cortisol participates in the stress response and modulates intermediary metabolism and immune functions. The inner layer zona reticularis produces androgens, which serve as precursors of testosterone and androstenedione; they play a role in the development of secondary sexual characteristics in females.

Biosynthesis of Adrenal Steroids

Cholesterol, the substrate for steroidogenesis is derived from dietary sources and endogenous synthesis. Uptake by the adrenal cortex is mediated by the low-density lipoprotein (LDL) receptor and is stimulated by adrenocorticotropic hormone

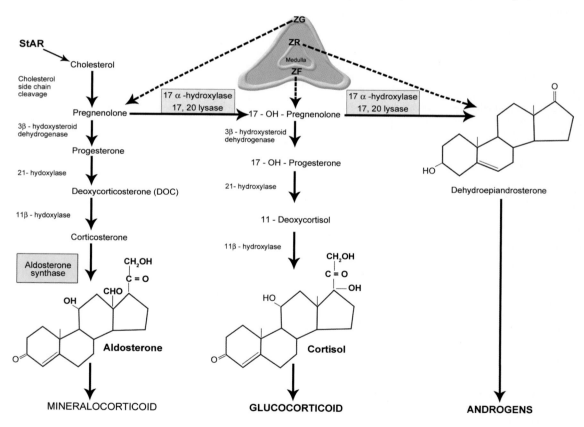

Fig. 2.1 Biosynthetic pathways for adrenal steroid production showing the zone specific synthesis of mineralocorticoid (aldosterone), glucocorticoid (cortisol) and androgen (DHEA). The organic structure of the final products is depicted. StAR – steroidogenic acute regulatory protein, ZG – zona glomerulosa, ZF – zona fasiculata, ZR- zona reticularis, DHEA – dehydroepiandrosterone

(ACTH) through a steroidogenic acute regulatory protein (StAR). Through a coordinated action of a series of cytochrome P450 enzymes (hydroxylases, dehydrogenases) specific hormones are synthesized in the three zones of the adrenal cortex (Fig. 2.1).

Steroid Transport

Cortisol circulates in the plasma as free and protein–bound cortisol, and cortisol metabolites. Free or unbound cortisol, which is approximately 5% of the total cortisol, is the physiologically active hormone acting at tissue sites. Cortisol is bound to cortisol-binding globulin (CBG), a high affinity low capacity α2-globulin produced in the liver. CBG is increased in high estrogen states (e.g. pregnancy, oral contraceptive administration) leading to elevated total plasma cortisol. However the free cortisol level remains normal and thus the manifestations of glucocorticoid excess are absent. The other low affinity, high capacity protein is albumin [1]. Cortisol metabolites are biologically inactive and bind only weakly to circulating plasma proteins. The circulating half–life of cortisol is 70–120 min. In contrast to cortisol, an ultra filtrate of plasma contains only 50% of circulating aldosterone bound to proteins.

Steroid Metabolism and Excretion

Glucocorticoids

The liver is the principal site of cortisol metabolism. Major enzymes involved in the regulation of cortisol metabolism are the two isoforms of 11β-hydroxysteroid dehydrogenase (11β-HSD). Hepatic 11β-HSD I converts the inactive cortisone to the active cortisol; hence mutations in this gene are associated with rapid cortisol turnover, leading to the activation of the hypothalamic- pituitary-adrenal (HPA) axis and increased adrenal androgen production. The 11β-HSD II isoform, which is co-expressed with the mineralocorticoid receptor (MR) in the kidney, colon and salivary gland inactivates cortisol to cortisone, permitting aldosterone to bind to the MR in vivo. If this mechanism is impaired cortisol can act as a mineralocorticoid explaining some forms of endocrine hypertension such as apparent mineralocorticoid excess.

Mineralocorticoids

The liver with subsequent conjugation with glucuronic acid primarily metabolizes aldosterone. The rate of inactivation is reduced in certain states such as congestive heart failure.

Adrenal Androgen

The chief androgens secreted by the adrenal cortex are dehydroepiandrosterone (DHEA) and its ester DHEAsulfate (DHEAS). They form more than half of circulating androgens in premenopausal females. Smaller amounts of androstenedione, 11β-hydroxyandrostenedione, and testosterone are secreted by the adrenal cortex. DHEA is metabolized to the urinary 17-ketosteroids.

Regulation of Hypothalamic-Pituitary-Adrenal Axis

ACTH, secreted and stored in the basophilic cells of the anterior pituitary gland regulates adrenal cortisol synthesis. The biological half-life of ACTH in the circulation is less than 10 min. ACTH stimulates cyclic AMP, which in turn promotes the synthesis of protein kinase enzymes, thus resulting in the phosphorylation of proteins that activate steroid biosynthesis.

ACTH is processed from a large precursor molecule propiomelanocortin (POMC) along with a number of other peptides including β-lipotropin, endorphins and melanocyte stimulating hormone. POMC is produced in the hypothalamus, anterior and posterior pituitary, liver, kidney, gonad, and placenta. Corticotropin- releasing hormone (CRH), produced in the hypothalamus stimulates the release of ACTH and its related peptides. Urocortin, a neuropeptide related to CRH, has many of the central nervous system effects of CRH such as appetite suppression and anxiety but its role in the regulation of ACTH is unclear (Fig. 2.2).

Factors Controlling the Release of ACTH

The following factors influence ACTH release – CRH, arginine vasopressin (AVP), circadian rhythm, stress, and free cortisol. CRH synthesized within the paraventricular nucleus of the hypothalamus is the principal stimulus for ACTH secretion. Hypothalamic neurotransmitters also regulate

Fig. 2.2 The hypothalamic-pituitary-adrenal axis. The main sites of feedback control for plasma cortisol - the pituitary gland, hypothalamus and higher centers of the brain. There is a short-feedback loop involving the inhibition of CRH by ACTH. There is negative feedback control of cortisol over the pituitary ACTH and hypothalamic CRH secretion. Inflammatory cytokines lead to increased cortisol secretion and the cortisol produced in turn suppress these proinflammatory cytokines-suppression, + stimulation. CRH – corticotropin releasing hormone, POMC – pro-opiomelanocortin, ACTH – Adrenocorticotropic hormone, DHEA – dehydroepiandrosterone, IL-1 – Interleukin-1, IL-6 – Interleukin-6, TNF-α – Tumor necrosis factor-α

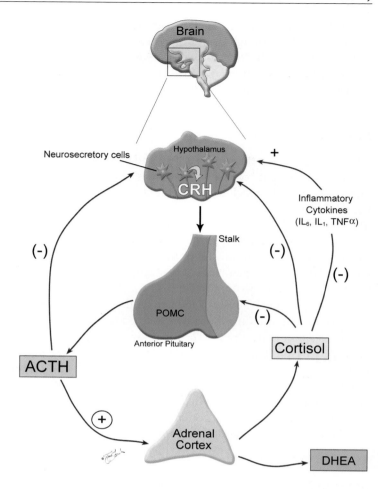

CRH: serotoninergic and cholinergic pathways stimulate while GABA inhibits CRH release [2]. ACTH has a pulsatile secretion pattern and follows a circadian rhythm with the peak levels prior to waking and nadir values in the late evening. The sleep-wake pattern, which is disturbed by long distance travel across time zones or by night shift working, takes about 2 weeks to reset. Stress such as fever, surgery, hypoglycemia, exercise and acute emotions trigger the release of CRH, AVP and subsequently ACTH; the sympathetic nervous system is also activated. Immune-endocrine interaction occurs when proinflammatory cytokines (particularly interleukin-1, interleukin-6 and tumor necrosis factor α) augment the effects of CRH and AVP on ACTH secretion (Fig. 2.2). Finally, negative feedback control of ACTH secretion is exerted by free plasma cortisol; whereby cortisol inhibits POMC

gene transcription in the anterior pituitary gland and CRH, AVP secretion in the hypothalamus. Cortisol also stimulates the higher brain centers (such as the hippocampus and reticular system) and inhibits the locus coerulus/sympathetic system. Chronic administration of corticosteroids suppresses the HPA axis, which persists for months after cessation of treatment.

Physiologic Actions of Glucocorticoids (GC)

Glucocorticoids play a prominent role in the intermediary metabolism of carbohydrate, protein and fat ultimately increasing the blood glucose concentration. In the liver they increase hepatic glycogen synthesis and stimulate gluconeogenesis. Glucocorticoids exert catabolic actions on protein metabolism, resulting in increased breakdown of protein and increased nitrogen excretion. Glucocorticoids exert an antiinsulin action in the peripheral tissues by reducing glucose uptake. In the adipose tissues lipolysis is stimulated through a glucocorticoid permissive effect on catecholamines and glucagon leading to elevated plasma free fatty acid levels. Consequently increased glucorticoid actions result in insulin resistance and an increase in blood glucose concentrations in the setting of increased protein and lipid catabolism.

Excess cortisol leads to increased deposition of adipose tissue centrally in the viscera as opposed to the periphery. Excess glucocorticoids cause muscle atrophy by catabolic actions as well as by reducing the protein synthesis in muscle. In the skeleton osteoblastic activity is inhibited leading to osteoporosis in GC excess. GC excess also induces a negative calcium balance by inhibiting intestinal calcium absorption and increasing renal calcium excretion.

Glucocorticoids cause lymphopenia as a result of redistribution of lymphocytes from the circulation to other compartments. Glucocorticoids increases neutrophil counts with depletion of the eosinophils. Changes in cortisol levels affect mood implicating the brain as an important target of this hormone.

Molecular Mechanisms of Cortisol Action

Free cortisol taken up from the circulation, binds to a specific intracellular glucocorticoid receptor (GR). The steroid receptor complex is transferred to the nucleus, where it binds to specific sites on steroid regulated genes, modifying levels of transcription. GR complex inhibits the transcription of nuclear factor kappa B (NFκ-B) and activating protein-1 (AP-1) thereby reducing the activity of various proinflammatory cytokine genes. Cortisol also inhibits POMC gene expression. Cortisol binds to the mineralocorticoid receptor (MR) with the same affinity as aldosterone but the local inactivation of cortisol to cortisone by 11β-HSD II results in mineralocorticoid specificity. Individuals who have inherited defects in the GR have resistance to glucocorticoid action with high levels of cortisol but no clinical manifestations of hypercortisolism.

Regulation of Renin-Angiotensin-Aldosterone Axis

Physiology of Renin-Angiotensin

Renin, part of aspartyl proteinase family of enzymes is formed in the juxtaglomerular cells (JG), located at the afferent arteriole of the glomerulus in the kidney. Renin acts on the substrate angiotensinogen (hepatic origin) to form the decapeptide angiotensin I. Angiotensin I is converted to octapeptide angiotensin II by angiotensin-converting enzyme (ACE) by the removal of the two C-terminal aminoacids. ACE is present in the endothelial cells throughout the vasculature but predominates in the pulmonary vascular endothelium. Angiotensin II is a potent vasoconstrictor and also stimulates the zona glomerulosa of the adrenal cortex to produce aldosterone secretion. The hexapeptide angiotensin III also acts as a potent secretagogue of aldosterone secretion. Angiotensin II binds to two classes of angiotensin receptors, AT1 and AT2. Angiotensin II operates primarily through the AT1 receptor to maintain normal extracellular volume (aldosterone secretion) and blood pressure. Studies have proposed that AT2 receptors have opposing actions to those of AT1. Angiotensin II is also produced in extrarenal sites (uterus, placenta, vascular tissue, heart, brain and adrenal cortex) where a paracrine role is likely.

Regulation of Renin Secretion

The juxtaglomerular cells are specialized myoepithelial cells, which act as intrarenal baroreceptors sensing renal perfusion pressure. A reduction in the blood volume leads to decrease in renal perfusion and afferent arteriolar pressure thus stimulating the JG cells to secrete renin (Fig. 2.3). This results in the formation of angiotensin II, which modulates the renal blood flow to maintain a constant glomerular filtration rate by constriction of the efferent arteriole in the nephron. The adrenal cortical glomerulosa is also stimulated to produce aldosterone which enhances renal sodium retention and expansion of the extracellular fluid volume [3].

A second control mechanism for the release of renin is found in the macula densa, a group of specialized distal convoluted tubular cells act as

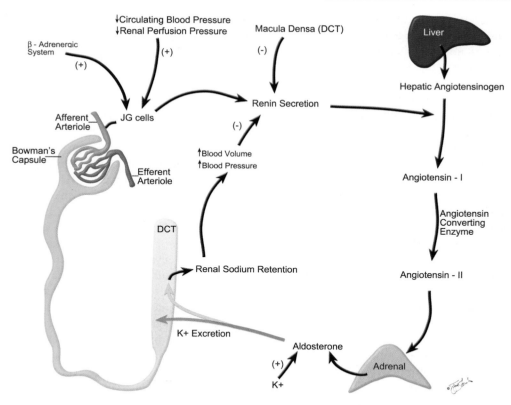

Fig. 2.3 The renin-angiotensin- aldosterone system. The interplay of various signals from the nephron (JG cells, Macula densa) in the kidney and adrenal gland form a feedback loop to maintain circulating blood volume. - suppression, + stimulation. DCT – distal convoluted tubule, K^+ – potassium, JG – juxtaglomerular

chemoreceptors for monitoring the sodium and chloride load in the distal tubule. Under conditions of increased delivery of filtered sodium to the macula densa, a signal is conveyed to juxtaglomerular cells to reduce the release of renin thereby modulating the glomerular filtration rate and the filtered load of sodium (Fig. 2.3).

The sympathetic nervous system stimulates the production of renin in response to upright posture. The other factors that control the release of renin include potassium, angiotensin II and atrial natriuretic peptide. Hypokalemia increases and hyperkalemia decreases renin secretion; in addition potassium also exerts a direct effect on the adrenal cortex to increase aldosterone secretion. Angiotensin II exerts a direct negative and feedback control on renin release. Atrial natriuretic peptide also inhibits renin release. Steady-state renin levels integrate all of these factors, with the intrarenal baroreceptor mechanism predominating.

Physiological Actions of Aldosterone

Aldosterone serves two important functions: regulation of extracellular fluid volume and potassium homeostasis [4]. These effects are mediated by the binding of aldosterone to the mineralocorticoid receptor (MR) in the epithelial cells of the renal collecting duct. Transport of the aldosterone/MR complex to the nucleus and binding to the targeted genes leads to increased expression of sodium and potassium channels. The result is a modification of the apical sodium channel due to an increase in ATPase resulting in sodium ion transport across the cell membrane. The sodium pump also provides the driving force for the excretion of potassium into the urine.

Chronic exposure to aldosterone leads to the "escape" phenomenon whereby after an initial period of sodium retention over 3–5 days, sodium balance is reestablished. As a result edema does not develop. The increase in atrial natriuretic peptide and interplay of renal hemodynamic factors, play a role in the "escape" from the sodium-retaining action of aldosterone. However it is important to realize that there is no escape from the potassium-losing effects of mineralocorticoids.

Non-epithelial action of aldosterone includes the expression of genes controlling tissue growth factors such as transforming growth factor β, plasminogen activator inhibitor type 1, adiponectin and leptin. Resultant actions include inflammation, necrosis (acutely) and subsequently fibrosis in a variety of tissues including the heart, kidney and vasculature. These pathophysiologic situations occur where aldosterone levels are inappropriately elevated on a high salt intake (primary aldosteronism).

Regulation of Aldosterone Secretion

The main mechanisms that control adrenal aldosterone secretion are the renin-angiotensin system, potassium and ACTH. The renin-angiotensin system controls extracellular fluid volume via regulation of aldosterone production. For example the renin-angiotensin-aldosterone system is suppressed when volume is expanded, resulting in a natriuresis. The potassium ion directly stimulates aldosterone secretion and also directly suppresses the renin-angiotensin system. ACTH stimulates aldosterone secretion acutely, but when ACTH is infused chronically, aldosterone secretion is not maintained beyond 48 h despite maintenance of increased cortisol secretion. Subjects receiving high dose glucocorticoid therapy, maintain normal aldosterone secretion. Neurotransmitters (such as serotonin) and endorphins stimulate while dopamine and atrial natriuretic peptide inhibit aldosterone release.

Adrenal Androgen Physiology

The principal adrenal androgens are dehydroepiandrosterone (DHEA), androstenedione and 11β-hydroxyandrostenedione. DHEA and androstenedione are weak androgens and exert their actions via peripheral conversion to the potent testosterone. ACTH positively regulates DHEA. In females androgenic effects such as sexual hair are primarily mediated by adrenal androgens.

In males the effects of the gonadal steroid testosterone overshadows the mild effects of adrenal androgens in regulating male secondary sexual characteristics.

Laboratory Evaluation of Adrenocortical Function

Random measurements of steroid hormones are usually not be useful to assess adrenocortical dysfunction. Circadian rhythm and pulsatile nature of hormone secretion affects random blood and urinary levels of steroid hormones. Therefore, endocrine testing using suppression and stimulation tests are needed to arrive at a diagnosis. Stimulation testing is needed to diagnose an adrenocortical deficiency states while suppression testing is used to diagnose a hypersecretion states. These tests are discussed in the relevant disease states.

Cushing's Syndrome

Cushing's syndrome is characterized by symptoms and signs of chronic exposure to elevated levels of glucocorticoids. Endogenous Cushing's syndrome is classified into ACTH dependent and independent causes [5]. However the most common cause of Cushing's syndrome is from exogenous corticosteroid therapy. Traditionally the term Cushing's syndrome is used for all hypercortisolism etiologies while Cushing's disease is reserved for individuals with the pituitary ACTH-dependent etiology.

ACTH-Dependent Causes

Cushing's Disease

An ACTH-producing pituitary adenoma results in bilateral adrenocortical hyperplasia with resultant overproduction of cortisol and androgens. Most individuals have a microadenoma (< 10 mm in diameter) but macroadenomas (>10 mm in diameter) or diffuse hyperplasia of the corticotrope cells are also seen. The primary abnormality is probably the de novo development of a pituitary neoplasm. The other theory is a defect in the hypothalamus and higher neural centers, which leads to chronic overproduction of CRH resulting in chronic stimulation of the corticotrophs (Fig. 2.4a).

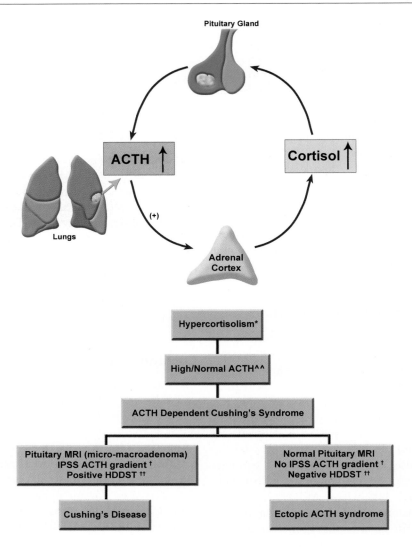

Fig. 2.4 Evaluation of ACTH- dependent causes of Cushing's syndrome. **a** Depicts sources of increased ACTH caused either by a pituitary tumor or an ectopic source stimulating the adrenal cortex to produce increased amounts of cortisol. **b** Alogarithm is a guide to evaluate ACTH dependent causes of Cushing's syndrome. *Failure of plasma cortisol to fall to <140 nmol/L after a standard low-dose dexamethasone suppression test (0.5 mg every 6 h for 2 days). ^^ ACTH levels range from 6 to 30 pmol/L (normal <14 pmolL) in pituitary microadenomas and may be greatly elevated >110 pmol/L in ectopic ACTH syndrome. † Inferior petrosal sinus sampling for ACTH. ACTH levels are measured at baseline, 2, 5, and 10 min after CRH injection (1 μg/kg IV). Peak petrosal: peripheral ACTH ratio >3 confirms a pituitary source of ACTH secretion. †† HDDST- High dose dexamethasone suppression test (2 mg every 6 h for 2 days). Positive response is ≥50% suppression of cortisol. MRI – magnetic resonance imaging, CRH – corticotropin releasing hormone, ACTH – adrenocorticotropic hormone, IPSS – inferior petrosal sinus sampling

Ectopic ACTH Syndrome

Classically a small cell carcinoma of the lung produces very high levels of ACTH leading to the acute onset of Cushing's syndrome. Here the prominent features are hypokalemic alkalosis with peripheral edema [6]. The typical signs and symptoms of Cushing's syndrome may be masked by weight loss and myopathy. Slower-growing ACTH-producing tumors such as bronchial carcinoid, pheochromocytoma and neuroendocrine tumors of pancreas have longer clinical course. As a result these patients present with typical cushingoid features. In ectopic ACTH syndrome, peripheral processing of POMC leads to increase in circulating α-MSH levels resulting in cutaneous hyper-pigmentation (Fig. 2.4a).

Other Causes

CRH production is a very rare cause of pituitary-dependent Cushing's syndrome and has been described in bronchial carcinoids, medullary thyroid and prostate carcinoma. Macronodular adrenal hyperplasia is thought to result from long-standing ACTH stimulation that subsequently results in autonomous cortisol production. These patients may be mistaken for adrenal adenomas.

ACTH-Independent Causes

Unilateral adrenal adenoma accounts for most cases with a gradual onset over months/years of clinical features. Adrenal carcinomas also produce Cushing's syndrome but with a more rapid clinical course. Carcinomas may additionally secrete androgen or mineralcorticoids. Hence in females additional features of virilization with hirsuitism, clitormegaly and severe acne may be present (Fig. 2.5a).

Other Etiologies

Macronodular adrenal hyperplasia may result from aberrant expression of receptors for ligands such as gastric-inhibitory peptide, lutenizing hormone,

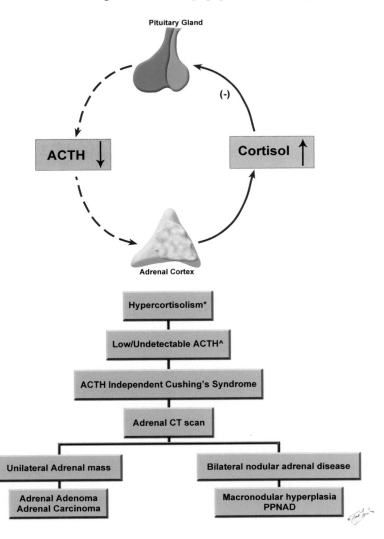

Fig. 2.5 Evaluation of ACTH- independent causes of Cushing's syndrome. **a** An adrenal tumor producing excess cortisol resulting in suppression of pituitary ACTH. **b** Algorithm shows the diagnostic pathway for evaluating ACTH-independent causes of Cushing's syndrome. *Failure of plasma cortisol to fall to <140 nmol/L after a standard low-dose dexamethasone suppression test (see Fig 2.4 (b)). ^ ACTH levels <14 pmol/L or undetectable. CT – computed tomography, PPNAD – primary pigmented nodular adrenal disease

vasopressin, catecholamines and serotonin. Another rare adrenal cause is primary pigmented nodular adrenal hyperplasia, either as isolated cases or as a part of the familial autosomal dominant condition called Carney complex. Cushing's syndrome has also been reported in McCune-Albright Syndrome where the more common manifestations include sexual precocity, growth hormone excess and skeletal fibrous dysplasia.

Clinical Features of Cushing's Syndrome

The classical features of Cushing's syndrome include truncal obesity, moon face, hirsuitism and facial plethora. Patients develop fat depots in characteristic sites such as the dorsocervical area (buffalo hump), supraclavicular fat pads, and the mesenteric bed. Signs of protein wasting are seen with thin skin, easy brusability, broad violaceous cutaneous striae and proximal myopathy. Myopathy and easy bruising are two characteristic features of Cushing's syndrome. Osteoporosis may occur with vertebral fractures. Hypercalciuria may be associated with renal calculi, but hypercalcemia is absent.

Glucose intolerance occurs owing to insulin resistance with overt diabetes mellitus in about 20% of the patients. Imaging studies show hepatic steatosis and increased visceral fat. Cortisol excess predisposes to hypertension and thereby increases the cardiovascular risk. Gonadal disturbances are common in both sexes and emotional dysfunction occurs in approximately 50% of patients. This may range from agitated depression, lethargy to overt psychosis with memory and cognitive disturbances. Wound infections are common and contribute to poor wound healing.

Diagnosis

Initial screening for Cushing's syndrome is to demonstrate increased cortisol production and/or failure to suppress cortisol secretion when exogenous glucocorticoid, (dexamethasone), is administered [7]. Once the diagnosis of hypercortisolism is ascertained the etiology should to be sought.

A sensitive screening test is the overnight dexamethasone suppression test (DST) (1 mg of dexamethasone at bedtime). A cortisol level greater than 140 nmol/L the next morning supports the diagnosis of Cushing's syndrome but false positive results are not uncommon. This maybe followed by the low-dose DST (0.5 mg every 6 h for 48 h), which has greater specificity. Failure of urinary cortisol to fall less than 25 nmol/day or of plasma cortisol to fall less than 140 nmol/L establishes the diagnosis of autonomous cortisol production [7].

Measurements of 24-h urinary free cortisol (along with urinary creatinine to ascertain the completeness of collection) are also useful to diagnose hypercortisolism. Normal values are less than 220–330 nmol/24 h depending on the assay. The normal circadian rhythm is lost in Cushing's syndrome; values of plasma midnight cortisol greater than 50 nmol/L are diagnostic [8]. Though this is a sensitive test, patients need hospitalization for this investigation and hence it is not a widely used screening test. Salivary cortisol also reflects the amount of free circulating cortisol; a midnight level can be a valuable test in the assessment of cyclic Cushing's syndrome [9, 10].

Investigations to Determine the Etiology of Cushing's Syndrome

Once a diagnosis of hypercortisolism is confirmed the next step is to confirm the etiology. The first step to differentiate between ACTH dependent and ACTH independent cause would be the measurement of a plasma ACTH level. A low or undetectable ACTH level (< 2 pmol/L) diagnose primary adrenal hypercortisolism. In pituitary macroadenomas and ectopic ACTH syndrome, ACTH values will be doubly elevated (>110 pmol/L) whereas in pituitary microadenomas (Cushing's disease) the levels are normal or modestly elevated (6–30 pmol/L).

High dose dexamethasone suppression test (HDDST) (2 mg every 6 h for 2 days) is used to diagnose Cushing's disease; there is suppression of greater than 50% of plasma cortisol in ACTH-secreting pituitary microadenomas, whereas there is no response with ectopic ACTH production. Nonetheless patients with carcinoid tumors may exhibit some suppression with high dose dexamethasone. On the other hand, ACTH-secreting pituitary macroadenomas usually show no suppression (Fig. 2.4b).

In patients with Cushing's disease there is an exaggerated rise in ACTH (greater than 50%) and cortisol (more than 20% of baseline value)

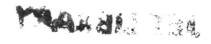

following a 100-μg intravenous dose of CRH. Though false positives can occur with ectopic ACTH syndrome this test has a specificity and sensitivity of 90%.

Imaging studies of the pituitary (CT scan or MRI with gadolinium) may not always demonstrate a pituitary lesion in patients with Cushing's disease. It is important to keep in mind that 10–20% of normal patients have non-functioning pituitary "incidentalomas". In the situation where a tumor is not visualized the best test, provided local expertise is available, would be inferior petrosal sinus sampling (IPSS). Blood from each half of the pituitary drains into ipsilateral inferior petrosal sinus, catherization and venous sampling of both the sinuses simultaneously would differentiate a pituitary source from an ectopic source. In pituitary ACTH-secreting tumor the ratio of ACTH concentrations from the inferior petrosal sinus to simultaneously drawn peripheral blood would be greater than 2.0. This test reaches a sensitivity of 97% and specificity of 100% when an ACTH petrosal sinus/peripheral ratio is enhanced after CRH injection. Hence IPSS is a highly sensitive test to distinguish between pituitary and nonpituitary sources of ACTH excess [11]. However IPSS is technically difficult and complications such as thrombosis can occur (Fig. 2.4b).

In cortisol-producing adrenal adenomas the ACTH level is low or undetectable. There is also suppression in plasma DHEAS as the adrenal androgens are reduced as a result of ACTH suppression. In adrenal carcinomas elevated androgen secretion is commonly seen along with an increase in urinary 17-ketosteroids. The steroid production in adrenal carcinoma is usually resistant to ACTH stimulation and dexamethasone suppression (Fig. 2.5b).

Radiological Evaluation of Cushing's Syndrome

The best radiological test to image the adrenal gland is a high resolution CT scan (Fig. 2.6). For Cushing's disease pituitary MRI with gadolinium is the investigation of choice bearing in mind that false positive results can occur (Fig. 2.7). To diagnose ectopic ACTH production, it would be reasonable to start with a CT scan of the chest and abdomen. PET scanning would be a second test if CT scanning were negative. Octreotide scanning can also be useful

to image ACTH-producing neuroendocrine tumors such as carcinoids. Inspite of meticulous investigations the cause for Cushing's syndrome can remain occult in about 5–15% of patients, and they would need constant follow-up.

Differential Diagnosis
Pseudo-Cushing's Syndrome

Obesity, chronic alcoholism and depression can mimic the biochemical abnormalities seen in Cushing's syndrome. Chronic alcohol intake and depression may cause mild elevation in urinary free cortisol, blunted circadian rhythm and resistance to suppression with dexamethasone. However these patients usually do not have the clinical features of Cushing's syndrome such as proximal myopathy and easy bruisability. Following discontinuation of alcohol or with improvement of depression steroid testing returns to normal.

Management
ACTH Dependent Causes

Treatment for Cushing's disease is transphenoidal resection of the pituitary adenoma. In the hands of an experienced surgeon the cure rates are 80%–90% for microadenomas and 50% for macroadenomas. After removal of the ACTH-producing pituitary adenoma the normal corticotrophes are suppressed; hence, patients need glucocorticoid treatment postoperatively until the HPA axis recovers. In the past bilateral adrenalectomy was performed for Cushing's disease; that led to the subsequent development of Nelson's syndrome in 10%–20% of patients – an aggressive ACTH-secreting pituitary macroadenoma. Pituitary irradiation is reserved for patients with postoperative recurrence and in Nelson's syndrome. In some centers gamma knife and stereotactic techniques have been used to treat pituitary adenomas.

Ectopic ACTH Syndrome

If the primary tumor is found and resected (e.g. bronchial carcinoid) it can lead to cure. However the prognosis remains poor for small cell lung tumors and medical therapy inhibit steroidogenesis is indicated for symptoms of cortisol excess.

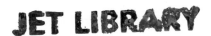
JET LIBRARY

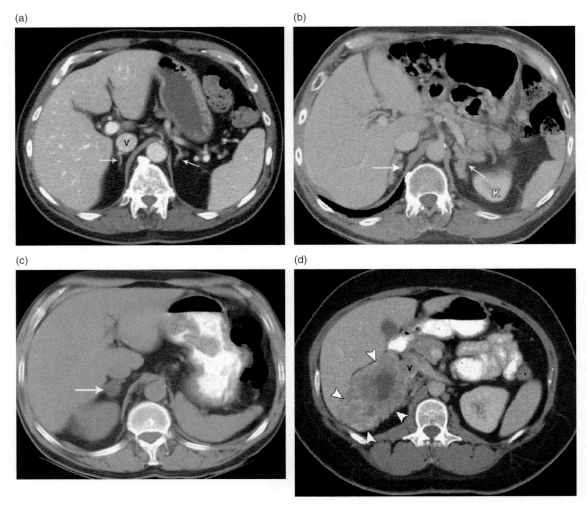

Fig. 2.6 Computed tomography (CT) is the preferred method for visualizing the adrenal glands. **A** The normal right adrenal gland is adjacent to the inferior vena cava (V). Usually the right adrenal gland appears as a linear structure extending posterior from the inferior vena cava into the space between the right lobe of the liver and the crus of the diaphragm. The normal left adrenal gland is shaped like an inverted V or Y and is found lateral to the left crus of the diaphragm and below the pancreas. **B** Both the adrenal glands are large and multilobular yet retaining their normal configurations suggesting bilateral adrenal hyperplasia. K – Kidney. **C** 1.5-cm right adrenal mass measuring −8 Hounsfield units (HU) seen in this oral contrast enhanced CT scan. **D** Oral and IV contrast enhanced CT scan in a patient with adrenal carcinoma. In contrast to the tumor in C, the right adrenal mass is large (12 cm) and heterogeneous. The mass is contiguous with the inferior vena cava and extends into the right lobe of the liver and the upper pole of the kidney

Adrenal Etiologies

Laparoscopic adrenalectomy is preferred for adrenal adenomas. Adrenal carcinomas carry a poor prognosis with dismal 5-year survival rates. Adrenal carcinomas are neither radiosensitive nor chemosensitive and the most important predictor of outcome is the ability to do a complete surgical resection.

Medical Therapies for Cushing's Syndrome

Drugs can be used to treat hypercortisolism – metyrapone, ketoconazole and mitotane. (Table 2.1) Metyrapone inhibits 11β-hydroxylase while ketaconazole blocks cytochrome P450-dependent enzymes. These drugs can be used preoperatively or as adjunctive

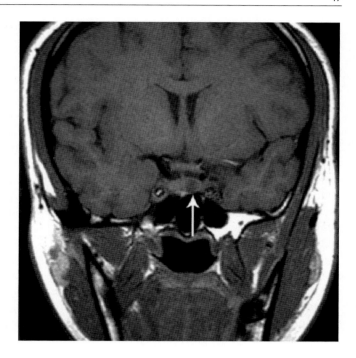

Fig. 2.7 IV Gadolinium-enhanced pituitary MRI of a patient with a pituitary microadenoma. A solitary rounded lesion measuring 5 mm is seen within the left anterolateral aspect of the pituitary gland; the microadenoma shows diminished enhancement in comparison to the rest of the gland. The optic chiasm is normal in appearance and the stalk is in the midline

Table 2.1 Medical management of Cushing's syndrome

Drug	Action	Indication
Metyrapone, ketaconazole, aminoglutethimide, etomidate (given intravenously)	Steroidogenic enzyme inhibitors	Metastatic ectopic ACTH production Cortisol- producing adrenal carcinoma (CPAC)
Mitotane	Steroidogenesis inhibitor and adrenolytic drug	CPAC
Mifepristone	Glucocorticoid receptor antagonist	CPAC; metastatic ectopic ACTH production

treatment following surgery or radiotherapy. Mitotane is an adrenolytic drug with delayed onset of action but long-lasting effect. Its use is primarily for adrenal carcinoma due to its potential cytotoxicity [12].

Mineralocorticoid Excess

Hyperaldosteronism

In primary hyperaldosteronism, autonomous aldosterone production leads to hypertension, hypokalemia and suppressed renin activity. An extra adrenal stimulus for increased renin secretion is found in secondary hyperaldosteronism. Recent studies suggest a prevalence of primary aldosteronism of 10% in the essential hypertensive population [13].

Primary Hyperaldosteronism

Etiology

Aldosterone-producing adenomas, (APA) (originally described by Conn) account for nearly one-third of cases of primary aldosteronism. These benign tumors are typically small (less than 2 cm). They usually occur between the ages of 30 and 50 and are twice as common in women as men. The prevalence of aldosterone-producing adenoma (APA) is 1% in the general hypertension population.

Bilateral idiopathic hyperplasia (IHA) is found in approximately two-thirds of cases of primary aldosteronism. The aldosterone excess is milder; therefore hypokalemia and suppression of plasma renin activity (PRA) is generally less severe [14].

A less common form of primary aldosteronism is Glucocorticoid-remediable aldosteronism (GRA), which is inherited in an autosomal dominant fashion. Increased levels of hybrid compound, 18-oxygenated cortisol and suppressibility with exogenous glucocorticoids characterizes this condition.

Clinical Features

Hypokalemia from renal potassium wasting is manifested as muscle weakness, cramps and fatigue. Aldosterone excess leads to increased distal tubular exchange of intratubular sodium for secreted potassium and hydrogen ions, leading to hypokalemic metabolic alkalosis. Polyuria and polydipsia result from the impaired urine concentrating ability as a result of hypokalemia-induced resistance to antidiuretic hormone (nephrogenic diabetes insipidus). Moderate to severe hypertension refractory to conventional antihypertensive agents is due to extracellular volume expansion. However despite high levels of aldosterone, patients rarely exhibit edema owing to the escape from the sodium-retaining effects of aldosterone.

Patients with APA more commonly exhibit hypokalemia compared to bilateral hyperplasia. In patients with primary aldosteronism regardless of etiology, left ventricular hypertrophy and renal proteinuria is greater than predicted based on the level of blood pressure.

Aldosterone and Cardiovascular Damage

Aldosterone can directly induce cardiovascular damage in animal models as a result of myocardial inflammation and fibrosis [15]. Studies have also revealed that small doses of mineralocorticoid antagonist can ameliorate such damage. In the RALES (randomized aldactone evaluation study) trial in patients with heart failure the low dose mineralocorticoid receptor (MR) antagonist spironolactone reduced cardiovascular mortality and hospitalizations by 30% after 3 years of therapy. More recently the EPHESUS (eplerenone post-acute myocardial infarction heart failure efficacy and survival study) trial showed that small doses of the MR antagonist eplerenone significantly reduced cardiovascular morbidity and mortality in individuals who developed congestive cardiac failure after acute myocardial infarction [16].

Diagnosis

Spontaneous hypokalemia (in the absence of potassium-wasting diuretics) in a hypertensive patient should alert the clinicians to suspect primary aldosteronism (PA). Recent studies, which have shown an increased prevalence of PA in normokalemic subjects, advocate screening of patients with treatment resistant hypertension [17]. Plasma renin activity is suppressed in PA; one caveat is that 25% of patients with essential hypertension also have low PRA. Hence, the concomitant demonstration of hyporeninism with an elevated plasma aldosterone is essential to diagnose primary aldosteronism.

The best screening test is the measurement of plasma aldosterone / plasma renin activity (PA/PRA) ratio. A ratio of 50 or more is strongly suggestive of diagnosis of primary aldosteronism while a ratio of greater than 30 is still consistent with the diagnosis [18]. Certain antihypertensive drugs, β-blockers and spironolactone, should be discontinued for 2–4 weeks prior to testing. For better accuracy this test is done after the correction of hypokalemia and without salt restriction. Typically younger hypertensive patients (< 50 years), with severe hypokalemia (< 3.0 mmol/L), high plasma aldosterone concentrations (>25 ng/dL) and a PA/PRA ratio >50 have a high probability of APA (Fig. 2.6). In situations when PA/PRA ratio is mildly abnormal (20–40), oral salt loading testing is done to confirm the presence of autonomous aldosterone production. Patients are instructed to take sodium chloride tablets (2 gm) with each meal for 3 days. On the fourth day a 24-hr urinary aldosterone excretion greater than 39 nmol/L, in the presence of urinary sodium excretion greater than 250 mmol/day, is diagnostic of autonomous aldosterone production (Fig. 2.8).

Radiographic studies should not be performed until after establishing a biochemical diagnosis of PA because of the high prevalence of non-functioning adrenal masses (see later). A high-resolution spiral CT scan is used to visualize the adrenal glands (Fig. 2.6). Regardless of the result of adrenal imaging, adrenal venous sampling (AVS) is usually done. This test is very specific to differentiate between APA and IHA. In APA the ratio of ipsilateral to contralateral aldosterone concentration is greater than 10:1. This procedure carries a small risk of venous thrombosis and adrenal hemorrhage.

Fig. 2.8 Algorithm for the diagnosis of primary aldosteronism. * Inadequate control of hypertension on three antihypertensive medications (including a diuretic). ^^ Oral salt loading – normal sodium intake and 2 gm of sodium chloride tablets with each meal for 4 days 24 h urinary aldosterone collected on day 4, abnormal response would be failure to normally suppress aldosterone production. IV saline infusion - 2 L (500 mL/h) of isotonic saline over 4 h intravenously. Plasma aldosterone is measured pre and post infusion. † dedicated adrenal protocol CT examination – see chapter, †† adrenal venous sampling (AVS) see text, APA – aldosterone- producing adenoma

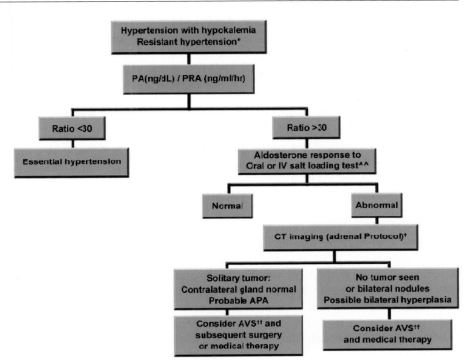

Differential Diagnosis

It is important to distinguish between an adenoma and idiopathic bilateral hyperplasia as the latter is medically managed. AVS is the gold standard to discriminate between these two conditions. Radiographic studies and biochemical testing have been shown to be inconclusive.

Management

Laparoscopic adrenalectomy is the recommended treatment for APA. Dietary sodium restriction, correction of hypokalemia and treatment with the MR antagonist (spironolactone or eplerenone) is recommended prior to surgery (Fig. 2.6). Postoperatively hypokalemia is corrected but persistent hypertension may remain due to chronicity or coexistence of essential hypertension. On the other hand IHA is managed medically usually with MR antagonists. In men chronic treatment with spironolactone is limited by gynecomastia, decreased libido and impotence. Eplerenone is

useful in this situation, as it has no antiandrogen actions. Another alternative is amiloride, a potassium-sparing diuretic, which acts by blocking the sodium epithelial channel.

Glucocorticoid-Remediable Aldosteronism

This is an autosomal dominant condition caused by chimeric gene duplication, a crossover between the homologous 11β-hydroxylase and aldosterone synthase genes. This result in ectopic expression of aldosterone synthase in the cortisol-producing zona fasiculata [19, 20]. GRA is characterized by early onset hypertension, hemorrhagic stroke and suppressed plasma renin levels. Prospective screening of GRA pedigrees can be done by mutational analysis using Southern blot techniques. Variable phenotype is exhibited in that many of the affected individuals are not hypokalemic and have only mild hypertension or normotension. Markedly elevated levels of the "hybrid" steroids 18-oxocortisol and 18-OH-cortisol can be demonstrated in a 24-h urine collection. Glucocorticoid treatment can usually reverse the syndrome; however, the smallest effective dose should be used to minimize the risk of Cushing's syndrome.

Secondary Hyperaldosteronism

Secondary hyperaldosteronism commonly occurs in the setting of an underlying edematous disorder where there is reduced effective circulating blood volume (e.g. cirrhosis, nephrotic syndrome and congestive cardiac failure) or with accelerated phase of hypertension. In some hypertensive states there is an overproduction of renin due to decreased renal perfusion. This may be due to narrowing of the major renal arteries from atherosclerosis or fibromuscular hyperplasia or small vessel vasoconstriction (such as vasculitis). Typically these patients have hypokalemic alkalosis, moderate to severe increases in plasma renin activity and aldosterone overproduction. However in Bartter and Gitelman's syndrome (see later) there is secondary hyperaldosteronism without edema or hypertension.

Other Causes of Increased Mineralocorticoid Action

Hypoaldosteronism with Low Plasma Renin Activity

Some etiologies of congenital adrenal hyperplasia (11β- or 17α-hydroxylase deficiencies) result in overproduction of the mineralocorticoid deoxycorticosterone (DOC). Such patients will have hypokalemia and suppressed levels of renin and aldosterone.

Apparent Mineralocorticoid Excess

This condition can occur in both heritable and acquired forms due to impaired activity of the enzyme 11β-hydroxysteroid dehydrogenase (11β-HSD II) [21]. This isoform of 11β-HSD inactivates cortisol in the kidney to cortisone, biologically inactive compound that cannot bind to the renal MR. Hence when the enzyme is deficient there is accumulation of cortisol in the kidney, which binds to the MR and exerts mineralocorticoid actions. The acquired form of this syndrome is caused by the ingestion of liquorice (active agent – glycyrrhizinic acid). Such patients exhibit hypertension, low PRA

levels, hypokalemia, normal plasma cortisol levels and low aldosterone levels. High potency glucocorticoids have been used to suppress the endogenous cortisol with some success.

Liddle's Syndrome

This autosomal dominant disorder is caused by gain-of-function mutations in the subunits of the renal sodium epithelial channel (ENaC). Congenital hypertension, hypokalemia and low renin/aldosterone levels result. This syndrome is treated with the ENaC antagonist's triamterene or amiloride.

Hyperaldosteronism with High Plasma Renin Activity

Bartter's Syndrome

This syndrome is caused by mutations in the loop of Henle Na-K-2Cl cotransporter gene, which results in renal wasting of sodium. Renal sodium loss stimulates renin and aldosterone production resulting in hypokalemic alkalosis; hypercalciuria, normal blood pressure and absence of edema also characterize this disorder.

Gitelman's Syndrome

Affected individuals have similar features to Bartter's syndrome except that they are hypocalciuric. Gitelman's syndrome results from loss-of-function mutations in the thiazide-sensitive Na-Cl co transporter in the distal convoluted tubule of the kidney.

Primary Adrenal Insufficiency

Primary adrenal insufficiency, often referred as Addison's disease, results from the loss of all zones of the adrenal cortex with deficiencies of aldosterone, cortisol and adrenal androgens. Secondary hypoadrenalism results from decreased ACTH production leading to reduced cortisol. The renin angiotensin axis maintains normal aldosterone production in such patients. Although Addison's disease is rare it carries significant morbidity and mortality if not diagnosed and treated.

Etiology

In the western world the most common cause of Addison's disease is autoimmune adrenalitis. In about 75% of these patients circulating adrenal antibodies are detected. Though the significance of these antibodies

Table 2.2 Etiologies of adrenal insufficiency

Primary adrenal insufficiency

Autoimmune
- Sporadic
- Autoimmune polyglandular syndromes (APS) I[a] & I I[b]

Infections
- Tuberculosis
- Fungal infections
- Cytomegalovirus
- HIV[d]

Hemorrhage
- Waterhouse–Friderichsen syndrome associated meningococcal septicemia
- Anticoagulant therapy
- Antiphospholipid syndrome

Metastatic disease

Bilateral adrenalectomy

Infiltrative disorders
- Amyloid, hemochromatosis

Drugs
- Enzyme inhibitors (metyrapone, ketoconazole, aminoglutethimide), adrenolytic agents (mitotane)

Miscellaneous
- Congenital adrenal hypoplasia
- Adrenoleukodystrophies
- ACTH[c] resistance syndromes
- Glucocorticoid resistance syndrome

Secondary adrenal insufficiency

Hypothalamic-pituitary diseases
- Pituitary tumors
- Pituitary surgery
- Postpartum pituitary infarction(Sheehan's syndrome)
- Lymphocytic hypophysitis
- Granulomatous disease – sarcoid, eosinophilic granuloma

Exogenous glucocorticoid therapy

[a]APS type I always includes Addison's disease and other autoimmune disorders such as, hypoparathyroidism and premature ovarian failure. The phenotype may also include chronic mucocutaneous candidiasis, dental enamel hypoplasia and alopecia
[b]APS type II may include Addison's disease but more commonly primary hypothyroidism, insulin dependent diabetes and primary hypogonadism. Additional disorders like pernicious anemia and vitiligo may be present.
[c]ACTH–Adrenocorticotropic hormone
[d]HIV – Human Immunodeficiency virus

in the pathogenesis of the disease remains unknown, the autoantibodies are usually directed towards 21-hydroxylase and side chain cleavage enzymes. Other autoimmune diseases (especially thyroid disease, type 1 diabetes and premature ovarian failure) also occur in patients with autoimmune adrenalitis. Primary adrenal insufficiency can occur as a part of autoimmune polyendocrine syndromes (APS) I and II [22].

In the developing world primary adrenal insufficiency is mainly due to infections, especially tuberculosis. Fungal infections such as histoplasmosis, coccidiomycosis and crytococcosis can also destroy the adrenal gland. Adrenal insufficiency can occur in patients with AIDS as a result of infection with cytomegalovirus or mycobacterium avium-intracellure; Kaposi's sarcoma may also result in adrenal destruction (Table 2.2).

Acute adrenocortical insufficiency as a result of hemorrhage can occur in children in the setting of septicemia with meningococcemia (Waterhouse-Friderichsen syndrome). In adults, anticoagulant therapy or hypercoagulable states can lead to bilateral adrenal hemorrhage [23].

Clinical Features

The clinical presentation in adrenal insufficiency depends on the rapidity of onset, duration and severity of adrenal hypofunction. Acute adrenal insufficiency when caused by adrenal hemorrhage presents as hypotension and acute circulatory failure [23]. Chronic adrenal insufficiency is manifested by symptoms of fatigability, weakness, anorexia, and nausea/vomiting. Cutaneous and mucous hyperpigmentation is usually seen in patients with chronic primary adrenal insufficiency (except in acute onset). Hyperpigmentation is typically seen in the sun-exposed areas, recent scars, palmar creases and buccal mucosa. Postural hypotension is frequently present as a result of salt wasting. Women may note loss of axillary and pubic hair, as a result of the adrenal androgen deficiency. Some patients can also show symptoms of memory impairment, excessive irritability, depression and psychosis. Weight loss and anorexia are common.

Diagnosis

Hyponatremia and hyperkalemia is often present in primary adrenal insufficiency. Aldosterone deficiency leads to renal sodium wasting which in turn depletes the extracellular fluid volume leading to postural hypotension. The compensatory elevated plasma vasopressin and angiotensin II levels result in decreased free water clearance. Hyperkalemia occurs due to a combination of aldosterone deficiency, impaired glomerular filtration and acidosis. The blood urea concentration is usually elevated and mild to moderate hypercalcemia is seen in some patients.

The best screening test is the ACTH stimulation test. 250 μg of cosyntropin is given intramuscularly or intravenously and the cortisol response is measured at 60 min. The normal response is a cortisol level greater than 495 nmol/L (18 μg/dL). If the cortisol response is abnormal then, measuring the plasma aldosterone level can differentiate primary and secondary adrenal insufficiency. Primary adrenal insufficiency is diagnosed when the plasma aldosterone increment is less than 150 pmol/L (5 ng/dL) following ACTH stimulation (30-min sample). A normal aldosterone increment is seen in secondary adrenal insufficiency. Moreover the morning plasma ACTH levels are elevated in primary adrenal insufficiency as opposed to secondary hypoadrenalism where the plasma ACTH values are low or "inappropriately" normal (Fig. 2.9).

Adrenal auto-antibodies (e.g. 21-hydroxylase) can be measured by radioimmunoassay to diagnose autoimmune adrenalitis. CT scan of the adrenal glands may show enlargement (e.g. hemorrhage) or calcification depending on the etiology of the adrenal failure.

Differential Diagnosis

Non-specific symptoms like fatigue, weakness and malaise can make the diagnosis difficult in adrenal insufficiency. When insidious in onset adrenal insufficiency is frequently mistaken as chronic fatigue syndrome. However hyperpigmentation, weight loss and gastrointestinal symptoms should alert the clinician to diagnose this disorder. It is also prudent to look for other organ specific autoimmune diseases in the context of autoimmune adrenal insufficiency.

Management

Replacement therapy should be directed to treat both the glucocorticoid and mineralocorticoid deficiencies. In case of adrenal crisis parenteral treatment with high doses of hydrocortisone should be initiated without any delay. After stabilization or in non-acute situations, replacement doses of oral

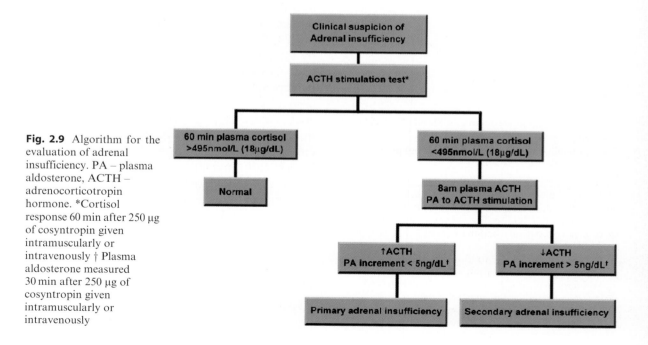

Fig. 2.9 Algorithm for the evaluation of adrenal insufficiency. PA – plasma aldosterone, ACTH – adrenocorticotropin hormone. *Cortisol response 60 min after 250 μg of cosyntropin given intramuscularly or intravenously † Plasma aldosterone measured 30 min after 250 μg of cosyntropin given intramuscularly or intravenously

hydrocortisone at a dose of 8–10 mg/m^2/day should be started. To follow the diurnal pattern of steroid secretion two-thirds of the total dose is given in the morning and one third is given in late afternoon with mealtime or snack.

Fludrocortisone is administered at a dose of 0.05–0.1 mg once a day orally. Plasma renin activity, blood pressure and serum electrolytes are useful parameters to titrate the dose of fludrocortisone. In female patients some studies have suggested the benefit of oral 25–50 mg per day of DHEA to improve sexual function and general well being [24, 25].

Patient education and daily replacement therapy forms a cornerstone in the management of primary adrenal insufficiency. During periods of intercurrent illness or surgery the dose of hydrocortisone should be increased. All patients should wear a med alert bracelet and should be instructed in parenteral self-administration of steroids if they cannot take their dosing orally.

Secondary Adrenocortical Insufficiency

Patients with secondary hypoadrenalism may have associated deficiencies of other pituitary hormones. They usually have some of the clinical features seen in primary adrenal insufficiency except for hyperpigmentation as the ACTH levels and α-MSH levels are low. They also have normal aldosterone secretion so that hyperkalemia is not seen. Pituitary MRI scans and assessment of anterior pituitary function are usually needed in these patients. To definitively diagnose secondary adrenal insufficiency insulin-induced hypoglycemia test can be used although the ACTH stimulation test is commonly used for screening.

Individuals receiving long-term high dose steroid therapy usually develop prolonged HPA suppression leading to adrenal atrophy. Recovery takes months to as long as one year after glucocorticoid withdrawal. ACTH stimulation testing is used to assess the adrenal recovery. Glucocorticoid therapy is similar to patients with primary adrenal insufficiency but mineralocorticoid therapy is not necessary.

Hypoaldosteronism

Aldosterone deficiency can result from impaired renin production, an inherited biosynthetic defect or renal resistance to aldosterone action. It can also occur in the setting of primary adrenal insufficiency or be drug induced such as following heparin administration.

Most cases of hyporeninemic hypoaldosteronism are often seen in the setting of mild renal impairment and longstanding diabetes mellitus. In such patients the degree of hyperkalemia and metabolic acidosis are typically is out of proportion to the degree of renal impairment. The cortisol response to ACTH stimulation is normal. The predilection for diabetic patients is unclear but plausible explanations in pathogenesis include autonomic dysfunction, renal disease, and defective conversion of renin precursors to active renin.

Hyporeninemic hypoaldosteronism has also been described in patients with AIDS, obstructive uropathy, those on chronic non-steroidal anti-inflammatory drugs and following removal of aldosterone-secreting adenomas. Treatment of the hyperkalemia involves either removal of the offending agent or treatment with fludrocortisone at an oral dose of 0.05–0.15 mg daily. Occasionally replacement with mineralocorticoid can be risky, as in patients with congestive heart failure.

Hyperreninemic hypoaldosteronism has been described in critically ill patients and is associated with a high mortality rate. It is speculated that stress-induced chronic ACTH stimulation shifts the steroidogenesis from mineralocorticoids to glucocorticoids. Another uncommon inherited disorder is pseudohypoaldosteronism, which is manifested by renal salt wasting, hyperkalemia and metabolic acidosis. These patients have a loss-of-function mutation in the epithelial sodium channel leading to renal tubular resistance to aldosterone; levels of both aldosterone and renin are elevated in such patients.

Congenital Adrenal Hyperplasia

Congenital adrenal hyperplasia (CAH) results from autosomal recessive mutations that cause enzymatic defects that result in deficient cortisol steroidogenesis. A block in cortisol secretion leads to increased ACTH secretion which results in increased adrenal androgen / mineralocorticoid synthesis, depending on the site of the enzyme block.

The most common enzyme defect in CAH is 21-hydroxylase deficiency. Decreased aldosterone secretion can occur along with cortisol deficiency. Early onset or classic CAH is usually associated with virilization in the female and isosexual precocity in the male.

Late-onset 21-hydroxylase deficiency from partial enzymatic defects results in hirsutism and oligomenorrhea in women. High levels of 17-hydroxyprogesterone characterize 21-hydroxylase deficiency, the steroid precursor prior to the enzymatic block. Adrenal androgen output is suppressed by glucocorticoid treatment. In adults with late onset CAH a single bedtime dose of a long-acting glucocorticoid is used to suppress adrenal hyperplasia (e.g. 5 mg of prednisone). Other enzyme deficiencies include 11β-hydroxylase, 17α-hydroxylase and 3β-hydroxy steroid dehydrogenase.

Adrenal "Incidentalomas"

An adrenal mass greater than 1 cm that is inadvertently discovered on radiological testing for other conditions that are not related to adrenal disease is known as an "incidentaloma" [26]. From autopsy studies the overall frequency of such adrenal adenomas is 6%; the prevalence increases as age advances [27].

When faced with adrenal incidentalomas two important issues needs to be addressed: first is the mass functional? and second, is it malignant?

It is important to take a careful history and a directed physical examination concentrating on signs and symptoms of adrenal hyperfunction. It is particularly important to note whether the patient is hypertensive and to ascertain when the patient has a prior history of malignancy. All the patients should undergo overnight dexamethasone suppression test to rule out "subclinical" Cushing's syndrome. Even though obvious stigmata for Cushing's syndrome are absent in these patients, they may exhibit metabolic features of hypercortisolism such as hypertension, diabetes mellitus and osteoporosis [28].

Measurement of plasma free metanephrines, a highly sensitive test, is recommended as a screening for phaeochromocytoma in all patients regardless of radiographic features. When the patient is hypertensive, screening should be done to rule out primary aldosteronism by

Table 2.3 Evaluation of adrenal incidentaloma

Clinical	- ?History of prior malignancy - ?Hypertension (±paroxysmal symptoms) - ?Cushingoid features - ?Hypokalemia
Hormonal	- Overnight dexamethasone suppression test - Plasma free metanephrines - Plasma aldosterone and plasma renin activity (if hypertensive) - DHEAS (female with signs of androgen excess)
Radiographic	Tumor phenotype - Size, regular/irregular margins and homo/heterogeneity - Attenuation coefficient (Hounsfield units) on unenhanced CT scan - Rapidity of washout of on contrast enhanced CT scan

DHEAS – dehydroepiandrosterone sulfate

measuring the PA/PRA ratio. If signs of androgen excess are noticed in females then testing for DHEAS and testosterone are indicated (Table 2.3).

Radiographic Evaluation

The following features need to be considered while assessing the mass radiographically: size, lipid content and washout of contrast medium with enhanced CT scanning [29].

Benign adrenal adenomas are typically less than 4 cm, homogeneous with smooth margins and low unenhanced CT values (<10 HU). They typically exhibit rapid washout on contrast enhanced CT scan. In contrast, malignant lesions are often larger than benign lesions with heterogeneity, irregular margins and sometimes hemorrhage and rarely tissue calcification. They have higher attenuation values, i.e. greater than 10 HU on unenhanced CT scan and have delayed washout of contrast material on an enhanced study. Similar features are noticed in chemical shift MRI. If biopsy is being considered, it is critical to rule out pheochromocytoma before undertaking FNA as the procedure may result in a hypertensive crisis [30]. An algorithm of adrenal mass characterization is suggested in Fig. 2.10.

Fig. 2.10 Algorithm for the evaluation of adrenal "incidentaloma". *An adrenal "incidentaloma" is an adrenal mass usually 1 cm or more in diameter that is incidentally discovered on imaging for indications other than an adrenal disorder. ^^ For evaluation of hormonal overproduction see Table 2.3. † Benign characteristics include size < 4 cm, homogeneous with smooth margins, ≤ 10 Hounsfield units, ≥ 50% washout of contrast medium at 10 min. †† Suspicious appearances include size > 4 cm, heterogeneity with irregular margins, > 10 Hounsfield units, < 50% washout at 10 min

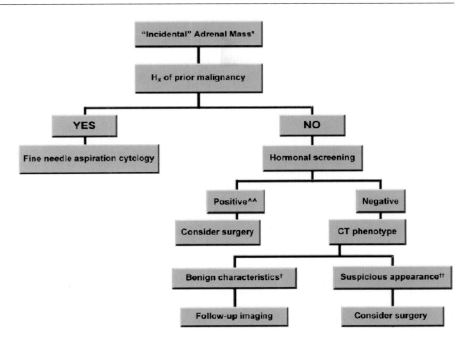

Follow Up

In patients with a small (< 4 cm) non-functional adrenal mass it would be prudent to repeat imaging studies at 6, 12, and 24 months [26]. Yearly hormonal screening for hypercortisolism and pheochromocytoma is recommended for 4 years. During the period of surveillance, if a mass enlarges by 1 cm or more over 1 year, develops worrying radiographic features, or if there is of evidence of hormonal production, then surgery may be recommended. However, benign adenomas have been noted to grow by 1–2 cm over several years of follow-up.

Summary Points

- Steroidogenesis in the adrenal cortex is regulated by negative feedback loops
  - Cortisol is regulated by the hypothalamic / pituitary ACTH axis
  - Aldosterone is regulated by the renin-angiotensin system
- Disorders of adrenal cortex include under and over production of the steroid hormones – aldosterone, cortisol and androgen.
- Suppression tests are helpful to diagnose hypersecretion states. Stimulation tests are used to diagnose hormone deficiencies.

- Imaging should be embarked upon only after biochemical confirmation to determine whether the demonstrated abnormality is primary (adrenal) or secondary (trophic regulatory hormones).
- Imaging the adrenal gland with high resolution CT in primary adrenal disorders is the imaging modality of choice.
- Imaging the pituitary gland with gadolinium-enhanced MRI in ACTH dependent cause of hypercortisolism is the preferred imaging modality.
- Venous sampling studies (IPSS and AVS) are used in special centers to definitively diagnose the location of hormonal hypersecretion.

References

1. Williams GH, Dluhy RG (2004) Disorders of the adrenal cortex. In: Kasper DL, Braunwald E, Fauci A, Hauser S, Longo D (eds) Harrison's principles of internal medicine. McGraw-Hill Professional
2. Stewart P (2003) The adrenal cortex. In: Kronenberg HM, Larsen R, Polonsky KS (eds) Williams textbook of endocrinology. Philadelphia, pp 491–548
3. Conlin PR, Dluhy RG, Williams GH (2002) Disorders of the renin-angiotensin-aldosterone system. In: Schrier RW (ed) Renal and electrolyte disorders, 6th edn. Lippincott Williams and Wilkins, Philadelphia, pp 303–341

4. Williams GH (2005) Aldosterone biosynthesis, regulation, and classical mechanism of action. Heart Fail Rev 10(1):7–13

5. Newell-Price J, Bertagna X, Grossman AB, Nieman LK (2006) Cushing's syndrome. Lancet 367(9522):1605–1617

6. Isidori AM, Kaltsas GA, Pozza C, Frajese V, Newell-Price J, Reznek RH et al. (2006) The ectopic adreno-corticotropin syndrome: clinical features, diagnosis, management, and long-term follow-up. J Clin Endocrinol Metab 91(2):371–377

7. Arnaldi G, Angeli A, Atkinson AB, Bertagna X, Cavagnini F, Chrousos GP et al. (2003) Diagnosis and complications of Cushing's syndrome: a consensus statement. J Clin Endocrinol Metab 88(12):5593–5602

8. Papanicolaou DA, Yanovski JA, Cutler GB Jr, Chrousos GP, Nieman LK (1998) A single midnight serum cortisol measurement distinguishes Cushing's syndrome from pseudo-Cushing states. J Clin Endocrinol Metab 83(4):1163–1167

9. Findling JW, Raff H (2006) Cushing's Syndrome: important issues in diagnosis and management. J Clin Endocrinol Metab 91(10):3746–3753

10. Mantero F, Scaroni CM, Albiger NM (2004) Cyclic Cushing's syndrome: an overview. Pituitary 7(4):203–207

11. Nieman LK, Ilias I (2005) Evaluation and treatment of Cushing's syndrome. Am J Med 118(12):1340–1346

12. Morris D, Grossman A (2002) The medical management of Cushing's syndrome. Ann N Y Acad Sci 970:119–133

13. Young WF (2007) Primary aldosteronism: renaissance of a syndrome. Clin Endocrinol (Oxf) 66(5):607–618

14. Mattsson C, Young WF Jr (2006) Primary aldosteronism: diagnostic and treatment strategies. Nat Clin Pract Nephrol 2(4):198–208; quiz, 1 p following 30

15. Williams GH (2003) Cardiovascular benefits of aldosterone receptor antagonists. Climacteric 6(Suppl 3):29–35

16. Pitt B, Remme W, Zannad F, Neaton J, Martinez F, Roniker B et al. (2003) Eplerenone, a selective aldosterone blocker, in patients with left ventricular dysfunction after myocardial infarction. N Engl J Med 348(14):1309–1321

17. Dluhy RG, Williams GH (2004) Aldosterone – villain or bystander? N Engl J Med 351(1):8–10

18. Mulatero P, Dluhy RG, Giacchetti G, Boscaro M, Veglio F, Stewart PM (2005) Diagnosis of primary aldosteronism: from screening to subtype differentiation. Trends Endocrinol Metab 16(3):114–119

19. McMahon GT, Dluhy RG (2004) Glucocorticoid-remediable aldosteronism. Cardiol Rev 12(1):44–48

20. Dluhy RG, Lifton RP (1999) Glucocorticoid-remediable aldosteronism. J Clin Endocrinol Metab 84(12):4341–4344

21. Draper N, Stewart PM (2005) 11beta-hydroxysteroid dehydrogenase and the pre-receptor regulation of corticosteroid hormone action. J Endocrinol 186(2):251–271

22. Eisenbarth GS, Gottlieb PA (2004) Autoimmune polyendocrine syndromes. N Engl J Med 350(20):2068–2079

23. Bouillon R (2006) Acute adrenal insufficiency. Endocrinol Metab Clin North Am 35(4):767–775, ix

24. Nair KS, Rizza RA, O'Brien P, Dhatariya K, Short KR, Nehra A et al. (2006) DHEA in elderly women and DHEA or testosterone in elderly men. N Engl J Med 355(16):1647–1659

25. Libe R, Barbetta L, Dall'Asta C, Salvaggio F, Gala C, Beck-Peccoz P et al. (2004) Effects of dehydroepiandros-terone (DHEA) supplementation on hormonal, metabolic and behavioral status in patients with hypoadrenalism. J Endocrinol Invest 27(8):736–741

26. Young WF Jr (2007) Clinical practice. The incidentally discovered adrenal mass. N Engl J Med 356(6):601–610

27. Bovio S, Cataldi A, Reimondo G, Sperone P, Novello S, Berruti A et al. (2006) Prevalence of adrenal incidentaloma in a contemporary computerized tomography series. J Endocrinol Invest 29(4):298–302

28. Mansmann G, Lau J, Balk E, Rothberg M, Miyachi Y, Bornstein SR (2004) The clinically inapparent adrenal mass: update in diagnosis and management. Endocr Rev 25(2):309–340

29. Grumbach MM, Biller BM, Braunstein GD, Campbell KK, Carney JA, Godley PA et al. (2003) Management of the clinically inapparent adrenal mass ("incidentaloma"). Ann Intern Med 138(5):424–429

30. Motta-Ramirez GA, Remer EM, Herts BR, Gill IS, Hamrahian AH (2005) Comparison of CT findings in symptomatic and incidentally discovered pheochromocytomas. AJR Am J Roentgenol 185(3):684–688

Contents

W.F. Young (✉)
Division of Endocrinology, Diabetes, Metabolism, Nutrition
and Internal Medicine, Mayo Clinic Rochester, 200 First
Street S.W., Rochester, MN 55905
E-mail: Young.William@Mayo.edu

Introduction

Catecholamine-secreting tumors that arise from chromaffin cells of the adrenal medulla are termed *pheochromocytomas*. Although pheochromocytomas are rare—annual incidence of 2–8 cases per million people [1]—it is important to suspect, confirm, localize, and resect these tumors because: there is the risk of a lethal paroxysm, the associated hypertension is curable with surgical removal of the tumor, and 5%–10% of the adrenal medullary neoplasms are malignant. These tumors occur with equal frequency in men and women, primarily in the third through fifth decades. Because of the widespread use of computerized imaging, up to half of pheochromocytomas are discovered incidentally in patients lacking symptoms related to the neoplasm [2, 3]. The remaining pheochromocytoma patients may present with symptoms and signs caused by the pharmacologic effects of catecholamine hypersecretion. The resulting hypertension may be sustained or paroxysmal. Episodic symptoms may occur in "spells", or paroxysms, that can be extremely variable in presentation but typically include forceful heartbeat, pallor, tremor, headache, and diaphoresis. Spells may be either spontaneous or precipitated by postural change, anxiety, medications (e.g., metoclopramide, anesthetic agents), exercise, medical procedures (e.g., colonoscopy) or maneuvers that increase intra-abdominal pressure. Although the types of spells experienced across all patients with pheochromocytoma are highly variable, spells tend to be stereotypical for each patient. However, a key point for all clinicians is that most patients with spells do not have a pheochromocytoma [4].

Additional clinical signs of pheochromocytoma include hypertension, hypertensive retinopathy, orthostatic hypotension, constipation (megacolon may be the presenting symptom), hyperglycemia, diabetes mellitus, hypercalcemia, and erythrocytosis. Some of the cosecreted hormones that may dominate the clinical presentation include adrenocorticotropin (Cushing's syndrome), parathyroid hormone-related peptide (hypercalcemia), vasoactive intestinal peptide (watery diarrhea), and growth hormone-releasing hormone (acromegaly). Cardiomyopathy, myocardial infarction with normal coronary arteries, and congestive heart failure are the symptomatic presentations that are perhaps most frequently unrecognized by clinicians to be caused by pheochromocytoma. Physical examination findings that are associated with genetic syndromes that predispose to pheochromocytoma include: retinal angiomas, marfanoid body habitus, café au lait spots, axillary freckling, subcutaneous neurofibromas, and mucocutaneous neuromas on the eyelids and tongue.

Syndromic Pheochromocytoma

Approximately 15%–20% of patients with pheochromocytoma have causative germline mutations (inherited mutations present in all cells of the body) [5]. The familial neurocristopathic syndromes associated with adrenal pheochromocytoma include multiple endocrine neoplasia (MEN) type 2A (pheochromocytoma, medullary thyroid carcinoma, and hyperparathyroidism) and type 2B (MEN 2B) (pheochromocytoma, medullary thyroid carcinoma, mucocutaneous neuromas, thickened corneal nerves, intestinal ganglioneuromatosis, and marfanoid body habitus); neurofibromatosis type 1 (NF1); von Hippel-Lindau disease (VHL) (pheochromocytoma, retinal angiomas, cerebellar hemangioblastoma, renal and pancreatic cysts, pancreatic islet cell tumors, and renal cell carcinoma); familial pheochromocytoma (specific mutations yet to be identified); and the succinate dehydrogenase (SDH; succinate:ubiquinone oxidoreductase) subunit mutations in *SDHD* and *SDHB*.

Diagnostic Investigation

Case Finding

Pheochromocytoma should be suspected in two general clinical settings:

- In patients with an incidentally discovered adrenal mass that has an imaging phenotype consistent with pheochromocytoma [3]
- In patients who have hypertension accompanied by one or more of the following: hyperadrenergic spells (e.g., self-limited episodes of non-exertional palpitations, diaphoresis, headache, tremor, and pallor); resistant hypertension; a familial syndrome that predisposes to catecholamine-secreting tumors (eg, MEN 2)

The single most reliable screening method for biochemically identifying a pheochromocytoma is measuring fractionated metanephrines in a 24-h urine collection [6–8]. If clinical suspicion is high, then urinary fractionated catecholamines (epinephrine, norepinephrine, and dopamine) are measured in addition to the 24-h urine fractionated metanephrines (Fig. 3.1) [9]. Plasma fractionated metanephrines, which are products of intrapheochromocytoma catecholamine metabolism, are also obtained in high clinical suspicion cases [3, 8, 10, 11]. The index of suspicion should be high for the following scenarios: resistant hypertension; pallor spells; a family history of pheochromocytoma; a genetic syndrome that predisposes to pheochromocytoma (eg, MEN 2); a past history of resected pheochromocytoma and present history of recurrent hypertension or spells; or an incidentally discovered adrenal mass that has imaging characteristics consistent with pheochromocytoma (e.g., increased CT attenuation, delayed CT contrast medium washout, high signal intensity on T_2-weighted MRI, cystic and hemorrhagic changes, and larger size [e.g., > 4 cm], or bilaterality). In addition, measuring plasma fractionated metanephrines is a good first-line test for children since obtaining a complete 24-h urine collection may be difficult. The clinician should recognize that the most common cause of increased levels of fractionated metanephrines and fractionated catecholamines is not pheochromocytoma, but rather, medication related (Table 3.1).

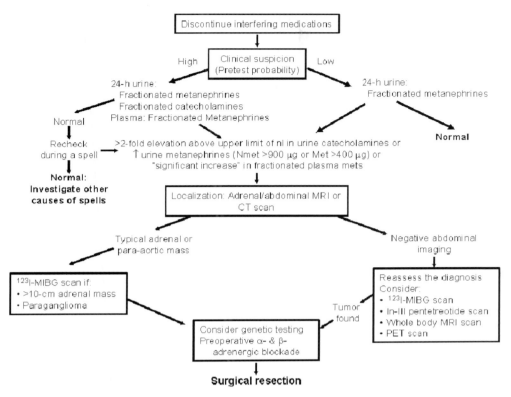

Fig. 3.1 Evaluation and treatment of catecholamine-secreting tumors. Clinical suspicion is triggered by the following: paroxysmal symptoms (especially hypertension); hypertension that is intermittent, unusually labile, or resistant to treatment; family history of pheochromocytoma or associated conditions; or incidentally discovered adrenal mass. The details are discussed in the text. CT, computed tomography; ^{123}I-MIBG, ^{123}I-metaiodobenzylguanidine; mets, metanephrines; MRI, magnetic resonance imaging; nl, normal; Nmet, normetanephrine; PET, positron emission tomography. (Modified from Young WF Jr: Pheochromocytoma: 1926–1993. Trends Endocrinol Metab 4:122, 1993; with permission)

Table 3.1 Medications that may increase measured levels of catecholamines and metanephrines

Tricyclic antidepressants

Levodopa

Drugs containing adrenergic receptor agonists
(e.g., decongestants)

Amphetamines

Buspirone and most psychoactive agents

Prochlorperazine

Reserpine

Withdrawal from clonidine and other drugs
(e.g., illicit drugs)

Ethanol

Acetaminophen (may increase measured levels of
fractionated plasma metanephrines in some assays)

Localization

Localization studies should not be initiated until biochemical studies have confirmed the diagnosis of a catecholamine-secreting tumor. Computer-assisted imaging of the adrenal glands and abdomen with MRI or CT should be the first localization test. Approximately 90% of catecholamine-secreting tumors are found in the adrenal glands and 98% are found in the abdomen and pelvis [12]. If the results of abdominal–pelvic imaging are negative, scintigraphic localization with 123I-metaiodobenzylguanidine (^{123}I-MIBG) is indicated. This radiopharmaceutical agent accumulates preferentially in catecholamine-producing tumors; however, this procedure is not as sensitive as initially hoped (sensitivity, 80%; specificity, 99%) [13]. In a study of 282 patients with catecholamine-secreting tumors that were surgically confirmed, the overall sensitivity was 89% for CT, 98% for MRI, and 81% for ^{131}I-MIBG [14]. If a typical (<10 cm) unilateral adrenal pheochromocytoma is found on CT or MRI, ^{123}I-MIBG scintigraphy is superfluous and the results may actually confuse the clinician [15, 16]. ^{123}I-MIBG scintigraphy is preferred over ^{131}I-MIBG because of more avid tumor uptake, shorter scan times, and the ability to perform single photon emission computed tomography. Performing preoperative ^{123}I-MIBG scintigraphy in patients with large (>10cm) adrenal pheochromocytomas may be indicated to identify metastatic disease; however, finding metastatic disease preoperatively does not usually change the initial surgical treatment plan. The clinician should be aware of the medications that may interfere with MIBG uptake and result on false negative scans (Table 3.2).

Table 3.2 Drugs that may interfere with metaiodobenzylguanidine (MIBG) uptake

Uptake-1 Inhibition (should be stopped at least 48-hours before MIBG administration)
Antiemetic (e.g., prochlorperazine)
Antipsychotics (e.g., chlorpromazine, haloperidol)
Cocaine
Labetalol
Phenylpropanolamine
Tricyclic antidepressants (e.g., amitriptyline, amoxapine, desipramine, doxepin, imipramine, nortriptyline)

Depletion of storage vesicle contents (should be stopped at least 72 h before MIBG administration)
Amphetamines (dextroamphetamine, fenfluramine, phentermine)
Dopamine
Labetalol
Reserpine
Sympathomimetics (e.g., ephedrine, phenylephrine, pseudoephedrine, salbutamol, terbutaline)

Inhibition of vesicular monoamine transporters (should be stopped at least 72 h before MIBG administration)
Reserpine

Unknown mechanism (should be stopped at least 48 h before MIBG administration)
Calcium channel blockers (e.g., diltiazem, nicardipine, nifedipine, nimodipine, verapamil)

Treatment

The treatment of choice for pheochromocytoma is complete surgical resection. Careful preoperative pharmacologic preparation is crucial for successful treatment. Most catecholamine-secreting tumors are benign and can be totally excised. Tumor excision usually cures hypertension in patients that lack a family history of essential hypertension.

Preoperative Management

Some form of preoperative pharmacologic preparation is indicated for all patients with catecholamine-secreting neoplasms. However, no randomized controlled trials have compared the different approaches. Combined α- and β-adrenergic blockade is one approach to control blood pressure and prevent intraoperative hypertensive crises [9]. α-Adrenergic blockade should be started at least 7–10 days preoperatively to normalize blood pressure and expand the contracted blood volume. Target blood pressure is low normal seated blood pressure for patient age; blood pressure target should be modified on the basis of comorbid disease. On the second or third day of α-adrenergic blockade, patients are encouraged to start a diet high in sodium content because of the catecholamine-induced volume contraction and the orthostasis associated with α-adrenergic blockade. After adequate α-adrenergic blockade has been achieved, β-adrenergic blockade is initiated, which typically occurs 2–3 days preoperatively.

α-Adrenergic Blockade
Phenoxybenzamine is the preferred drug for preoperative preparation to control blood pressure and arrhythmia. It is an irreversible, long-acting, nonspecific α-adrenergic blocking agent. The initial dosage of 10 mg once or twice daily, and the dose is increased by 10–20 mg every 2–3 days as needed to control blood pressure and prevent spells. The final target dosage of phenoxybenzamine is typically 20–100 mg daily. The patient should be warned about the orthostasis, nasal stuffiness, and fatigue that occur in almost all patients. With their more favorable side-effect profile, selective α_1-adrenergic blocking agents (e.g., prazosin, terazosin, and doxazosin) are preferable to phenoxybenzamine when long-term pharmacologic treatment is indicated (e.g., for metastatic pheochromocytoma). However, treatment with selective α_1-adrenergic blocking agents is not routinely used preoperatively because of incomplete α-adrenergic blockade.

β-Adrenergic Blockade
The β-adrenergic antagonist should be only administered after α-adrenergic blockade is effective because with β-adrenergic blockade alone hypertension may be more severe from the unopposed α-adrenergic stimulation. Preoperative β-adrenergic blockade is

indicated to control the tachycardia associated with both the high concentrations of circulating catecholamines and the α-adrenergic blockade. The clinician should exercise caution if the patient is asthmatic or has congestive heart failure. Chronic catecholamine excess can produce a myocardiopathy, this may become evident with the initiation of β-adrenergic blockade, resulting in acute pulmonary edema. Therefore, when the β-adrenergic blocker is administered, it should be used cautiously and at a low dose. For example, a patient is usually given 10 mg of propranolol every 6 h to start; on the second day of treatment, the β-adrenergic blockade (assuming the patient tolerates the drug), propranolol is converted to a single long-acting dose. The dose is then increased as necessary to control the tachycardia (goal heart rate is 60–80 beats/min).

Catecholamine Synthesis Inhibitor

α-Methyl paratyrosine (metyrosine) should be used with caution and only when other agents have been ineffective or when significant tumor manipulation is anticipated. Although some centers have used this agent preoperatively, most reserve it primarily for patients who cannot be treated with the typical combined α- and β-adrenergic blockade protocol for of cardiopulmonary reasons. Metyrosine inhibits catecholamine synthesis by blocking the enzyme tyrosine hydroxylase. Metyrosine's side effects can be disabling, and they include sedation, depression, diarrhea, anxiety, nightmares, crystalluria and urolithiasis, galactorrhea, and extrapyramidal signs.

Calcium Channel Blockers

Calcium channel blockers, which block norepinephrine-mediated calcium transport into vascular smooth muscle, have been used successfully at several medical centers to preoperatively prepare patients with pheochromocytoma [17–19]. Nicardipine is the most commonly used calcium channel blocker in this setting. It is given orally to control blood pressure preoperatively and is given as an intravenously infusion intraoperatively. When calcium channel blockers are used as the primary mode of antihypertensive therapy, they appear to be just as effective as α- and β-adrenergic blockade [17–19].

Acute Hypertensive Crises

Acute hypertensive crises may occur before or during an operation, and they should be treated intravenously with sodium nitroprusside, phentolamine, or nicardipine. Sodium nitroprusside is an ideal vasodilator for intraoperative management of hypertensive episodes because of its rapid onset of action and short duration of effect. It is administered as an intravenous infusion at 0.5–5.0 μg/kg/min; the maximal dose should not exceed 800 μg/min. Phentolamine is available in lyophilized form in 5-mg vials; the initial infused dose should be 1 mg, followed by repeat 5-mg boluses or a continuous infusion. Nicardipine can be started at an infusion rate of 2.5 mg/h and titrated for blood pressure control (maximum dose is 15 mg/h).

Anesthesia and Surgery

Surgical resection of a catecholamine-secreting tumor is a high risk surgical procedure, and an experienced surgeon/anesthesiologist team is required. The last oral doses of α- and β-adrenergic blockers can be administered orally early in the morning on the day of the operation. Fentanyl, ketamine, and morphine should be avoided because they can potentially stimulate catecholamine release from a pheochromocytoma [20]. Also, parasympathetic nervous system blockade with atropine should be avoided because of the associated tachycardia. Anesthesia may be induced with intravenous injection of propofol, etomidate, or barbiturates in combination with synthetic opioids [20]. Most anesthetic gases can be used, but halothane and desflurane should be avoided [20]. Cardiovascular and hemodynamic variables must be monitored closely. Continuous measurement of intra-arterial pressure and heart rhythm is required. If the patient has congestive heart failure or decreased cardiac reserve, monitoring of pulmonary capillary wedge pressure is indicated. Surgical survival rates are 98%–100%. Four perioperative deaths occurred in a series of 165 patients operated on in Paris, France, from 1975 to 1997 [21]. The preoperative and perioperative treatment approach outlined here is the same for adults and children [22, 23].

In the past, an anterior midline abdominal surgical approach was generally used for resecting adrenal pheochromocytoma. However, the laparoscopic approach to the adrenal gland is currently the procedure of choice for patients with solitary intra-adrenal pheochromocytomas less than 8–10 cm in diameter [24]. If the pheochromocytoma is in the adrenal gland, the entire gland should be removed. Laparoscopic adrenalectomy for pheochromocytoma should be converted to open adrenalectomy for difficult dissection, invasion, adhesions, or surgeon inexperience [25]. If the tumor is malignant, as much of the tumor should be removed as possible. If a bilateral adrenalectomy is planned preoperatively, the patient should receive glucocorticoid stress coverage while awaiting transfer to the operating room. Glucocorticoid coverage should be initiated in the operating room if unexpected bilateral adrenalectomy is necessary. Cortical-sparing bilateral adrenalectomies have been used to treat patients with MEN 2 and VHL disease [26–28]. However, with MEN 2 patients, there is a concern of leaving residual adrenal medullary tissue behind and, thus increase the risk of recurrent pheochromocytoma. An anterior midline abdominal surgical approach is indicated for abdominal paragangliomas.

Hypotension may occur after surgical resection of the pheochromocytoma, and it should be treated with fluids and small, intermittent doses of intravenous pressor agents. Postoperative hypotension is less frequent in patients who have had an adequate pre-operative α-adrenergic blockade. If both adrenal glands were manipulated during surgery, adrenocortical insufficiency should be considered as a potential cause of postoperative hypotension. Because hypoglycemia can occur in the immediate postoperative period, blood glucose levels should be monitored and fluid given intravenously should contain 5% dextrose.

Blood pressure is usually normal by the time of hospital discharge. Some patients remain hypertensive for up to 4–8 weeks postoperatively. Long-standing, persistent hypertension does occur and may be related to inadvertent ligation of a polar renal artery, resetting of baroreceptors, hemodynamic changes, structural changes of the blood vessels, altered sensitivity of the vessels to pressor substances, functional or structural renal changes, or coincident primary hypertension.

Long-Term Postoperative Follow-up

Approximately 1–2 weeks after surgery, catecholamines and metanephrines should be measured by collecting urine for 24 h. If the levels are normal, the resection of the pheochromocytoma should be considered complete. The survival rate after removal of a benign pheochromocytoma is nearly that of age- and sex-matched normal controls. Increased levels of catecholamines and metanephrines detected postoperatively are consistent with residual tumor, either a second primary lesion or occult metastases. If bilateral adrenalectomy was performed, life-long glucocorticoid and mineralocorticoid replacement therapy is prescribed. Twenty-four hour urinary excretion of fractionated metanephrines and catecholamines or plasma fractionated metanephrines should be checked annually for life. Annual biochemical testing assesses for metastatic disease, tumor recurrence in the adrenal bed, or delayed appearance of multiple primary tumors. Recurrence rates are highest for patients with familial disease, right-sided adrenal pheochromocytoma, or a paraganglioma [29]. Follow-up imaging with CT or MRI is not needed unless the fractionated metanephrine and/or catecholamine levels become elevated or the original tumor was associated with minimal catecholamine excess.

The clinician should consider genetic testing for patients with one or more of the following: a family history of pheochromocytoma, paraganglioma, or any sign that suggests a genetic cause (e.g., retinal angiomas, axillary freckling, café au lait spots, cerebellar tumor, MTC, hyperparathyroidism) [30]. In addition, all first-degree relatives of a patient with pheochromocytoma should have biochemical testing (e.g., 24-h urine for fractionated metanephrines and catecholamines). If mutation testing in a patient is positive, first-degree relatives should have stepwise (e.g., parents first) germline screening.

Malignant Pheochromocytoma

Distinguishing between benign and malignant catecholamine-secreting tumors is difficult on the basis of clinical, biochemical, or histopathologic characteristics. Malignancy is rare in patients with an adrenal familial syndrome, but is common in those with familial paraganglioma caused by mutations in *SDHB*. Although the 5-year survival rate for patients with malignant pheochromocytoma is less than 50%, the prognosis is variable: approximately 50% of patients have an indolent form of the disease, with a life expectancy of more than

20 years, and the other 50% of patients have rapidly progressive disease, with death occurring within 1–3 years. Metastatic sites include local tissue invasion, liver, bone, lung, and lymph nodes. Metastatic lesions should be resected if possible. Skeletal metastatic lesions that are painful or threaten structural function can be treated with external radiotherapy or cyroablation therapy. External radiotherapy can also be used to treat unresectable soft tissue lesions.

Local tumor irradiation with therapeutic doses of ^{131}I-MIBG has produced partial and temporary responses in approximately one-third of patients [31–34]. Thrombotic therapy for large unresectable liver metastases and radiofrequency ablation for small liver metastases are options to be considered. In selected cases, long-acting octreotide has been beneficial. If the tumor is considered aggressive and the patient's quality of life is affected, combination chemotherapy may be considered. In a nonrandomized, single-arm trial, the efficacy of chemotherapy (CVD protocol: cyclophosphamide 750 mg/m^2 body surface area on day 1; vincristine, 1.4 mg/m^2 on day 1; and dacarbazine 600 mg/m^2 on days 1 and 2 and every 21 days) was studied in 14 patients with malignant pheochromocytoma [35]. The combination CVD protocol produced a complete and partial response rate of 57%. Complete and partial biochemical responses were seen in 79% of patients. All responding patients had objective improvement in performance status and blood pressure. Management of a patient who has malignant pheochromocytoma can be frustrating because curative options are limited. Clearly, innovative prospective protocols are needed to seek new treatment options for this neoplasm [36].

Summary

- Although pheochromocytomas are rare, it is important to suspect, confirm, localize, and resect these tumors because: there is the risk of a lethal paroxysm, the associated hypertension is curable with surgical removal of the tumor, and 5%–10% of the adrenal medullary neoplasms are malignant.
- Because of the widespread use of computerized imaging, up to half of pheochromocytomas are discovered incidentally in patients lacking symptoms related to the neoplasm.
- Pheochromocytoma should be suspected in two general clinical settings: in patients with an incidentally discovered adrenal mass that has an imaging phenotype consistent with pheochromocytoma and in patients who have hypertension accompanied by one or more of the following: hyperadrenergic spells (e.g., self-limited episodes of non-exertional palpitations, diaphoresis, headache, tremor, and pallor); resistant hypertension; a familial syndrome that predisposes to catecholamine-secreting tumors (e.g., MEN 2).
- The single most reliable screening method for biochemically identifying a pheochromocytoma is measuring fractionated metanephrines in a 24-h urine collection.
- Imaging characteristics consistent with pheochromocytoma include increased CT attenuation, delayed CT contrast medium washout, high signal intensity on T_2-weighted MRI, cystic and hemorrhagic changes.
- Approximately 90% of catecholamine-secreting tumors are found in the adrenal glands and 98% are found in the abdomen and pelvis.
- Some form of preoperative pharmacologic preparation is indicated for all patients with catecholamine-secreting neoplasms—combined α- and β-adrenergic blockade is one approach to control blood pressure and prevent intraoperative hypertensive crises.
- Surgical resection of a catecholamine-secreting tumor is a high risk surgical procedure, and an experienced surgeon/anesthesiologist team is required.
- The laparoscopic approach to the adrenal gland is currently the procedure of choice for patients with solitary intra-adrenal pheochromocytomas less than 8–10 cm in diameter.
- After surgery, patients should have annual biochemical testing assesses for metastatic disease, tumor recurrence in the adrenal bed, or delayed appearance of multiple primary tumors.

References

1. Stenstrom G, Svardsudd K (1986) Phaechromocytoma in Sweden, 1958-81. An analysis of the National Cancer Registry Data. Acta Med Scand 220:225–232
2. Motta-Ramirez GA, Remer EM, Herts BR, Gill IS, Hamrahian AH (2005) Comparison of CT findings in symptomatic and incidentally discovered pheochromocytomas. Am J Roentgenol 185:684–688

3. Young WF Jr (2007) The incidentally discovered adrenal mass. N Engl J Med 356(6):601–610

4. Young WF Jr, Maddox DE (1995) Spells: in search of a cause. Mayo Clin Proc 70:757–765

5. Neumann HP, Bausch B, McWhinney SR et al. (2002) Germ-line mutations in nonsyndromeic pheochromocytoma. N Engl J Med 346:1459–1466

6. Kudva YC, Sawka AM, Young WF Jr (2003) Clinical review 164: The laboratory diagnosis of adrenal pheochromocytoma: the Mayo Clinic experience. J Clin Endocrinol Metab 88:4533–4539

7. Perry CG, Sawka AM, Singh R, Thabane L, Bajnarek J, Young WF Jr (2007) The diagnostic efficacy of urinary fractionated metanephrines measured by tandem mass spectrometry in detection of pheochromocytoma. Clin Endocrinol 66:703–708

8. d'Herbomez M, Forzy G, Bauters C et al. (2007) An analysis of the biochemical diagnosis of 66 pheochromocytomas. Eur J Endocrinol 156(5):569–575

9. Young WF Jr (1993) Pheochromocytoma: 1926-1993. Trends Endocrinol Metab 4:122–127

10. Lenders JW, Pacak K, Walther MM et al. (2002) Biochemical diagnosis of pheochromocytoma: which test is best? JAMA 287:1427–1434

11. Sawka AM, Prebtani AP, Thabane L et al. (2004) A systematic review of the literature examining the diagnostic efficacy of measurement of fractionate plasma free metanephrines in the biochemical diagnosis of pheochromocytoma. BMC Endorc Disord 4:2

12. van Gils APG, Falke THM, van Erkel AR et al (1991) MR imaging and MIBG scintigraphy of pheochromocytomas and extraadrenal functioning paragangliomas. Radiographics 11:37–57

13. Shapiro B, Gross MD, Fig L et al. (1990) Localization of functioning sympathoadrenal lesions. In: Biglieri EG, Melby JC (eds) Endocrine hypertension. Raven Press, New York, pp 235–255

14. Jalil ND, Pattou FN, Combemale F et al. (1998) Effectiveness and limits of preoperative imaging studies for the localisation of pheochromocytomas and paragangliomas: a review of 282 cases. French Association of Surgery (AFC) and The French Association of Endocrine Surgeons (AFCE). Eur J Surg 164:23–28

15. Miskulin J, Shulkin BL, Doherty GM et al. (2003) Is preoperative iodine 123 meta-iodobenzylguanidine scintigraphy routinely necessary before initial adrenalectomy for pheochromocytoma? Surgery 134:918–922

16. Taieb D, Sebag F, Hubbard JG et al. (2004) Does iodine-131 meta-iodobenzylguanidine (MIBG) scintigraphy have an impact on the management of sporadic and familial phaeochromocytoma? Clin Endocrinol (Oxf) 61:102–108

17. Bravo EL (2002) Pheochromocytoma: an approach to antihypertensive management. Ann N Y Acad Sci 970:1–10

18. Combemale F, Carnaille B, Tavernier B et al. (1998) Exclusive use of calcium channel blockers and cardioselective beta-blockers in the pre- and per-operative management of pheochromocytomas. 70 cases. Ann Chir 52:341–345

19. Lebuffe G, Dosseh ED, Tek G et al. (2005) The effect of calcium channel blockers on outcome following the surgical treatment of phaeochromocytomas and paragangliomas. Anaesthesia 60:439–444

20. Memtsoudis SG, Swamidoss C, Psoma M (2005) Anesthesia for adrenal surgery. In: Linos D, van Heerden JA (eds) Adrenal glands: diagnostic aspects and surgical therapy. Springer, Berlin Heidelberg New York, pp 287–297

21. Plouin PF, Duclos JM, Soppelsa F et al. (2001) Factors associated with perioperative morbidity and mortality in patients with pheochromocytoma: analysis of 165 operations at a single center. J Clin Endocrinol Metab 86:1480–1486

22. Hack HA (2000) The perioperative management of children with phaeochromocytoma. Paediatr Anaesth 10:463–476

23. Reddy VS, O'Neill JA Jr, Holcomb GW III et al. (2000) Twenty-five-year surgical experience with pheochromocytoma in children. Am Surg 66:1085–1091

24. Grant C (2005) Pheochromocytoma. In: Clark O, Duh Q-Y, Kebebew E (eds) Textbook of endocrine surgery. Elsevier Saunders, Philadelphia, pp 621–633

25. Shen WT, Sturgeon C, Clark OH et al. (2004) Should pheochromocytoma size influence surgical approach? A comparison of 90 malignant and 60 benign pheochromocytomas. Surgery 136:1129–1137

26. Lee JE, Curley SA, Gagel RF et al. (1996) Cortical-sparing adrenalectomy for patients with bilateral pheochromocytoma. Surgery 120:1064–1071

27. Walther MM, Keiser HR, Choyke PL et al. (1999) Management of hereditary pheochromocytoma in von Hippel-Lindau kindreds with partial adrenalectomy. J Urol 161:395–398

28. Diner EK, Franks ME, Behari A, Linehan WM, Walther MM (2005) Partial adrenalectomy: the National Cancer Institute experience. Urology 66(1):19–23

29. Amar L, Servais A, Gimeniz-Roqueplo AP et al. (2005) Year of diagnosis, features at presentation, and risk of recurrence in patients with pheochromocytoma or secreting paraganglioma. J Clin Endocrinol Metab 90:2110–2116

30. Pawlu C, Bausch B, Reisch N, Neumann HP (2005) Genetic testing for pheochromocytoma-associated syndromes. Ann Endocrinol (Paris) 66:178–185

31. Sisson JC (2002) Radiopharmaceutical treatment of pheochromocytomas. Ann N Y Acad Sci 970:54–60

32. Safford SD, Coleman RE, Gockerman JP et al. (2003) Iodine-131 metaiodobenzylguanidine is an effective treatment for malignant pheochromocytoma and paraganglioma. Surgery 134:956–962

33. Rose B, Matthay KK, Price D et al. (2003) High-dose 131I-metaiodobenzylguanidine therapy for 12 patients with malignant pheochromocytoma. Cancer 98:239–248

34. Loh KC, Fitzgerald PA, Matthay KK et al. (1997) The treatment of malignant pheochromocytoma with iodine-131 metaiodobenzylguanidine (131I-MIBG): a comprehensive review of 116 reported patients. J Endocrinol Invest 20:648–658

35. Averbuch SD, Steakley CS, Young RC et al. (1988) Malignant pheochromocytoma: effective treatment with a combination of cyclophosphamide, vincristine, and dacarbazine. Ann Intern Med 109:267–273

36. Eisenhofer G, Bornstein SR, Brouwers FM et al. (2004) Malignant pheochromocytoma: current status and initiatives for future progress. Endocr Relat Cancer 11:423–436

The Adrenals in Oncology

4

Claire E. Higham, John J. Coen, Giles W.L. Boland, Peter J. Trainer

Contents

Adrenal Anatomy for Oncology 65

Adrenal Physiology for Oncology 66

Adrenals and Cancer – Overview 66

Adrenal Cortical Carcinomas 67
Epidemiology 67
Natural History 67
Clinical Presentation 67
Diagnostic Workup and Staging 68
Endocrinology 68
Imaging Characteristics of ACC 68
Pathologic Classification 68
General Management 69
Surgery 69
Chemotherapy 69
Radiation Therapy Techniques 70

Adrenal Medulla Tumors 71
Epidemiology 71
Natural History 71
Clinical Presentation 72
Diagnostic Work-up and Staging 72
Pathological Classification 72
General Management 73

Conclusion and Summary 73

References 74

G.W.L.Boland (✉)
Division of Abdominal Imaging and Intervention,
Department of Radiology, Massachusetts General Hospital,
Boston, MA 02114
E-mail: gboland@partners.org

Adrenal Anatomy for Oncology

The paired suprarenal (adrenal) glands are located between the superomedial aspects of the kidney and the diaphragmatic crura. They are surrounded by connective tissue containing perinephric fat. The glands are enclosed by renal fascia, but separated from the kidneys by fibrous tissue. The triangular right gland relates to the diaphragm posteriorly, and the inferior vena cava and liver anteriorly. The semilunar left adrenal gland is positioned in the middle of the left crux of the diaphragm. The omental bursa separates it from the stomach. It is also related to the spleen and pancreas [1].

The endocrine function of the adrenal glands necessitates an abundant blood supply. The superior suprarenal arteries are derived from the inferior phrenic artery, the middle suprarenal arteries from the abdominal aorta near the origin of the superior mesenteric artery and the inferior suprarenal arteries from the renal artery. A large central vein leaves the anterior surface of the gland at the hilum. The shorter right suprarenal vein drains into the inferior vena cava and the longer left suprarenal vein into the left renal vein [1].

The lymphatic drainage follows the arterial supply and is predominantly to lumbar lymph nodes. The superior lymphatic trunks end in aortocaval lymph nodes located near the origin of the celiac plexus. The inferior lymphatic trunks end in lateroaortic nodes above the renal pedicle. Some trunks may pass through the diaphragm,

M.A. Blake, G. Boland (eds.), *Adrenal Imaging*, DOI 10.1007/978-1-59745-560-2_4,
© 2009 Humana Press, a part of Springer Science+Business Media, LLC

65

following the splanchnic nerves, ending in retro-aortic nodes in the posterior mediastinum. On the right, some lymphatic trunks may penetrate the liver [2].

The adrenal gland is composed of a central catecholamine-producing medulla enveloped by the steroid-secreting cortex. Although they are in intimate contact, they represent two functionally separate organs with different embryologic origins, the cortex being derived from the embryonic mesoderm and the medulla from the ectoderm.

Adrenal Physiology for Oncology

The adrenal cortex consists of three layers, each secreting distinct steroid hormones. The exterior layer, zona glomerulosa produces mineralocorticoids, most importantly, aldosterone, regulating salt and water metabolism. The middle layer or zona fasciculata produces the glucocorticoids, particularly cortisol and the innermost layer, zona reticularis, the adrenal androgens DHEA, DHEAS-S and androstenedione. All these steroids are produced from the common precursor, pregnenolone, available throughout the cortex and the functional zonation is maintained by the differing availability and inhibition of enzymes catalyzing conversion reactions.

The adrenal medulla in contrast is derived from ectoderm, which forms part of the sympathochromaffin system and includes the sympathetic nervous system. The medullary chromaffin cells produce epinephrine and norepinephrine from tyrosine and secrete mainly epinephrine into the circulation under the control of preganglionic sympathetic nerves. Epinepherine and norepinepherine are metabolized into metanepherine and normetanepherine, which can be measured in the serum and urine.

Adrenals and Cancer – Overview

Tumors of the adrenal gland are discovered in 4%–9% of abdominal CT scans, the incidence increasing with age [3–5]. These "incidentalomas" are usually benign adenomas, although more rarely can represent metastatic disease, adrenocortical carcinomas or primary lymphomas. The investigation and management of incidentalomas is discussed in detail in Chap. 8.

Patients with adrenal adenomas of the cortex may present with clinical symptoms and signs related to excess aldosterone (Conn's syndrome) or cortisol (Cushing's syndrome). A recent overview of 13 studies involving 2005 patients with asymptomatic incidentalomas reported that 5%–6% of these also secrete cortisol autonomously [3]. These tumors will not be considered further in this chapter.

Metastases to the adrenals are another cause of adrenal masses and are a relatively frequent occurrence in patients with advanced solid tumors. In autopsy series, up to 20% of gastric cancer, 40% of bronchogenic cancer and 60% of breast and malignant melanoma patients had evidence of adrenal infiltration [6–8]. Metastatic infiltration can be in the form of small, micro deposits or larger macro deposits and the prevalence of metastases correlates with the stage of the disease [9]. Hypoadrenalism is a possible, but rare consequence of bilateral adrenal metastases and occurs particularly in those with metastases greater than 4 cm in diameter [9].

With improvements in scanning techniques, it is becoming apparent that the adrenal glands in patients with cancer can be bilaterally and uniformly enlarged without evidence of metastases [10, 11]. The enlargement most likely represents hypertrophy and is associated with altered HPA (hypothalamic-pituitary-axis) axis function and it was originally reported in the early 1990s in a large group of patients with lymphoma, lung carcinoma, tumors of the GI tract and gynaecological malignancies [10]. The finding has since been confirmed in further studies, adenocarcinomas of the GI tract (rectal, oesophageal, pancreatic, renal) and adenocarcinoma and carcinomatosis of unknown primary [11]. One case report describes the discovery of bilateral adrenal enlargement on CT scanning as the presenting feature of a gastric carcinoma [12]. The presence or degree of enlargement did not correlate with the site of the primary malignancy or the stage of the disease in these studies.

This hypertrophy is associated with activation of the HPA and indeed most of these patients demonstrated a degree of non-suppression of the HPA axis assessed by the cortisol response to dexamethasone suppression [11, 12]. The activation is a likely result of cytokine release as a result of tumor although psychological factors may contribute.

Interestingly the patients do not demonstrate any clinical signs or symptoms of glucocorticoid excess, suggesting that the activation is accompanied by a relative cortisol resistance and therefore the significance of this phenomenon remains uncertain.

The remainder of this chapter will focus on malignant tumors of the adrenal cortex and pheochromocytomas arising from the adrenal medulla.

Adrenal Cortical Carcinomas

Epidemiology

Adrenal cortical carcinomas (AAC) are very rare, with an incidence of about 1–2 per million per year worldwide and lead to 0.1%–0.2% of all cancer deaths [13]. Although the cancer can follow a variable and unpredictable course, prognosis is usually dismal, with a 30%–40% 5 year survival described in most series [14, 15].

There is a bimodal age distribution with disease peaks before the age of five and in the fourth to fifth decade of life and overall adrenocortical carcinoma is slightly more common in women than men. Nonfunctional carcinomas occur in an older age population (>30 years old) and are more common in men (3:2 male:female ratio), while functional tumors are more common in women (7:3 female:male ratio) and younger patients. As they frequently present with symptoms related to hormone production, functional tumors are detected at an earlier stage.

Although most cases of adrenocortical carcinoma are sporadic, it has been described as a component of several hereditary cancer syndromes including Li-Fraumeni syndrome (breast cancer, soft tissue and bone sarcoma, brain tumors and ACC associated with a mutation in TP53 gene) [16], Beckwith-Wiedemann syndrome (Wilms' tumor, neuroblastoma, hepatoblastoma and ACC) [17], Multiple Endocrine Neoplasia type I (parathyroid, pituitary and pancreatic neuroendocrine tumors, and adrenal adenomas and carcinomas associated with mutations in the menin gene) and SBLA syndrome (sarcoma, breast, lung, ACC and other tumors) [18–20]. A role for somatic mutations of TP53 has also been determined in at least 25% of sporadic cases of ACC [21–23].

Natural History

A review of 87 published series of adrenal cortex carcinoma demonstrated that 59% of adrenal cortex carcinomas secrete detectable levels of hormones (hypersecretory tumors). The left:right ratio is approximately 1:1, and 2.4% are bilateral [24]. Diagnosis is frequently delayed due to the rarity of disease and the deep retroperitoneal location of the adrenals [25].

Non-hypersecretory adrenocortical carcinomas typically present as larger tumors, with a diameter of greater than 6 cm. Hypersecretory tumors are more commonly discovered at an earlier stage as a result of clinical symptomatology. Adrenocortical carcinoma is an aggressive malignancy, which frequently violates the tumor capsule and invades surrounding tissues. It metastasizes to lungs, liver, brain and regional lymph nodes. Many patients present with widespread metastasis, most of whom die within 6 months of diagnosis. This is especially common in the pediatric population.

Clinical Presentation

The most frequent presentation of ACC in adults is a rapidly progressive Cushing's syndrome combined with evidence of hyperandrogenemia; hirsuitism, oligomenorrhoea and sometimes frank virilisation. Hypercortisolemia in isolation cannot distinguish between an adrenal adenoma and ACC but the excess secretion of more than one class of hormone is indicative of ACC. Children are more likely to present with virilisation alone. More rarely, estrogen-secreting tumors in men present with gynecomastia accompanied by testicular atrophy whereas tumors secreting cortisol and/or aldosterone lead to resistant hypertension and hypokalemia [13–15].

In contrast, patients with clinically non-hypersecretory tumors are more likely to present with nonspecific symptoms related to tumor burden including abdominal fullness, early satiety, pain, weight loss, weakness, fever or an abdominal mass [26]. Although these tumors do not present with symptoms relating to hormone excess, the majority do secrete non-bioactive steroid precursors. Non-hypersecretory ACCs are more common in older patients and tend to progress more rapidly.

Diagnostic Workup and Staging

The differentiation of benign adenoma from ACC is not always straightforward and is based on a combination of features including hormonal evaluation, imaging characteristics and behavior of the tumor with regards to size and growth rate. Histology is of limited value in this differentiation.

Endocrinology

It is vital to incorporate a comprehensive evaluation of adrenal steroid secretion in the workup of ACC. This assists with diagnosis (the excess secretion of more than one class of hormone being very suggestive of carcinoma) and possible determination of an appropriate tumor marker for monitoring of treatment.

Production of excess amounts of ACTH-independent cortisol is the most common biochemical abnormality detected in ACC, although in itself cannot differentiate between carcinoma or adenoma. Excess cortisol production is established by measurement of 24-h urinary free cortisol levels, non-suppression of serum cortisol following dexamethasone (overnight or 48-h low dose testing) and low/undetectable serum ACTH levels. Mineralocorticoid (aldosterone) and sex steroid (estrogen and testosterone) levels should also be measured. Levels of adrenal steroid precursors, serum DHEAS and 17-OHP are frequently raised, even in asymptomatic patients and can be used to monitor disease. Finally, it is important to exclude pheochromocytomas on biochemical testing as imaging is unreliable at distinguishing this from ACC.

Imaging Characteristics of ACC

Computed tomography (CT) of the abdomen with thin cuts through the adrenal gland is the imaging test of choice for the evaluation of adrenal tumors. Carcinomas can mimic adenomas but are characterized by larger size (> 6 cm), irregular margins, and heterogeneous enhancement. NIH criteria advise removal of tumors > 6 cm and therefore it is probably more important although more difficult, to determine the nature of lesions intermediate in nature (4–6 cm). Carcinomas are more likely to demonstrate tumor necrosis and cystic degeneration. Advanced disease may be more straightforward to detect as local invasion, tumor extension into the vena cava, lymph node or other metastases are often seen.

Compared to adenomas which often have a high lipid content, ACCs usually demonstrate greater attenuation on unenhanced CT, >10 and commonly >25 Hounsfield units. Pheochromocytomas and metastatic disease also demonstrate this property and non-contrast CT has a sensitivity and specificity of approximately 71% and 98% respectively for distinguishing adenomas from non-adenomas [27]. The specificity can be increased by considering other factors such as size, irregularity and heterogeneous density.

In the event of CT imaging being equivocal, adrenal MRI imaging could prove helpful. Adrenocortical carcinomas are in general hyperintense on T2-weighted images, (although there is a significant overlap between benign and malignant lesions), show similar signal intensity on in phase and out of phase images as a result of low lipid content (and in contrast to many adenomas) and venous invasion is better imaged on MRI. Adenomas enhance vigorously and washout quickly on enhanced MRI as on CT and this is a sensitive method for distinguishing adenoma from non-adenoma.

Overall, imaging methods that determine intracellular lipid content and differences in vascular enhancement can distinguish adenomas from non-adenomas with most specificity.

There is increasing evidence that FDG-PET is useful in differentiating benign from malignant lesions [28–30]. It may also serve as an additional staging study for patients with known ACC or for detection of residual disease. A chest CT should also be performed for patients with ACC for staging purposes.

Pathologic Classification

The pathologic classification of tumors of the adrenal gland is outlined in Table 4.1. Tumors greater than 6 cm are more likely carcinomas, although some smaller tumors may be malignant.

At present histological examination of surgical adrenal samples is not usually able to distinguish between benign and malignant disease with certainty although certain pathological features make the diagnosis of ACC more likely. Careful

Table 4.1 Classification of adrenal tumors

Adrenal cortex
Adenoma
    Functioning
    Nonfunctioning
Carcinoma
Adrenal medulla
Ganglioneuroma
Pheochromocytoma
Neuroblastoma
Mixed type (ganglioneuroblastoma)
Connective tissue tumors
Myelolipomas
Lipomas
Myomas
Angiomas
Fibromas
Fibrosarcoma

macroscopic examination is essential; most ACC's weigh more than 100 g [31] and measure greater than 6 cm in diameter [32]. Several systems have been proposed to help discriminate between ACC and adenoma at a histological level, these include criteria for tumor architecture, venous and capsule invasion and mitotic rate, although none are 100% sensitive [33–35]. Finally, immunohistochemical techniques are under development. Staining for the Ki-67 proliferation index is established as a diagnostic marker for malignancy [36, 37]. Cyclin E and B-catenin staining can also distinguish between benign adenomas and malignant tumors, with P53 and IGF-2 positive staining more specific for ACCs [36]. The role of these new markers in diagnosis remains to be determined. Increasing tumor size, mitotic rate and staining for Ki-67 and cyclin E are poor prognostic markers in ACC [38].

General Management

Management of ACCs must address both management of tumor mass and control of excess hormone secretion.

Surgery

Surgery is the primary treatment for adrenocortical carcinoma and should be carried out using an open approach by an experienced surgeon within a multidisciplinary team setting. Complete resection (R0 resection of stages I–III ACC) is the only treatment that offers long-term disease free survival, but is not always feasible. For patients with a macroscopically complete resection, a margin free resection is a strong predictor for survival. Efforts to avoid tumor spillage are warranted and the tumor capsule should remain intact. Endoscopic removal should be avoided to prevent seeding of malignant cells. Stage II disease requires upper peri-renal fat resection and locoregional lymphadenectomy whereas stages III and IV with invasion or adherence of adjacent structures often necessitate en bloc resection of the kidney or spleen, partial hepatectomy or pancreatectomy [39].

Patients with glucocorticoid secreting tumors are at risk of hypoadrenalism due to an atrophic contralateral adrenal gland following removal of tumor. These patients must be adequately treated with exogenous steroids (100 mg, four times a day via intramuscular injection) throughout the operative period. Indeed, failure of patients to become hypoadrenal following surgery for a glucocorticoid secreting tumor suggests the presence of residual disease.

The role of tumor debulking in the presence of metastatic disease is not clear. Incomplete resection of the primary tumor or metastatic disease not amenable to surgery is associated with a poor prognosis. Still, tumor debulking may help control hormonal oversecretion or relieve local symptoms in certain cases. Even with a complete resection, local recurrence and metastatic disease is common.

Chemotherapy

Almost 50% of patients have invasive or metastatic disease at the time of diagnosis and recurrence occurs in more than half of those undergoing "curative" surgery. The need for effective treatment of these patients is pressing but analysis of chemotherapeutic agents have been limited due to lack of consistent end-points across studies and the small number of patients involved. Large scale randomized control trials are needed in this field.

Mitotane, a chemical conger of the insecticide DDT, is an adrenolytic compound with specific activity on the adrenal cortex. It is the chemotherapeutic agent most commonly used in the management of adrenocortical carcinoma as it is both adrenolytic and inhibits cortisol secretion. In patients with measurable disease, overall response rates of 14%–36% have been reported, but most studies have shown no significant survival benefit [40]. Responses are usually partial and transient with only an occasional complete remission [24]. The role of mitotane as adjuvant therapy after complete surgical resection is controversial [41, 42]. Despite limited supporting data, it is frequently employed in this setting given the high rates of locoregional and distant recurrence. Serum levels of mitotane are monitored in order to optimize therapy as objective response in the metastatic setting was associated with higher serum levels (>14 mg/L). Unfortunately, increased toxicity is also associated with higher serum levels. Side effects are predominantly gastrointestinal, particularly nausea but anorexia and diarrhea also occur. Though less common, CNS toxicity can include lethargy, somnolence, ataxia, dizziness or confusion. It is generally agreed that it has an anti-tumoral effect, however, no survival benefit has been demonstrated for its use in ACC although the studies addressing this were observational, non-randomized and retrospective.

Single agent chemotherapy has also proven disappointing in the management of adrenocortical carcinoma. Doxorubicin and cisplatin have both been evaluated as single agent therapy and in combination with mitotane. Neither drug was efficacious [43]. Multiagent chemotherapy has shown more promise. A multicenter phase II study by the Italian Group for the Study of Adrenal Cancer demonstrated 49% overall response rate using a regimen of etoposide, doxorubicin and cisplatin (EDP) in combination with mitotane. The regimen was well tolerated with the most common side effects being gastrointestinal. The time to progression in responding patients was 2 years [44]. Inclusion of mitotane in a multidrug regimen is rational as adrenocortical carcinomas are prone to multidrug resistance mediated by the MDR-1/P glycoprotein drug pump whose mechanism is inhibited by mitotane. However, this observation has never been proven in a clinical setting.

The small number of patients involved in these studies means the relative efficacies of the regimes are very difficult to determine. The international FIRM-ACT trial (www.firm-act.org) was established in 2004 to overcome this, the aim is to recruit 150 patients with stage III-IV ACC into each of the two arms of this randomized, prospective controlled open label study comparing etoposide, doxorubicin, cisplatin and mitotane with streptozotocin and mitotane.

There are isolated reports of the use of thalidomide as a potentially effective chemotherapeutic agent in ACC [45] and newer therapeutic modalities such as monoclonal antibodies and tyrosine kinase inhibitors are promising developments.

Patients with advanced disease can be very debilitated as a consequence of uncontrolled steroid hormone secretion from the tumor leading to significant reductions in quality of life. Agents such as metyrapone, ketoconazole, aminoglutathimide and etomidate block steroidogenic enzymes and potentially have some anti-proliferative properties. These agents can be used to successfully reduce steroid hormone levels but use must be carefully monitored to avoid adrenal insufficiency.

Radiation Therapy Techniques

The role of radiation in the management of adrenocortical carcinoma is not well defined. It has been proposed as adjuvant therapy after complete resection or as management of microscopic residual disease. One series reports a 10-year crude survival rate of 33% for surgical resection followed by adjuvant radiation [46]. External radiation results in good response rates and effective palliation in patients with residual macroscopic disease or bone or nodal metastases [47, 48].

In the primary management of adrenocortical carcinoma, external radiation may play a role either pre-operatively for unresectable tumors, post-operatively for patients with residual disease or high risk of local failure, or as definitive therapy for patients medically unfit for surgery. Radiation is also effective in the palliative setting for bone and nodal metastases.

For patients with macroscopic or unresectable disease, doses of 50–60 Gy delivered over 5–6 weeks should be considered. Initial fields should encompass the gross tumor with adequate margins as well as the regional lymph nodes, which should include the contralateral para-aortic lymph nodes. Dose to regional nodes can be limited to 45 Gy when they are not macroscopically involved. Care should be taken to limit dose to the spinal cord, kidneys, liver and small bowel. For macroscopic disease where high dose is desired, conformal techniques and intensity modulated radiation should be considered. For patients receiving post-operative treatment for high risk or microscopic disease doses of 45–54 Gy are appropriate.

There may also be a role for radiotherapy in all ACC patients post surgery as approaching 60% of patients develop local tumor recurrence within 5 years of apparently complete tumor resection and there is some evidence that radiotherapy can reduce this. A recent review of adjuvant tumor bed irradiation in patients from the German ACC registry following seemingly curative surgery revealed local tumor recurrence in 11/14 patients who did not receive the adjuvant radiotherapy compared to only 2/14 patients in those irradiated [49].

In the palliative setting, doses of 30-40 Gy given over the course of 2–3 weeks are reasonable. In patients with painful bone metastases, hypofractionated regimens should be considered for patients with poor performance status or otherwise limited life expectancy.

Adrenal Medulla Tumors

Epidemiology

Pheochromocytomas and paragangliomas (extraadrenal pheochromocytomas) as discussed in Chap. 3 are rare tumors that arise from chromaffin cells in the adrenal medulla and elsewhere. They secrete catecholamines that can cause intermittent, episodic or sustained hypertension. Pheochromocytomas have an estimated prevalence of 0.1% in hypertensive patients and are an often overlooked cause in this group [50]. In autopsy series, there is a 0.01%–0.1% prevalence of unsuspected pheochromocytomas. Estimates of the incidence of malignancy in pheochromocytoma ranges from 5% to 46% in different series [51, 52]. Extraadrenal tumors are more commonly malignant [53].

Medical dogma has previously dictated that a hereditary cause for pheochromocytoma is found in 10% of cases. Recent discoveries in germ-line mutations however have revealed this hereditary disposition to be closer to 20%–30% of all tumors particularly in those <50 years of age [54].

Pheochromocytomas are a component of multiple endocrine neoplasia type IIa (MEN IIA) syndrome (pheochromocytoma, medullary thyroid carcinoma, and parathyroid hyperplasia as a result of mutations in the RET protooncogene) or MEN IIB syndrome in which they are associated with medullary thyroid carcinoma, parathyroid hyperplasia, marfanoid habitus and mucosal neuromas. Patients with MEN IIA and B have an approximately 40% lifetime risk of developing a pheochromocytoma. Pheochromocytomas occur in 10%–20% of patients with Von Hippel-Lindau's disease (characterized by multiple hemangioblastomas, retinal angiomas, renal cell cancer and renal/pancreatic cyst as a result of mutations in the VHL gene, those with a missense mutation in this gene are more likely to develop pheochromocytoma) and less than 1% of patients with neurofibromatosis type 1 (peripheral neuroblastomas, café au lait spots, intertriginous freckling, Lisch nodules, optic gliomas and bony abnormalities) [55, 56]. Recently, mutations in the succinate dehydrogenase subunits B and D have been discovered that are associated with familial non syndromic pheochromocytomas and extra adrenal paragangliomas [57, 58]. Lifetime risk of developing pheochromocytomas in these two conditions is currently unknown.

Natural History

Sporadic pheochromocytomas are generally unilateral; when associated with MEN II syndromes, 80% are bilateral. Children and young adult patients with pheochromocytoma present as a result of catecholamine induced symptoms, older patients may have tumor detected as an incidental finding on imaging. Very rarely symptoms of tumor mass can be the presenting feature. A tumor larger than 5 cm more commonly has a malignant course than a smaller lesion. Serum and urinary catecholamines, catecholamine metabolites and vanillylmandelic acid levels are elevated in 90% of pheochromocytomas.

Malignant pheochromocytomas exhibit a similar pattern of spread to ACC but also metastasize to bone. They are equally common in men and women. The average age of presentation is 40–50 years, but they may also occur in children. Patients with

SDH-B mutations are at high risk for developing malignant disease and patients with familial disease tend to present with malignant and non-malignant disease at an earlier age.

Clinical Presentation

Patients with pheochromocytomas present with a range of symptoms resulting from catecholamine excess, from mild labile hypertension to sudden cardiac death secondary to hypertensive crisis, myocardial infarction or cerebrovascular accident. The classic triad of symptoms consists of episodic headaches, diaphoresis and tachycardia [59, 60]. About half of patients have paroxysmal hypertension, while others have sustained hypertension. It may also present with normal blood pressure in 5%–15%. Other symptoms may include pallor, palpitations, panic attack symptoms or generalized weakness. Orthostatic hypertension may occur in association with hypovolemia. Early diagnosis as a result of incidental imaging findings and screening in those with a genetic predisposition has meant an increase in pheochromocytoma diagnosis in the absence of symptoms.

Diagnostic Work-up and Staging

Endocrinology

Diagnosis of pheochromocytoma relies on detection of excess catecholamine synthesis and secretion. There has been much recent discussion with regards to the optimal biochemical test for diagnosis and screening of this condition. There are various methods available; urinary testing for catecholamines, metanephrines and VMA and plasma testing of catecholamines and metanephrines. The consensus is that urinary and plasma metanephrines are the most sensitive and specific method as they are secreted continuously leading to more consistently stable levels compared to the episodic secretion of catecholamines [60].

Biochemical confirmation of catecholamine excess should lead to evaluation of the adrenals using imaging techniques and consideration of an underlying familial cause. There are some who advocate genetic screening in all patients with pheochromocytoma, however testing of patients who are below 50 years with multiple, extra adrenal or malignant tumors and a positive family history is far more likely to yield a genetic defect [60].

Imaging

Either CT or MRI of the abdomen will detect the majority of pheochromocytomas larger than1 cm as discussed in Chaps. 6 and 7. A CT scan should be performed with thin cuts through the adrenal gland. On MRI, pheochromocytomas appear hyperintense on T2-weighted images as opposed to other lesions which are frequently isointense with the liver on these images [61]. Occasionally, CT or MRI may fail to reveal a lesion despite biochemical evidence of a pheochromocytoma. This is more common in the setting of an inherited disorder.

In this case, functional imaging with ^{123}I-metaiodobenzylguanidine, a radiolabeled analog of norepinephrine, (MIBG) scintigraphy may identify the location of the tumor [59]. The major drawback of this study is that there is normal adrenal gland uptake of the compound. MIBG can also be useful when there are multiple lesions or a high risk of metastasis [62]. Additionally, it is used to follow patients after surgical resection. MIBG has less than optimal sensitivity however, particularly for the detection of metastases and recent functional imaging using PET (6-[18F]-flourodopamine, [18F]-dihydroxyphenylalanine, [11C]-hydroxyephedrine or [11C]-epinephrine) appears promising.

There is also an important role for imaging in screening of asymptomatic patients harboring mutations. The most effective mode for this has yet to be established, particularly in those with SDH B mutations where extradrenal, malignant and aggressive tumors are more common. A balance needs to be sought between excessive radiation dosage in young patients by CT and labor intensive analysis of multiple MRI slices from whole-body scans whilst ensuring optimal detection rate.

Pathological Classification

Pheochromocytomas have malignant features in fewer than 10% of cases. Macroscopically, they tend to be encapsulated with areas of cystic change, hemorrhage and necrosis. The capsule is frequently invaded, but that does not constitute malignant change. Benign and malignant pheochromocytomas may appear identical histologically. The only absolute criteria for malignancy is metastasis [63]. Histologically, cell size, nuclear size and arrangement of cells are variable. A twisted cell cord pattern, basophilic or cytophilic staining with fine intracytoplasmic pigment granules and periodic acid-Schiff staining of secretory droplets aid in the diagnosis.

General Management

Surgery

Surgical resection is the definitive management of pheochromocytoma, achieving cure in >90% of patients but can be a high-risk procedure. Cardiovascular and hemodynamic parameters must be monitored closely. Pre-operative medical therapy is aimed at controlling hypertension and expanding intravascular volume. Preoperative pharmacologic preparation typically includes alpha-blockade to counter the effects of released catecholamines and beta-adrenergic blockade if tachyarrythmias occur, but only once adequate alpha-blockade is attained. A recent series reported mortality rates of 2.4% in a group of patients who underwent careful alpha-blockade and volume expansion prior to surgery.

In patients with undiagnosed pheochromocytomas who undergo surgery for other reasons, surgical mortality rates are high due to lethal hypertensive crisis and multiorgan failure [64]. In the largest series of 147 patients undergoing surgery for pheochromocytoma, perioperative mortality and morbidity rates were 2.4% and 24%, respectively [65]. Although it results in rapid symptomatic control, surgical removal of a pheochromocytoma does not always lead to a long time cure. In a large series of 176 patients, pheochromocytoma recurred in 16% of patients [66]. In patients with bilateral pheochromocytomas, usually in the setting of an inherited syndrome, bilateral adrenalectomy is recommended. Adequate steroid hormone replacement will be necessary in this setting although there has been recent interest in the success of cortical sparing surgery in these cases. Although not curative, debulking surgery for control of symptoms is the primary therapy for malignant pheochromocytoma.

Malignant pheochromocytoma has a poor prognosis, with an overall survival rate between 34% and 60%. The radioisotope ^{131}I-MIBG is the most valuable addition to surgical treatment in the management of this condition. Investigators have reported partial responses, based upon biochemical response as well as decreased tumor volume, ranging from 18% to 82% [67–70]. Symptomatic improvement was observed in responding patients with regards to both painful metastases and manifestations of increased catecholamine levels. Partial remissions are usually temporary with some patients relapsing between doses of MIBG. In other patients, sustained partial remissions have been noted with durable palliation extending 2 to 3 years [71, 72]. Prolonged survival has been associated with measurable responses and higher administered doses of MIBG (>500 mCi) [69]. Toxicity includes bone marrow toxicity (particularly thrombocytopenia), nausea and vomiting. Further, larger studies are required with regards to the optimal use of this treatment.

Combination chemotherapy with cyclophosphamide, vincristine and dacarbazine has shown efficacy in a small study. In 14 treated patients, the clinical and biochemical response rates were 57% and 79%, respectively although these were relatively short-lived. Response was associated with objective improvement in performance status and blood pressure. Treatment was well tolerated [73].

Conclusion and Summary

1. Cancer may affect the hypothalamic-pituitary-adrenal axis. This includes stimulation of the axis with increased cortisol secretion and anatomical bilateral adrenal enlargement on adrenal imaging or, more rarely, bilateral adrenal metastases (generally >4 cm) causing hypoadrenalism. Bilateral smooth and uniform enlargement usually represents altered HPA axis function and not malignant disease.

2. The adrenal gland is a common site for adrenal neoplasms but in the absence of a known primary malignancy, lesions detected by imaging are usually cortical adenomas.

3. Conversely, enlargement of the adrenals in patients with a known extra-adrenal malignancy, often represents metastatic disease. The management of metastatic adrenal disease will depend on the type and grade of the primary extraadrenal malignancy.

4. For larger lesions (particularly in patients with Cushing's Syndrome), adrenal cortical carcinoma should be considered. ACC most commonly

presents as either a result of mass effects or as rapidly progressive Cushing's syndrome, although tumours can express any or a combination of adrenal steroids and precursors. The excess secretion of more than one steroid hormone from an adrenal mass is indicative of ACC.

5. All patients with an ACC should have a comprehensive evaluation of adrenal steroid secretion (cortisol production, aldosterone, sex steroid (oestrogen and testosterone) and precursor molecules (17-OHP, DHEAS)) to aid diagnosis and treatment and provide potential biomarkers for follow-up.

6. Surgery for a cortisol-producing ACC leaves the patient susceptible to hypoadrenalism secondary to an atrophic contralateral adrenal. These patients should be adequately covered with intramuscular hydrocortisone during the procedure. In such patients, failure to become hypoadrenal following surgery is indicative of residual disease.

7. In patients with pheochromocytoma, patients usually present with the appropriate clinical and biochemical findings, in the presence of an adrenal mass. Pheochromocytomas typically present as hypertension and the triad of episodic headaches, diaphoresis and tachycardia. Urinary and plasma metanephrines are the most sensitive and specific diagnostic indicators.

8. Surgery is the definitive management of pheochromocytoma. It is essential that during treatment of pheochromocytomas adequate alpha blockade precedes beta-blockade.

References

1. Moore K, Agur A (2002) Essential clinical anatomy. Lippincott Williams and Wilkins, pp 182–185
2. Rouvière H (1932) Anatomie des lymphatiques de l'homme. Masson
3. Young WF (2000) Management approaches to adrenal incidentalomas: a view from Rochester, Minnesota. Endocrinol Metab Clin North Am 29:159–185
4. Kloos RT, Gross MD, Francis IR, Korobkin M, Shapiro B (1995) Incidentally discovered adrenal masses. Endocr Rev 16:460–484
5. Bovio S, Cataldi A, Reimondo G, Sperone P, Novello S, Berruti A, Borasio P, Fava C, Dogliotti L, Scagliotti GV, Angeli A, Terzolo M (2006) Prevalence of adrenal incidentaloma in a contempory computerised tomography series. J Endocrinol Invest 29:298–302
6. Abrams HL, Spiro R, Goldstein N (1950) Metastases in carcinoma. Cancer 3:74–84
7. Glomset DA (1938) The incidence of metastases of malignant tumours to the adrenals. Am J Med Sci 226:521–530
8. Cedermark BJ, Blumenson LE, Pickren JW, Elias EG (1977) The significance of metastasis to the adrenal gland from carcinoma of the stomach and oesophegus. Surg Gynaecol Obstet 145:41–48
9. Lutz A, Stojkovic M, Schmidt M, Arlt W, Allolio B, Reincke M (2000) Adrenocortical function in patients with macrometastases of the adrenal gland. Eur J Endocrinol 143:91–97
10. Vincent JM, Morrison ID, Armstrong P, Reznek RH (1994) Computed tomography of diffuse, non-metastatic enlargement of the adrenal glands in patients with malignant disease. Clin Radiol 49:456–460
11. Jenkins PJ, Sohaib SA, Trainer PJ, Lister TA, Besser GM, Reznek R (1999) Adrenal enlargement and failure of suppression of circulating cortisol by dexamethasone in patients with malignancy. Br J Cancer 80:1815–1819
12. Biswas M, Smith JC, Davies JS (2004) Bilateral adrenal enlargement and non-suppressible hypercortisolism as a presenting feature of gastric cancer. Ann Clin Biochem 41:494–497
13. Wajchenberg BL, Albergaria-Pereira MA, Medonca BB, Latronico AC, Campo-Carneiro P, Alves VA, Zerbini MC, Liberman B, Carlos-Gomes G, Kirschner MA (2000) Adrenocortical carcinoma: clinical and laboratory observations . Cancer 88:711–736
14. Abiven G, Coste J, Groussin L, Anract P, Tissier F, Legmann P, Dousset B, Bertagna X, Bertherat J (2006) Clinical and biological features in the prognosis of adrenocortical cancer: poor outcome of cortisol-secreting tumors in a series of 202 consecutive patients. J Clin Endocrinol Metab 91:2650–2655
15. Allolio B, Fassnacht M (2006) Clinical review: adrenocortical carcinoma: clinical update J Clin Endocrinol Metab 91:2027–2037
16. Li FP, Fraumeni JF, Mulvihill JJ, Blattner WA, Dreyfus MG, Tucker MA, Miller RW (1988) A cancer family syndrome in twenty-four kindreds. Cancer Res 48:5358–5362
17. Wiedemann H (1964) Complexe malformatif familial avec hernie ombilicale et macroglossie, un "syndrome nouveau" J Genet Hum 13:223
18. Sidhu S, Sywak M, Robinson B, Delbridge L (2004) Adrenocortical cancer: recent clinical and molecular advances. Curr Opin Oncol 16:13–18
19. Koch CA, Pacak K, Chrousos GP (2002) The molecular pathogenesis of hereditary and sporadic adrenocortical and adrenomedullary tumors. J Clin Endocrinol Metab 87:5367–5384
20. Lynch HT, Mulcahy GM, Harris RE, Guirgis HA, Lynch JF (1978) Genetic and pathologic findings in a kindred with hereditary sarcoma, breast cancer, brain tumors, leukemia, lung, laryngeal, and adrenal cortical carcinoma. Cancer 41:2055–2064
21. Ohgaki H, Kleihues P, Heitz PU (1993) p53 mutations in sporadic adrenocortical tumours. Int J Cancer 54:408–410
22. Reincke M, Karl M, Travis WH, Mastorakos G, Allolio B, Linehan HM, Chrousos GP (1994) p53

mutations in human adrenocortical neoplasms: immunohistochemical and molecular studies. J Clin Endocrinol Metab 78:790–794

23. Barzon L, Chilosi M, Fallo F, Martignoni G, Montagna L,
Palu G, Boscaro M (2001) Molecular analysis of
CDKN1C and TP53 in sporadic adrenal tumors. Eur J
Endocrinol 145:207–212

24. Wooten MD, King DK (1993) Adrenal cortical carcinoma. Epidemiology and treatment with mitotane and a
review of the literature. Cancer 72:3145–3155

25. Haak HR, Hermans J, van de Velde CJ et al. (1994)
Optimal treatment of adrenocortical carcinoma with
mitotane: results in a consecutive series of 96 patients
[see comment]. Br J Cancer 69:947–951

26. Norton J (1997) Adrenal tumors. Cancer: Principles and
Practice of Oncology. Lippincott-Raven, Philadelphia,
vol 1659, p77

27. Boland GW, Lee MJ, Gazelle GS, Halpern EF,
McNicholas MM, Mueller PR (1998) Characterisation
of adrenal masses using unenhanced CT: an analysis of
the CT literature. AJR Am J Roentgenol 171:201–204

28. Boland GW, Goldberg MA, Lee MJ, Mayo-Smith WW,
Dixon J, McNicholas MM, Meuller PR (1995) Indeterminate adrenal mass in patients with cancer: evaluation
at PET with 2-[F-18]-fluoro-2-deoxy-D-glucose. Radiology 194:131–134

29. Maurea S, Mainolfi C, Bazzicalupo L, Panico MR,
Imparato C, Alfano B, Ziviello M, Salvatore M (1999)
Imaging of adrenal tumours using FDG PET: comparison of benign and malignant lesions. AJR Am J Roentgenol 173:25–29

30. Kumar R, Xiu Y, Yu JQ, Takalkar A, El-Haddad G,
Potenta S, Kung J, Huang H, Alavi A (2004) 18F-FDG
PET in evaluation of adrenal lesions in patients with lung
cancer. J Nucl Med 45:2058–2062

31. Saeger W (2000) Histopathological classification of adrenal tumours. Eur J Clin Invest 30(Suppl 3):58–62

32. Ross NS, Aron DC (1990) Hormonal evaluation of the
patient with an incidentally discovered adrenal mass.
N Eng J Med 323:1401–1405

33. Weiss LM (1984) Comparative histologic study of
43 metastasising and nonmetasising adrenocortical
tumours. Am J Surg Pathol 8:163–169

34. Hough AJ, Hollifield JW, Page DL, Hartmann WH
(1979) Prognostic factors in adrenal cortical tumours. A
mathematical analysis of clinical and morphological
data. Am J Clin Path 72:390–399

35. Aubert S, Wacrenier A, Leroy X, Devos P, Carnaille B,
Proye C, Wemeau JL, Lecomte-Houcke M, Leteurte E
(2002) Weiss system revisited: a clinicopathologic and
immunohistochemical study of 49 adrenocortical
tumours. Am J Surg Pathol 26:1621–1629

36. McNicol AM, Nolan CE, Struthers AJ, Farquharson MA,
Hermans J, Haak HR (1997) Expression of p53 in adrenocortical tumours: clinicopathological correlations. J Pathol
181:146–152

37. Wachenfield C, Beuschlein F, Zwermann O, Mora P,
Fassnacht M, Allolio B, Reincke M (2001) Discerning
malignancy in adrenocortical tumours: are molecular
markers useful? Eur J Endocrinol 145:335–341

38. Tissier F, Louvel A, Grabar S, Hagnere AM, Bertherat J,
Vacher-Lavenu MC, Dousset B, Chapuis Y, Bertagna X,
Gicquel C (2004) Cyclin E correlates with malignancy
and adverse prognosis in adrenocortical tumours. Eur J
Endocrinol 150:809–817

39. Dousset B, Gaujoux S, Thillois J-M (2006) Surgical
treatment of adrenal cortical carcinoma. In: Bertagna X
(ed) Adrenal cancer. John Libbey Eurotext, pp 71–95

40. Pommier RF, Brennan MF (1992) An eleven-year
experience with adrenocortical carcinoma: Surgery
112(6):963–970; discussion 970–971

41. Luton JP, Cerdas S, Billaud L et al. (1990) Clinical
features of adrenocortical carcinoma, prognostic factors,
and the effect of mitotane therapy [see comment]. N Engl
J Med 322:1195–1201

42. Vassilopoulou-Sellin R, Guinee VF, Klein MJ et al.
(1993) Impact of adjuvant mitotane on the clinical course
of patients with adrenocortical cancer [see comment].
Cancer 71:3119–3123

43. Ahlman H, Khorram-Manesh A, Jansson S et al. (2001)
Cytotoxic treatment of adrenocortical carcinoma. World
J Surg 25:927–933

44. Berruti A, Terzolo M, Sperone P et al. (2005) Etoposide,
doxorubicin and cisplatin plus mitotane in the treatment
of advanced adrenocortical carcinoma: a large prospective phase II trial. Endocr Rel Cancer 12:657–666

45. Chacon R, Tossen G, Loria F, Chacon M (2005) CASE
2. Response in a patient with metastatic adrenal cortical carcinoma with thalidomide. J Clin Oncol 1 23:
1579–1580

46. Magee BJ, Gattamaneni HR, Pearson D (1987) Adrenal
cortical carcinoma: survival after radiotherapy. Clin
Radiol 38:587–588

47. Percarpio B, Knowlton AH (1976) Radiation therapy of
adrenal cortical carcinoma. Acta Radiol Ther Phys Biol
15:288–292

48. Markoe AM, Serber W, Micaily B, Brady LW (1991)
Radiation therapy for adjunctive treatment of adrenal
cortical carcinoma. Am J Clin Oncol 14:170–174

49. Fassnacht M, Hahner S, Polat B, Koschker AC,
Kenn W, Flentje M, Allolio B (2006) Efficacy of adjuvant radiotherapy of the tumor bed on local recurrence
of adrenocortical carcinoma J Clin Endocrinol Metab
91:4501–4504

50. Cryer PE (1985) Phaeochromocytoma. Clin Endocrinol
Metab 14:203–220

51. Beierwaltes WH, Sisson JC, Shapiro B (1986) Malignant
potential of pheochromocytoma. Proc AACR 27:617

52. Melicow MM (1987) One hundred cases of pheochromocytoma (107 tumors) at the Columbia-Presbyterian Medical Center, 1926–1976: a clinicopathological analysis.
Cancer 40:1987–2004

53. Neumann HP, Bausch B, McWhinney SR, Bender BU,
Gimm O, Franke G, Schipper J, Klisch J, Altehoefer C,
Zerres K, Januszewicz A, Eng C, Smith WM, Munk R,
Manz T, Glaesker S, Apel TW, Treier M, Reineke M,
Walz MK, Hoang-Vu C, Brauckhoff M, Klein-Franke A,
Klose P, Schmidt H, Maier-Woelfle M, Peczkowska M,
Szmigielski C, Eng C (2002) Freiburg-Warsaw-Columbus
Pheochromocytoma Study Group. 2002 Germ-line

mutations in nonsyndromic pheochromocytoma N Engls J Med 346:1459–1466

54. Nakagawara A, Ikeda K, Tsuneyoshi M, Daimaru Y, Enjoji M (1985) Malignant pheochromocytoma with ganglioneuroblastoma elements in a patient with von Recklinghausen's disease. Cancer 55:2794–2798

55. Loughlin KR, Gittes RF (1986) Urological management of patients with von Hippel-Lindau's disease. J Urol 136:789–791

56. Astuti D, Latif F, Dallol A, Dahia PL, Douglas F, George E, Skoldberg F, Husebye ES, Eng C, Maher ER (2001) Gene mutations in the succinate dehydrogenase subunit SDHB cause susceptibility to familial pheochromocytoma and to familial paraganglioma Am J Hum Genet 69:49–54

57. Astuti D, Douglas F, Lennard TW, Aligianis IA, Woodward ER, Evans DG, Eng C, Latif F, Maher ER (2001) Germline SDHD mutation in familial phaeochromocytoma Lancet 357:1181–1182

58. Stein PP, Black HR (1991) A simplified diagnostic approach to pheochromocytoma. A review of the literature and report of one institution's experience. Medicine 70:46–66

59. Bravo EL (1991) Pheochromocytoma: new concepts and future trends. Kidney Int 40:544–556

60. Pacak K, Eisenhofer G, Ahlman H, Bornstein SR, Gimenez-Roqueplo AP, Grossman AB, Kimura N, Mannelli M, McNicol AM, Tischler AS (2005) International Symposium on Pheochromocytoma. 2005 Pheochromocytoma: recommendations for clinical practice from the First International Symposium Nat Clin Pract Endocrinol Metab 3:92–102

61. Bravo EL (1994) Evolving concepts in the pathophysiology, diagnosis, and treatment of pheochromocytoma. Endocr Rev 15:356–368

62. Whalen RK, Althausen AF, Daniels GH (1992) Extraadrenal pheochromocytoma. J Urol 147:1–10

63. Cotran A, Kumar V, Robbins SL (1994) Robbins pathologic basis of disease, 5th edn. WB Saunders, Philadelphia, pp 1161–1164

64. Lo CY, Lam KY, Wat MS, Lam KS (2000) Adrenal pheochromocytoma remains a frequently overlooked diagnosis. Am J Surg 179:212–215

65. Plouin PF, Duclos JM, Soppelsa F, Boublil G, Chatellier G (2001) Factors associated with perioperative morbidity and mortality in patients with pheochromocytoma: analysis of 165 operations at a single center [see comment]. J Clin Endocrinol Metab 86:1480–1486

66. Amar L, Servais A, Gimenez-Roqueplo AP, Zinzindohoue F, Chatellier G, Plouin PF (2005) Year of diagnosis, features at presentation, and risk of recurrence in patients with pheochromocytoma or secreting paraganglioma. J Clin Endocrinol Metab 90:2110–2116

67. Shapiro B, Gross MD, Shulkin B (2001) Radioisotope diagnosis and therapy of malignant pheochromocytoma. Trend Endocrinol Metab 12:469–475

68. Schlumberger M, Gicquel C, Lumbroso J et al. (1992) Malignant pheochromocytoma: clinical, biological, histologic and therapeutic data in a series of 20 patients with distant metastases. J Endocrinol Invest 15:631–642

69. Safford SD, Coleman RE, Gockerman JP et al. (2003) Iodine -131 metaiodobenzylguanidine is an effective treatment for malignant pheochromocytoma and paraganglioma. Surgery 134:956–962

70. Rose B, Matthay KK, Price D et al. (2003) High-dose 131I-metaiodobenzylguanidine therapy for 12 patients with malignant pheochromocytoma. Cancer 98:239–248

71. Loh KC, Fitzgerald PA, Matthay KK, Yeo PP, Price DC (1997) The treatment of malignant pheochromocytoma with iodine-131 metaiodobenzylguanidine (131I-MIBG): a comprehensive review of 116 reported patients. J Endocrinol Invest 20:648–658

72. Shapiro B, Sisson JC, Wieland DM et al. (1991) Radiopharmaceutical therapy of malignant pheochromocytoma with [131I]metaiodobenzylguanidine: results from ten years of experience. J Nucl Biol Med 35:269–276

73. Averbuch SD, Steakley CS, Young RC et al. (1988) Malignant pheochromocytoma: effective treatment with a combination of cyclophosphamide, vincristine, and dacarbazine. Ann Intern Med 109:267–273

Adrenal Surgery

5

Antonia E. Stephen, Alex B. Haynes, Richard A. Hodin

Contents

Introduction

The adrenal glands, also known as the suprarenal glands, are located in the retroperitoneum superomedial to the kidneys. They consist of an outer cortex and inner medulla and secrete hormones essential for normal physiologic function. Surgical removal of one or both of the adrenal glands is performed for tumor, hormone hypersecretion, or a combination of both. The specific indications for adrenal resection are complex, and have evolved dramatically in recent years with the introduction of increasingly sophisticated imaging techniques. The unique anatomy of the adrenal glands, including their location, intra-abdominal relationships, and blood supply has led to creative operative strategies over the years, most recently sophisticated minimally invasive techniques. Patients undergoing surgery for adrenal tumors with excess hormonal secretion require specific pre, post, and intraoperative management. These topics, as well as an historical overview of adrenal surgery, are included in this chapter.

The History of Adrenal Anatomy and Surgery

History of the Adrenal Glands – Form and Function

The adrenals were first described as a distinct entity in 1552 by Bartholomaeus Eustachius, a Roman anatomist who labeled them 'glandulae renibus incumbentes' (translation: 'glands lying on the

A.E. Stephen (✉)
Division of Surgical Oncology, Massachusetts General Hospital Cancer Center, 55 Fruit Street, YAW 7, Boston, MA 02114

M.A. Blake, G. Boland (eds.), *Adrenal Imaging*, DOI 10.1007/978-1-59745-560-2_5,
© 2009 Humana Press, a part of Springer Science+Business Media, LLC

kidneys') [1]. In an interesting historical note, he correctly contradicted the famous anatomist Andreas Vesalius who had described dog kidneys and neglected description of the adrenal glands [2]. With a detailed examination of the human retroperitoneal organs, Eustachius ascertained that the adrenal gland consisted of two parts, an outer cortex of mesodermal origin and inner medulla derived from neuroendocrine tissue. He also noted additional adrenal tissue at the aortic bifurcation, now known as the Organ of Zukerkandl [3]. It was many years following the anatomic description that the physiologic function of the adrenals was elucidated. In 1855, Thomas Addison of London published a report of patients with dark skin color, anemia, and general malaise who at autopsy were noted to have severely diseased adrenal glands [4]. One year later, French physiologist Charles Brown-Sequard reported that bilateral adrenalectomy in dogs led to a similar illness and was eventually fatal [5]. These reports established the importance of the adrenal gland hormone secretions, but the exact nature of the secretions was unknown until almost a century later, when a group from the Mayo Clinic extracted the components of the adrenal cortex and described them as glucocorticoids and mineralocorticoids. Epinephrine, or adrenaline, and norepinephrine were also extracted from the adrenal glands in the mid-1900s and described in reports of hormonally productive adrenal tumors published by Rabin [6] and Holton [7]. With the discovery of the secreted hormones, biochemical testing soon became available, and with that the ability to diagnose hypersecreting tumors. It was not, however, until the introduction of computed tomography in the 1970s that adrenal imaging and the pre-operative identification of adrenal tumors became possible.

Early Adrenal Surgery

Prior to the relatively modern techniques of adrenal imaging and hormonal biochemical testing, indications for adrenalectomy were limited to symptomatic tumors large enough for detection on physical examination. The first such surgery was performed via a transabdominal incision, similar to those used for removal of intra-abdominal organs such as the gallbladder [1, 8]. The early approaches to adrenalectomy were modeled

after abdominal surgical incisions, such as those used for cholecystectomy and gastrectomy. It soon became evident that these approaches were less than ideal due to the superior retroperitoneal location of the adrenals high up under the costal margin. In order to gain better access, a posterior, transdiaphragmatic approach was described in 1932 by Lennox Broster of London [1, 9]. The flank approach was popularized by George Crile of the Cleveland Clinic [10], and Charles Mayo described removing a pheochromocytoma via a flank approach just a few years later in 1927 [11]. In 1936, Hugh Young of Baltimore described a posterior approach for exposure of both adrenal glands, a method to avoid an abdominal incision [12]. This wide array of patient positioning and method of access to the adrenal glands continued in its evolution throughout the latter half of the twentieth century, culminating in the introduction of laparoscopic adrenal surgery.

Review of Adrenal Anatomy and Histology
General Adrenal Anatomy

Each of the adrenal glands, in their normal size and configuration, measure approximately 3–5 cm in length, 4–6 mm in thickness and weigh approximately 4–5 g [13]. They maintain close approximation to the superiomedial aspect of the kidneys, and are surrounded on their surface by a fibrous capsule of connective tissue. The position and appearance of normal adrenal glands as seen on a CT scan is shown in Fig. 5.1. Outside of the layer of loose connective tissue is abundant perinephric and retroperitoneal fat. The adrenal glands are distinguished from the surrounding fat by their rich and bright yellow color and more nodular and fibrous consistency. Despite this, however, small tumors can often be difficult to find intraoperatively in obese patients with abundant intraabdominal and retroperitoneal fat. The adrenal glands have an abundant blood supply and hence are a common site for tumor metastases. They receive their arterial blood supply from three main sources, the inferior phrenic artery, the aorta, and the renal artery. These three arteries provide several subsegmental branches which divide into smaller channels over the capsule of the gland [13]. It is uncommon to identify three discrete adrenal arteries at surgical exploration, although the subsegmental branches

Fig. 5.1 Coronal CT scan demonstrating normal right and left adrenal glands (*arrows*) with inverted "Y" and "V" shapes respectively located above both kidneys

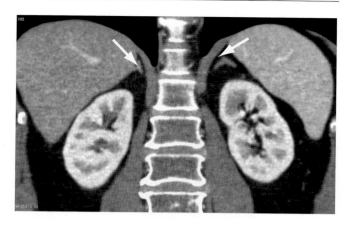

can become significantly enlarged in patients with sizable adrenal tumors. The arteries form a rich plexus within the gland and coalesce into a single draining vein. Additional smaller accessory veins follow the anatomic course of the subsegmental arteries. The specific anatomic relationships of the right and left adrenal glands are described separately, and are outlined in list form in Table 5.1 [13, 14]; a schematic diagram of the adrenal glands and their blood supply is shown in Fig. 5.2. Despite the known anatomic relationships of the adrenal glands described in the following paragraphs, the exact location of the glands and their associated tumors can be quite variable and detailed pre-operative imaging is invaluable in ensuring a good operative outcome.

Anatomy of Right Adrenal Gland

The right adrenal gland is located directly inferior to the medial portion of the right diaphragm and poster-omedial to the liver. The lateral and inferior edges are closely apposed to the right kidney. The inferior vena cava is just medial to the kidney, and the right adrenal vein drains directly into the vena cava and measures approximately 6 mm [15]. Dissection and control of the right adrenal vein during adrenalectomy can be challenging due to the relatively short length and its direct connection to the inferior vena cava.

Anatomy of Left Adrenal Gland

The left adrenal gland is slightly thicker and larger than the right, and although it is primarily located

Table 5.1 Detailed adrenal anatomic relationships

Margin	Region	Relation
Right gland		
Anterior	Medial	No peritoneal covering; IVC anterior
	Lateral	Upper contacts inferomedial bare area of the liver; lower covered by peritoneum from the coronary ligament
Posterior	Upper	Lies against the diaphragm
	Lower	Contacts upper anterior right kidney
Medial		Right inferior phrenic artery and celiac ganglion
Left gland		
Anterior	Upper	Covered by omental bursa peritoneum
	Lower	No peritoneal covering; contacts pancreatic tail and splenic artery
Posterior	Medial	Contacts left diaphragmatic crus
	Lateral	Right kidney
Medial		Left inferior phrenic and gastric arteries, and left celiac ganglion

Adapted from Mihai R, Farndon JR. Surgical embryology and anatomy of the adrenal glands. In: Clark OH, Duh QY (eds) Textbook of endocrine surgery. Philadelphia Saunders, 1997, p 452 and from Udelsman R. Adrenal. In: Norton JA et al. (eds) Surgery: basic science and clinical evidence, pp 897–917

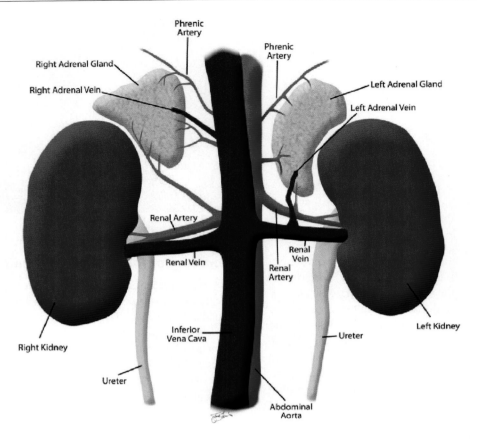

Fig. 5.2 Schematic representation of the blood supply of the adrenal glands

at the superomedial aspect of the kidney, it extends alongside the medial edge of the kidney more inferiorly than on the left [1]. It is closely apposed to and usually directly posterior to the tail of the pancreas, although its exact relationship to the pancreas can be somewhat variable. It lies just inferior to the diaphragm, and because if its medial location, it is often closely associated with the left crus. The spleen is anterior and superior to the left adrenal gland, and the left kidney directly lateral. As described later in the chapter, mobilization of the spleen is a key step in exposing the left adrenal gland. The aorta is just medial, and the renal vein and artery inferior. The left adrenal vein measures approximately 30 mm and drains into the left renal vein. During surgery, it is typically located at the inferomedial aspect of the adrenal gland, and its dissection significantly less risky than on the right due to its longer length and greater distance from the inferior vena cava.

Adrenal Gland Histology

The cortex and medulla comprise the adrenal gland, and each have separate functions and embryologic origin. The adrenal cortex is the outer layer of the gland, arises from the mesoderm during embryologic development, and accounts for the majority of the gland weight. The cortex has three separate layers, or zones. The outermost layer is the zona glomerulosa, and secretes the mineralocorticoid known as aldosterone. The middle layer and inner regions of the cortex, the zona fasciculata and zona reticularis, secrete glucocorticoids (cortisol) and androgens. The most inner portion of the adrenal gland is the adrenal medulla, which is derived from the same neural crest cells that compose the sympathetic ganglia. The adrenal medulla is innervated by preganglionic fibers of the sympathetic nervous system [16], and secretes catecholamines (epinephrine and norepinephrine).

Adrenal Hormonal Function

Each hormone secreted by the adrenal gland has a specific function and is essential for normal human physiology. Fortunately, the presence of two adrenal glands makes it possible to remove one gland, when diseased, with essentially no physiologic consequences. Removal of both adrenal glands, however, necessitates hormone replacement therapy and in the untreated state is eventually fatal. Of the three hormones secreted by the adrenal, glucocorticoids are the most essential to life [13]. The synthesis and secretion of cortisol is controlled by the pituitary gland via adrenocorticotropin (ACTH) and controls cellular functions by binding to steroid receptors which are present throughout the body. The physiologic effects of cortisol include stimulation of hepatic gluconeogenesis, inhibition of protein synthesis, increased protein catabolism, and lipolysis of adipose tissue [16]. Aldosterone, the primary mineralocorticoid, regulates the extracellular fluid balance through its effect on sodium and potassium excretion. The secretion of aldosterone is controlled primarily by three different sources, the renin-angiotensin-aldosterone axis, ACTH, and increased serum potassium. The adrenal sex steroids, dehydroepiandrosterone (DHEA) and DHEA sulfate, are converted to testosterone in the periphery and account for only a small fraction of androgens in the body, the majority of which are secreted by the testes in males.

Diagnosis of Adrenal Pathology

Adrenal tumors and/or hormone overproduction becomes evident in three ways: an incidental radiologic finding, a syndrome of hormonal excess, or less frequently in this current era, a symptomatic or palpable abdominal mass.

Differential Diagnosis of an Adrenal Mass

Regardless of how the tumor is discovered, it is essential when evaluating a patient with an adrenal tumor to consider the differential diagnosis. In doing so, a number of factors should be considered such as the size of the mass, the presence of a known malignancy or a history of hypertension, or a family history of pheochromocytoma or MEN II. A complete list of the differential diagnosis for an adrenal mass is provided in Table 5.2 [17, 18]. The

Table 5.2 Differential diagnosis and frequency of incidentally discovered adrenal masses

Adenoma		
	No cancer history	36%–94%
	Cancer history	7%–68%
	Cortisol producing	2%–15%
	Aldosteronoma	0%–2%
Adrenocortical Carcinoma		0%–25%
Pheochromocytoma		0%–11%
Metastasis		
	No cancer history	0%–21%
	Cancer history	32%–73%
Cyst		4%–22%
Ganglioneuroma		0%–6%
Myelolipoma		7%–15%
Hematoma		0%–4%

Adapted from Kloos RT, Korobkin M, Thompson NW, Francis IR, Shapiro B, Gross MD (1997) Incidentally discovered adrenal masses. Cancer Treat Res 89:263–292 and from Brunt LM, Moley JF (2001) Adrenal incidentaloma. World J Surg 25:905–913

variation in percentages is due to the fact that the data was assembled from different patient populations. Most notable is the fact that the majority of adrenal tumors are benign, nonproductive, cortical adenomas that require no intervention.

Adrenal Incidentaloma

Adrenal tumors are extremely common in the general population; autopsy studies estimate an incidence of 3%–5% in persons over the age of 50 [19]. In this era of the widespread use of CT scans and other imaging modalities, adrenal tumors are frequently discovered as incidental abnormalities on radiologic studies performed for an unrelated reason. These incidental adrenal tumors are noted at an estimated rate of 1%–2% in patients undergoing a radiologic study of the abdomen [20, 21]. With the continued refinement and improvement in scanning techniques, this number is expected to increase, and may approach that noted on autopsy studies [22]. In the past decade, many publications have investigated and attempted to address the question of how to evaluate and treat incidental adrenal masses, and most specifically, determine when surgery is indicated [20]. A consensus statement issued forth from the National Institute of Health in 2002, as summarized from a conference of experts on adrenal disease, further defined the entity of "adrenal incidentaloma" and assembled recommendations for evaluation and treatment. In this statement, adrenal incidentalomas are defined as "clinically inapparent adrenal masses discovered inadvertently in the course of diagnostic testing or treatment for other clinical conditions that are not related to suspicion of adrenal disease" (NIH consensus statement). Once an adrenal mass is noted, there are two key questions that need to be addressed: 1. Is the mass hormonally productive and therefore causing a syndrome of hormonal excess? and 2. Is the mass malignant, or perhaps more accurately worded, what is the risk of malignancy? The answers to these two specific questions will then determine whether or not surgery is indicated.

Syndromes of Hormonal Excess

Hormonally active adrenal tumors are either discovered in the course of a work-up for a constellation of signs and/or symptoms (escalating hypertension, features of Cushing's syndrome, etc.) in which case the biochemical work-up leads to an abdominal CT scan to evaluate the adrenals, or the opposite, whereby an incidentally noted adrenal mass is discovered and biochemical screening is initiated. In the latter cases, retrospective questioning often notes the patient to be hypertensive, or have classic symptoms of a pheochromocytoma. In some cases, however, such as subclinical Cushing's Syndrome, the hormonally active mass is completely asymptomatic.

Aldosterenoma (Conn's Syndrome)

The overproduction of aldosterone causes the retention of sodium and water, and the excretion of potassium, leading to hypertension and hypokalemia. It is thought to be a common cause of secondary hypertension. The diagnosis of primary hyperaldosteronism is based on elevated serum aldosterone levels in conjunction with a suppressed renin level with a ratio of aldosterone/renin >20 highly suggestive of the diagnosis [23]. This can be confirmed with a 24-h urine alsosterone level after salt loading (which should suppress aldosterone secretion in the normal physiologic state). The majority (70%) of syndromes of aldosterone excess are caused by a aldosterone producing tumor and the remainder bilateral cortical hyperplasia [24]. It is essential for the clinician to distinguish these, as surgery is the treatment of choice for an isolated adenoma and medical management is indicated for bilateral cortical hyperplasia. Further complicating matters is the fact that aldosterone producing tumors are often quite small, measuring 1–2 cm, making the distinction between a solitary adrenal mass and bilateral hyperplasia more difficult. Adrenal vein sampling for aldosterone levels is an option in these patients to determine if there is unilateral overproduction. This is discussed in more detail in Chap. 12.

Cortisol-producing Adenoma

Cushing's syndrome is a constellation of signs and symptoms resulting from an overproduction of cortisol. These signs and symptoms include hypertension, glucose intolerance, easy bruisability, and obesity with a classic central fat distribution. The overproduction of cortisol is most commonly the result of a pituitary adenoma, whereby the excess cortisol production is secondary and stimulated by adrenocorticotropin from the pituitary gland. Approximately 20% of cases, however, are caused by an adrenal tumor [18]. First line screening tests for hypercortisolism include a morning serum cortisol level and a 24-h urine cortisol. This level of testing, however, may not be adequate in asymptomatic patients with an incidentaloma. It is estimated that 2%–15% of patients with an adrenal incidentaloma will have subtle abnormalities in cortisol regulation as detected in a dexamethasone suppression test. These patients can be more susceptible to hypertension and diabetes and hence may benefit from surgical excision. It is therefore recommended that patients with an adrenal incidentaloma undergo a dexamethasone suppression test in addition to the general screening tests for cortisol overproduction. The appearance of a left sided cortisol producing adrenal adenoma on CT scan and grossly following surgical resection is shown in Fig. 5.3.

Pheochromocytoma

A pheochromocytoma is a neuroendocrine tumor arising from the cells of the adrenal medulla. The adrenal medullary cells are responsible for the secretion of

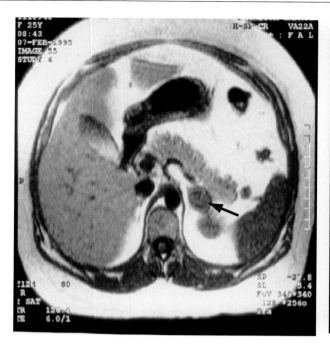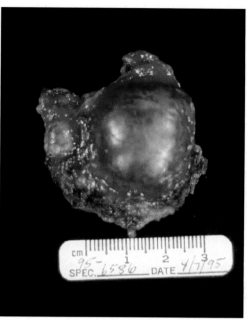

Fig. 5.3 Left sided cortisol-producing adrenal adenoma (*arrow*) on axial TIW MRI and corresponding surgical specimen

catecholamines (epinephrine and norepinephrine). The overproduction of catecholamines from the pheochromocytoma often results in episodes of hypertension, flushing, palpitations, tremor, diaphoresis, and headache. Not every patient experiences these classic symptomatic episodes; patients can also have sustained hypertension that is often difficult to control, requiring multiple antihypertensive medications. The diagnosis of a pheochromocytoma is primarily based on serum and urine measurements of the catecholamine metabolites metanephrine and normetanephrine. Pheochromocytomas also tend to be large (>3 cm) and demonstrate a bright signal intensity on T2-weighted MRI imaging. It is of paramount importance to accurately diagnose an incidentaloma as a pheochromocytoma pre-operatively, as surgery can precipitate a potentially lethal hypertensive crisis. These patients also require pre-operative preparation with alpha-blocking agents and careful intra-operative monitoring and blood pressure control to avoid hyper and hypotension during tumor manipulation and dissection. The specifics regarding the pre and intraoperative management of pheochromocytoma patients is discussed further later in this chapter.

Sex Hormone Secreting Tumors

Adrenal tumors productive of sex hormones are quite rare, and are often malignant. Patients may note virilizing or feminizing symptoms, but are frequently asymptomatic. It is generally recommended that DHEA sulfate levels are checked in patients with an adrenal incidentaloma [25].

Hormonal Work-up for Adrenal Incidentaloma

Despite the fact that the syndromes described above should be clinically evident, this is not always the case. Patients with aldosteronomas can be normokalemic, and their elevated blood pressure is often attributed to essential hypertension. Classic symptoms of pheochromocytoma can be varied, and symptomatic episodes labeled "anxiety attacks". Subclinical Cushing's Syndrome can be particularly difficult to diagnose, with routine biochemical testing often normal and specialized testing in order. Because a patient with an incidentally discovered adrenal mass may fit into one of these categories, it is recommended that all patients with adrenal

Table 5.3 Biochemical work-up of an incidental adrenal mass

Blood tests
Am blood cortisol
ACTH
Renin (plasma renin activity)
Aldosterone
Plasma metanephrines
Dexamethasone suppression test
24-h urine
Creatinine
Aldosterone
Cortisol
Catecholamines
Vanillylmandelic acid (VMA)
Metanephrines

incidentalomas undergo biochemical screening, regardless of overt signs or symptoms. A comprehensive list of the biochemical tests for an adrenal mass is listed in Table 5.3; this may be tailored for each individual patient depending of their history, physical exam, and appearance of the mass on radiologic studies.

Surgical Approaches to Adrenalectomy

After an adrenal mass has been identified and the decision has been made to proceed with adrenalectomy, the next step is to decide upon the optimal procedure. Surgery can be performed with either open or endoscopic techniques, with the patient in supine, prone, or lateral decubitus position approaching the adrenal gland transabdominally or retroperitoneally. There are advantages and disadvantages to each procedure and position. The choice of technique depends upon the nature and size of the tumor, the patient's body habitus and previous procedures, as well as surgeon preference.

In 1992, Gagner, Lacroix, and Bolte published a description of laparoscopic adrenalectomy in the New England Journal of Medicine [26]. They described a lateral, transabdominal laparoscopic technique for resection of pheochromocytoma and aldosteronoma. This began an era of marked change in adrenal surgery with new minimally invasive options. Additional endoscopic procedures for adrenalectomy have subsequently been introduced, including anterior transabdominal laparoscopy and posterior retroperitoneoscopy. Indications for

laparoscopic adrenalectomy have expanded beyond those described by Gagner et al., but these approaches do not replace open techniques, but rather serve as additional tools in the armamentarium of the adrenal surgeon.

Laparoscopy (as well as other endoscopic approaches) decreases the morbidity of adrenal surgery [27]. Hospital stays are much shorter, with some even advocating laparoscopic adrenalectomy as day surgery in selected patients. Recovery is shortened, as well, with greatly decreased postoperative pain. Modern fiberoptic instruments also provide excellent visualization of the operative field without the extensive mobilization and retraction required for open surgery. On the other hand, laparoscopy is inadequate for the en bloc resections often required for malignant tumors of the adrenal glands. In addition, inadvertent injury to surrounding structures, including large vessels, can necessitate emergent conversion to an open procedure.

Retroperitoneal Adrenalectomy

Retroperitoneal approaches, both open and endoscopic, are sometimes employed for adrenalectomy. These techniques avoid entering the peritoneum, which can be highly advantageous in patients who have undergone multiple previous abdominal procedures. Posterior retroperitoneal adrenalectomy was first performed in 1936 [12]. This procedure uses an approach over the 12th rib, with the patient in a prone position. Bilateral adrenalectomy can be performed without repositioning. This was once the preferred technique for urologists, as the exposure is similar to that used in much urologic surgery. However, only moderate sized tumors (up to 6 cm) can be removed through this incision, as the working area is confined. Many patients also suffered from prolonged postoperative incisional pain due to injury to the subcostal nerve.

The advantages of posterior adrenalectomy (ease of bilateral exposure, avoidance of the peritoneal cavity) combined with minimally invasive techniques led to the development of posterior retroperitoneoscopic adrenalectomy (Fig. 5.4). First described by Mercan and colleagues in 1995 [28], and further popularized by Siperstein at the Cleveland Clinic [29], this approach allows minimally invasive adrenalectomy to be performed without the risk to abdominal organs. Access

Fig. 5.4 Laparoscopic posterior retroperitoneal adrenalectomy. Four trocars are inserted below the costal margin as indicated and the localization of the kidney and adrenal gland are guided by transabdominal ultrasound

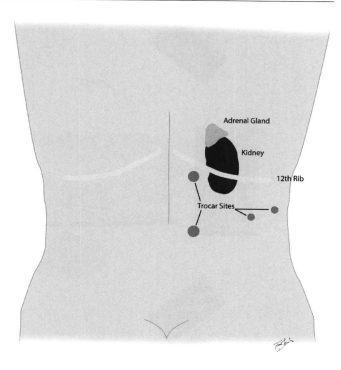

is obtained under direct vision into Gerota's fascia. A balloon dissection is used to develop a working space, followed by insufflation of carbon dioxide. Especially when combined with laparoscopic ultrasound, this has proven to be an effective technique for removal of adrenal tumors. However, anatomic considerations preclude the use of this technique for tumors greater than six centimeters in size. Employing endoscopy for posterior adrenalectomy avoids the troubling incidence of sensory nerve issues and chronic pain issues found with open posterior techniques.

Open Adrenalectomy

Open transabdominal adrenalectomy still has a role in modern endocrine surgical practice, despite the appeal of minimally invasive surgery. Although there are reports of very large tumors being removed laparoscopically, tumor size greater than 8 cm is a relative indication for open adrenalectomy. Any tumor with evidence of invasion of surrounding structures or intravascular tumor thrombus necessitates approach through an open operation. En bloc resection of tumor can be achieved, the only hope for cure in adrenal malignancy. The most common

incision employed is a subcostal incision, but surgeon preference or the specifics of the tumor anatomy may lead to the use of vertical midline, flank, or thoracoabdominal incisions in order to achieve appropriate exposure and margins.

Lateral Laparoscopic Adrenalectomy

In most institutions, lateral laparoscopic adrenalectomy has become the preferred procedure for extirpation of adrenal masses. It is a technique that is readily learned by surgeons with laparoscopic experience. The equipment necessary is part of standard laparoscopic supplies. This includes a camera (typically with a 30° angled telescope) and standard dissectors, clip appliers, staplers, and hemostatic devices of the surgeon's preference. Many surgeons find ultrasonic shears to be particularly useful in mobilizing the adrenal glands, as there are a multitude of small blood vessels surrounding the gland. A specimen retrieval bag is essential for the safe removal of the adrenal gland from the abdominal cavity without rupture.

The patient is brought to the operating room and general endotracheal anesthesia is induced in the supine position. The patient is then repositioned in

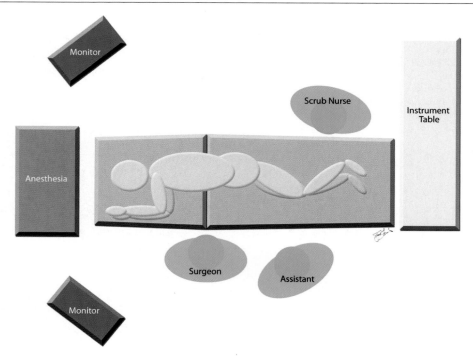

Fig. 5.5 Patient and surgeon positioning for the lateral transperitoneal approach to laparoscopic adrenalectomy. The recommended operating room positioning of the monitors and the staff including surgeon, assistant and nurse for a left sided adrenalectomy. The patient is in the lateral decubitus postion with the side up that is to be operated upon

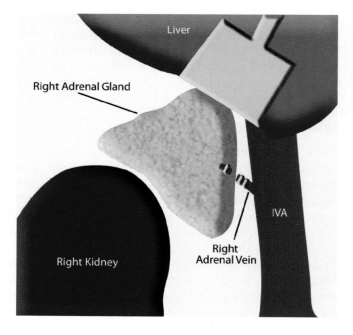

Fig. 5.6 Exposure and dissection of the right adrenal gland in the lateral transperitoneal approach. The right lobe of the liver is mobilized and retracted medially and superiorly to gain access to the right adrenal gland. The adrenal gland is circumferentially mobilized, and the adrenal vein is located along the medial edge of the gland

the lateral decubitus position with the affected gland up. Pneumoperitoneum is obtained with either the closed technique, using a Veress needle or an open technique. This site serves as the camera port. Additional ports are placed in a fashion that will allow free movement of instruments and comfortable dissection at the operative site. Care is taken to not place ports too closely to the costal margin, as this has a great impact on postoperative pain. Two or three additional working ports are then placed under direct vision. Four ports are almost always necessary for right adrenalectomy, as retraction of the liver is essential to obtaining adequate exposure, while some surgeons prefer to use three ports for left-sided procedures. See Fig. 5.5 for patient positioning in lateral laparoscopic adrenalectomy.

Right adrenalectomy begins with the division of the triangular ligament of the right lobe of the liver. Generous mobilization allows the liver to fall away from the retroperitoneum, exposing the vena cava, kidney and adrenal gland. The peritoneum is incised and the retroperitoneal space is entered. Once the gland is identified, dissection can begin from either the lateral or medial border. An illustration of the dissection for a right adrenalectomy is shown in Fig. 5.6. Historically, it has been thought advantageous to divide the adrenal vein as the first maneuver when operating for pheochromocytoma to prevent an adrenergic surge. However, with modern pharmaceutical preparation and intraoperative monitoring, this concern has lessened. The right adrenal vein is relatively short and wide and is controlled with clips before division. On the other hand, the arterial blood supply to the gland is from multiple small branches from the aorta and the phrenic and renal arteries. These can generally be controlled either through electric or ultrasonic coagulation, although clips may be used. Once dissected free, the specimen is placed in a retrieval bag and removed. This may require enlargement of one of the port sites, as it is advantageous to remove the specimen intact for appropriate histologic evaluation. The fascia is closed at the extraction site and the skin closed in a standard fashion after pneumoperitoneum is released.

Left adrenalectomy involves a somewhat more complicated dissection. The port placement is shown in Fig. 5.7. Care must be taken to avoid injury to the spleen, colon, pancreas, and other nearby organs. The

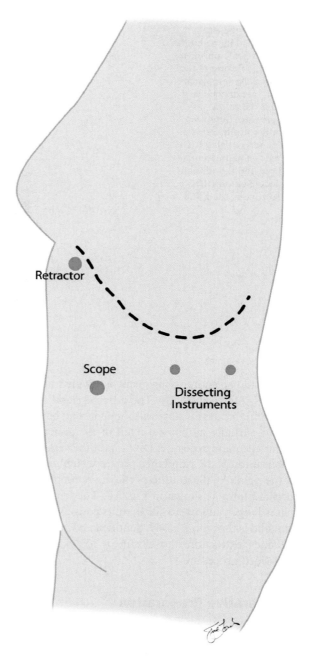

Fig. 5.7 Port placement for lateral transperitoneal approach to the left laparoscopic adrenal resection. The fourth and most lateral port is often not necessary on the left side, as the spleen does not usually require instrument retraction

procedure commences with a generous mobilization of the splenic flexure of the colon, taking care to leave the kidney and adrenal in the retroperitoneum. Once the colon has fallen away, allowing visualization of the

Fig. 5.8 Exposure and dissection of the left adrenal gland in the lateral transperitoneal approach. The splenic flexure of the colon and the splenorenal ligament are divided to mobilize the colon inferiorly and the spleen medially to gain access to the left adrenal gland. The adrenal is circumferentially localized and the adrenal vein located along the medial edge of the gland

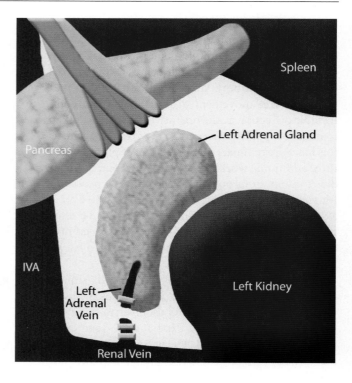

kidney, the splenorenal ligament is divided and the spleen is rotated medially. The adrenal gland should be identifiable at this stage, although it may be necessary to partially mobilize the tail of the pancreas to obtain adequate exposure. Division of the vessels and mobilization of the gland then proceeds similarly as to on the right. An illustration of the dissection for a left adrenalectomy is shown in Fig. 5.8. The left adrenal vein is longer and narrower than its congener on the right and is thus more easily identified and controlled. Specimen extraction and closure is identical to the right-sided procedure.

Preoperative Preparation

All patients undergoing adrenalectomy should have a standard preoperative workup, including laboratory, electrocardiographic and radiographic evaluation, as fits their age and medical comorbidities. Patients with invasive malignancies requiring en bloc excision should be evaluated for tolerance of organ resection, such as liver function. Pneumococcal, meningococcal, and *Hemophilus influenzae* vaccinations should be administered if the possibility of splenectomy is entertained.

Patients with pheochromocytomas require special care in preoperative preparation. The mainstay of this is alpha-blockade, control of hypertension and volume repletion. An alpha-adrenergic antagonist such as phenoxybenzamine is begun several weeks prior to surgery. Therapy is instituted at low dose and titrated up. The goal is for the patient to be normotensive and mildly orthostatic. As the chronic vasoconstriction is relieved, patients will require fluid repletion. This can usually be accomplished through increased oral intake in the days leading up to surgery, although anesthesiologists must be acutely aware of the potential for hypovolemia. Once adequate alpha blockade has been established, a beta-blocker is often added to control tachycardia. Careful intraoperative management of blood pressure and intravascular volume is imperative, often necessitating invasive cardiovascular monitoring.

Other hormonally active tumors also necessitate special perioperative care. Aldosteronomas lead to hypertension and hypokalemia. Correction of these conditions is necessary for safe surgery. This can be accomplished through a variety of pharmacologic means, including diuretics, most commonly spironolactone. These tumors do not create the same sort of hemodynamic lability as pheochromocytoma and can usually be managed without arterial or central venous catheters.

Glucocorticoid secreting tumors mandate that stress-dose steroid be administered intraoperatively. They also require prolonged administration of glucocorticoid replacement therapy postoperatively, often for many months to one year. This is due to the state of relative adrenal insufficiency created when a dominant adrenal adenoma is removed. The contralateral gland will eventually produce more than ample steroid, but it can take a great deal of time to resume physiologic activity.

Conclusions and Summary

Adrenal surgical resection is generally performed for tumor, hormone hypersecretion, or a combination of both. The specific indications for adrenal resection are varied and often complicated, and have evolved dramatically with the advent of highly structurally detailed and functional imaging techniques. The history of adrenal surgery is illuminating and many creative adrenal operative strategies have been developed over the years, most recently sophisticated minimally invasive techniques. Patient positioning and method of access vary for different patient indications and types of adrenal surgery. Large tumor size or with evidence of invasion of surrounding structures or intravascular tumor thrombus necessitates approach through an open operation. Patients undergoing surgery for functional adrenal tumors require specific and expert pre, post, and intraoperative care.

References

1. Sadler GP, Wheeler MH (2002) Open anterior right adrenalectomy. Oper Tech Gen Surg 4:279–287
2. Fahrer M (2003) Bartholomeo Eustachio - the third man: Eustachius published by Albinus. Aust NZ J Surg 73:523–528
3. Norton JA (2001) History of endocrine surgery. In: Norton JA et al. (eds) Surgery: basic science and clinical evidence. Springer, Berlin Heidelberg New York, pp 849–855
4. Addison T (1855) On the constitutional and local effects of disease of the suprarenal capsules. Samuel Highly, London
5. Brown-Sequard E (1856) Recherches experimentales sur la physiologie et al pathologie des capsules surrenales. Arch Gen Med (Paris) ;8:385–401
6. Rabin CB (1929) Chromaffin cell tumor of the suprarenal medulla. Arch Pathol 7:228–243
7. Holton P (1949) Noradrenaline in tumors of the adrenal medulla. J Physiol 108:525–529
8. Thorton JK (1890) Abdominal nephrectomy for large sarcoma of the left suprarenal capsule. Clin Soc Trans (London) 23:150–153
9. Broster LR, Hill HG, Greenfield JG (1932) Adreno-genital syndrome and unilateral adrenalectomy. Br J Surg 19:557–570
10. Crile GW (1923) Clinical studies of adrenalectomy and sympathectomy. Ann Surg 88:470–473
11. Mayo CH (1927) Paroxysmal hypertension with tumor of retroperitoneal nerve. J Am Med Assoc 89:1047–1049
12. Young HH (1936) A technique for simultaneous exposure and operation on the adrenals. Surg Gynecol Obstet 54:179–188
13. Udelsman R (2001) Adrenal. In: Norton JA et al. (eds) Surgery: basic science and clinical evidence. Springer, Berlin Heidelberg New York, pp 897–917
14. Mihai R, Farndon JR (1997) Surgical embryology and anatomy of the adrenal glands. In: Clark OH, Duh QY (eds) Textbook of endocrine surgery. Saunders, Philadelphia, p 452
15. Quinn TM, Rubino F, Gagner M (2002) Laparoscopic adrenalectomy. In: ACS surgery: principles and practice. WebMD, Inc
16. Brunt LM, Halverson JD (1996) The endocrine system. In: O'Leary JP (ed) The physiologic basis of surgery. William and Wilkins, , pp 312–348
17. Kloos RT, Korobkin M, Thompson NW, Francis IR, Shapiro B, Gross MD (1997) Incidentally discovered adrenal masses. Cancer Treat Res 89:263–292
18. Brunt LM, Moley JF (2001) Adrenal incidentaloma. World J Surg 25:905–913
19. National Institute of Health (2002) Management of the clinically inapparent adrenal mass (incidentaloma). National Institute of Health State-of-the-Science Conference Statement
20. Barry MK, van Heerden, Farley DR et al. (1998) Can adrenal incidentalomas be safely observed? World J Surg 22:599–603
21. Belldegrun A, Hussain S, Seltzer SE et al. (1986) Incidentally discovered mass of the adrenal gland. Surg Gynecol Obstet 163:203–208
22. Bovio S, Cataldi A, Reimondo G et al. (2006) Prevalence of adrenal incidentaloma in a contemporary computerized tomography series. J Endocrinol Invest 29:298–302
23. Young WF Jr, Hogan MJ, Klee GG et al. (1990) Primary aldosteronism: diagnosis and treatment. Mayo Clin Proc 65:96–110
24. Ganguly A (1998) Primary aldosteronism. NEJM 339:1828–1834
25. Kloos RT, Gross MD, Francis IR (1995) Incidentally discovered adrenal masses. Endocr Rev 16:460–484
26. Gagner M, Lacroix A, Bolte E (1992) Laparoscopic adrenalectomy in Cushing's Syndrome and pheochromocytoma. N Eng J Med 327:1003
27. Gonzalez R, Smith CD, McClusky DA III et al. (2004) Laparoscopic approach reduces likelihood of perioperative complications in patients undergoing adrenalectomy. Am Surg 70(8):668–674
28. Mercan S, Seven R, Ozarmagan S, Tezelman S (1995) Endoscopic retroperitoneal adrenalectomy. Surgery 118:1071–1076
29. Siperstein AE, Berber E, Engle KL et al. (2000) Laparoscopic posterior adrenalectomy. Arch Surg 135:967–971

Imaging Adrenal Dysfunction

6

Anju Sahdev and Rodney H. Reznek

Contents

A. Sahdev (✉)
Department of Diagnostic Imaging, St Bartholomew's
Hospital, West Smithfield, London EC1A 7BE, UK
E-mail: Anju.Sahdev@bartsandthelondon.nhs.uk

Introduction

Disorders of adrenal function are usually suspected clinically and confirmed biochemically. The role of imaging is to identify the site of the lesion, to determine whether the disease is unilateral or bilateral, to characterise any focal lesions and to plan therapy.

Hyperfunction of the zona glomerulosa within the adrenal cortex leading to excess glucocorticoid production results in Cushing's syndrome, excess mineralcorticoid production from the zona fasciculate and reticularis results in Conn's syndrome and excess androgen production in virilization. Adrenal medullary hyperfunction in adults is usually due to phaeochromocytomas, rarely due to medullary hyperplasia and in children and young adults neuroblastomas or ganglioblastomas. Adrenal hypofunction has many causes but in the developed world, is most frequently due to primary adrenal atrophy. This chapter will discuss the imaging appearances of the adrenal glands in these syndromes.

Adrenal Cortical Hyperfunction

Cushing's Syndrome

Cushing's syndrome is the associated symptoms and signs that result from long-term inappropriate elevation of free circulating glucocorticoid levels with an incidence of about 30 per 1,000,000. Although the outlook of the condition has improved greatly over the years, it remains a physically and psychologically disabling condition, even though the disease is suspected and investigated much earlier now in those

M.A. Blake, G. Boland (eds.), *Adrenal Imaging*, DOI 10.1007/978-1-59745-560-2_6,
© 2009 Humana Press, a part of Springer Science+Business Media, LLC

who present with diabetes, hypertension, osteoporosis, psychiatric and gynaecological disorders. Imaging has come to play a central role in the early diagnosis of these patients.

In 80%–85% of cases, CS is ACTH dependent usually secondary to a pituitary ACTH secreting tumour (Cushing's disease). Less frequently ACTH secretion is from non-pituitary sources or ectopic secretion (10%) [1]. In the remaining 15%–20% of patients the syndrome is ACTH-independent due to primary adrenal pathology. The treatment of Cushing's syndrome depends on distinguishing between ACTH-dependent and ACTH-independent disease. Imaging now plays an extremely important role in identifying the cause. In ACTH-independent disease, the role of imaging is to identify and localise adrenal masses. In ACTH-dependent Cushing's disease imaging is important to identify an anterior pituitary adenoma or to identify a source of ectopic ACTH.

ACTH-Dependent Cushing's Syndrome

Having confirmed a biochemical diagnosis of ACTH dependent Cushing's, it is imperative to identify the source of ACTH production. Clinically and biochemically it may be difficult to distinguish between a pituitary or occult ectopic ACTH secreting tumour. Chronic ACTH hyperstimulation of the adrenal glands usually results in bilateral

enlargement evident on CT and MRI. The largest glands, usually nodular in outline, result from an ectopic rather than pituitary ACTH source. Two types of hyperplasia are seen pathologically and on CT: smooth (diffuse) or nodular [2, 3]. Smooth hyperplasia is more common than nodular hyperplasia, accounting for 83% (Fig. 6.1). In 30% of cases with histo-pathological hyperplasia, the adrenal glands appear normal on CT [2]. A normal CT therefore does not exclude the diagnosis. Pathologically, nodular hyperplasia can be micro or macronodular. In macronodular hyperplasia there is bilateral enlargement of adrenal glands with one or more nodules visible on CT (Fig. 6.2). A dominant nodule may reach up to 4 cm and can be misinterpreted as an apparently hyperfunctioning adenoma, conflicting with biochemical evidence of ACTH-dependence. Usually, however the underlying macronodular hyperplasia is suspected by the enlargement and nodularity of the remainder of the ipsilateral and contralateral adrenal glands (Fig. 6.2).

Identifying an Ectopic ACTH Source

Investigation of patients with 'occult' ectopic ACTH production represents a major challenge since clinical, biochemical and radiological features are often indistinguishable from pituitary dependent Cushing's disease [4]. In our experience, the commonest

(a)

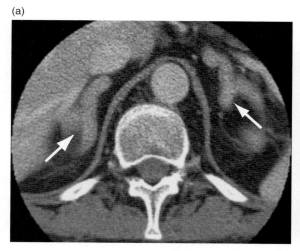

(b)

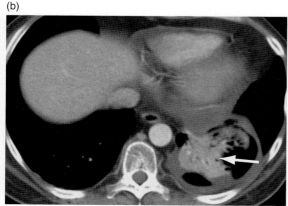

Fig. 6.1 A Contrast enhanced CT of the adrenal glands showing ACTH dependent bilateral smooth hyperplasia. **B** Contrast enhanced CT of the chest with left lower lobe

collapse (*arrow*) secondary to an endo-bronchial carcinoid tumour which was the source of the ectopic ACTH

Fig. 6.2 Contrast enhanced CT of the adrenal glands demonstrating ACTH-dependent bilateral macronodular hyperplasia (*arrow heads*). The underlying adrenal gland between the nodules is hyperplastic and enlarged (*arrows*)

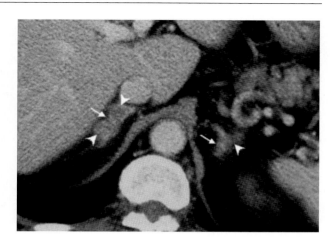

site of origin is the lung (48%) with the majority of cases being bronchial carcinoids tumours (30%) (Fig. 6.1) and less often a small cell lung cancer (SCLC) (18%). Other sources of excess ACTH production include neuroendocrine tumours of the thymus, bowel and pancreas, medullary carcinoma of the thyroid, pheochromocytomas and mesotheliomas. In approximately 12%–20% of patients, despite repeated biochemical and radiological investigations the source of the ectopic ACTH production remains undiscovered [1, 5].

CT of the chest, abdomen and pelvis with intravenous injection of contrast medium is the most sensitive imaging modality for the identification of the ectopic source. Bronchial carcinoids are small, typically between 3 mm and 15 mm in size and may be difficult to distinguish from granulomas and hamartomas [4]. ACTH producing small cell lung cancers (SCLC) and neuroendocrine tumours of the pancreas and colon have radiological features similar to non-ACTH producing tumours. Thus in patients with unexplained ectopic ACTH production, all small intrapulmonary lesions should be viewed with suspicion. MRI is useful in resolving equivocal CT findings or where CT is negative and a high index of suspicion persists particularly for tumours within the abdomen. In the chest, MRI is of limited value in identifying bronchial carcinoids but may be of value in imaging the mediastinum for thymic lesions. In the abdomen, MRI may identify small islet cell tumours of the pancreas not seen on CT. Overall, two large studies have found ^{111}In-octreotide scintigraphy and whole body venous sampling generally unhelpful in localising the source of

ectopic ACTH [1, 5]. [18]Fluorodeoxyglucose positron emission tomography (FDG PET) has been recently evaluated and shown to be inferior to CT and MRI in the detection of ectopic ACTH sources. The hyperstimulated, hyperplastic adrenal glands also obscure the detection of any ACTH secreting adrenal lesion like a phaeochromocytoma [6].

Pituitary Dependent Cushing's Disease
Cushing's disease is secondary to a secretory pituitary adenoma. Imaging of the pituitary is discussed elsewhere.

ACTH-Independent Cushing's Syndrome
ACTH-independent Cushing's syndrome is always due to autonomous primary adrenal pathology producing cortisol. Adrenal adenomas and carcinomas account for 95% of the cases. Rarely primary pigmented nodular adrenal dysplasia (PPNAD) and ACTH independent macronodular hyperplasia (AIMAH) are responsible.

Adrenal Adenomas
Hyperfunctioning ACTH secreting adenomas, which account for up to 65% of the cases, have imaging features similar to other benign non hyperfunctioning adrenal adenomas. They are best demonstrated on CT, are between 2 cm and 7 cm in size and have low or soft tissue attenuation usually enhancing after contrast administration. As in our experience 95% of these hyperfunctioning adenomas are lipid rich, they have non-contrast CT attenuation values of 10 HU or lower [7] (Fig. 6.3). MRI also readily demonstrates adrenal adenomas as low homogenous signal on T1-weighted images

Fig. 6.3 Contrast enhanced CT showing a left adrenal cortisol producing adenoma (*arrow*). The adenoma is low attenuation, lipid rich with an attenuation value of 2 HU. The contralateral right adrenal is atrophic due to the suppressed ACTH levels

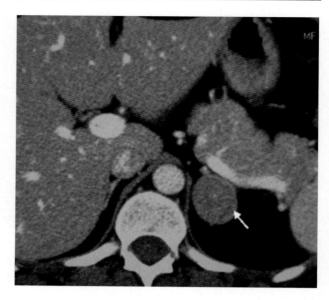

and a signal intensity equivalent or higher than the liver on T2-weighted images. Chemical shift imaging will readily identify the lipid rich adenomas with signal loss on the out-of-phase images [7] (Fig. 6.4). The remainder of the adrenal gland and the contralateral adrenal are either normal or atrophic due to low circulating ACTH levels [7]. Rarely, cortisol producing adenomas may be bilateral or occur simultaneously with PPNAD [8–10]. Heterotopic adrenal tissue can be found along the embryological migration path of the adrenal glands. Although in the majority this is normal accessory adrenal tissue, secretory adenomas causing Cushing's syndrome have been reported [11, 12].

Adrenal Carcinoma

Adrenal carcinomas are rare with an incidence approximately 0.6–1.67 cases per million persons per year. The female-to-male ratio is approximately 2.5–3:1. Male patients tend to be older and have a worse overall prognosis than female patients. Female patients are more likely to have an associated endocrine syndrome. Non-functional carcinomas are distributed equally between the sexes. Adrenal carcinoma occurs in two major peaks: in the first decade of life and again in the fourth to fifth decades. Approximately 75% of the children with adrenal carcinoma are younger than 5 years. Functioning tumors are more common in children with

(a)

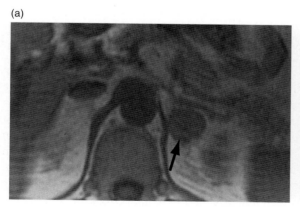

(b)

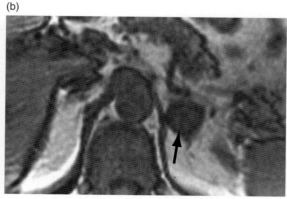

Fig. 6.4 **A** In-phase chemical shift imaging of the adrenals showing a left sided adrenal mass (*arrow*) in a patient with elevated cortisol levels. **B** Out-of-phase chemical shift imaging shows loss of signal intensity in the mass (*arrow*) relative to splenic signal intensity indicating a functioning lipid rich adenoma

resultant Cushing's syndrome or virilization, while non-functional tumors are more common in adults [7]. In adults, 30%–40% of adrenal carcinomas are hyperfunctioning. Hypercortisolism and virilization is the most common endocrine manifestation although trace amounts of other hormones may be produced. In our series, carcinomas accounted for 27% of ACTH-independent Cushing's syndrome [8] (Fig. 6.5).

CT typically shows a unilateral mass, usually over 6 cm in size with necrosis, haemorrhage, fibrosis and calcification. Smaller carcinomas may resemble adenomas. Recent studies combining non-enhanced, delayed enhancement CT attenuation and percentage of contrast enhancement washout attenuation values at 10 min showed adrenal carcinomas all behaved as non-adenomas. Using these criteria adenomas were distinguished from adrenal carcinomas and phaeochromocytomas with a sensitivity and specificity of 100% [13, 14]. As with renal tumours, careful assessment of the draining venous structures is essential on imaging together with identification of direct infiltration of adjacent viscera such as the liver, kidney or spleen. Venous invasion occurred in 40% of our series [8].

Multiplanar imaging using MRI or multidetector CT allows better assessment of invasion into adjacent structures, important for surgical planning. Metastases to the liver and lungs is not infrequent. A large mass, high suspicion of malignancy and surrounding invasion preclude laproscopic adrenelectomy which may be suitable for small unilateral benign adenomas.

Primary Pigmented Nodular Adrenocortical Disease (PPNAD)

This is a rare cause of Cushing's syndrome in infants, children and young adults. The disease may be familial and frequently associated with the Carney complex (spotty skin pigmentation, endocrine hyperfunction, testicular tumours and myxomas). On imaging, adrenal glands in PPNAD may be normal or minimally hyperplastic with multiple, unilateral or bilateral benign cortical nodules (Fig. 6.6). The adrenal nodules are macroscopically pigmented and due to this pigmentation, the nodules demonstrate lower T1 and T2 signal intensity on MRI compared to surrounding atrophic cortical tissue. The nodules do not normally exceed 5 mm but in older patients may be 1–2 cm [15].

(b)

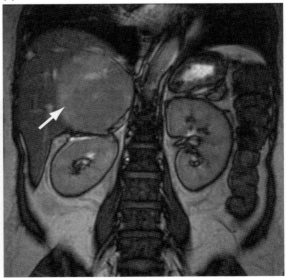

(a)

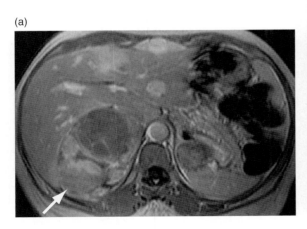

Fig. 6.5 A Axial T1-weighted post gadolinium enhanced MRI showing a heterogenous right sided adrenal mass (*arrow*) with central cystic changes and solid enhancing peripheral tissue in a patient with Cushing's and virilization. **B** Coronal T2-weighted image showing the right adrenal mass (*arrow*) with central areas of high T2 signal intensity. The MR features suggest an adrenal carcinoma, confirmed histologically

Fig. 6.6 Non-contrast enhanced CT demonstrating bilateral multiple small adenomas (*arrows*) in a 20-year-old patient. Note the intervening cortex is not hyperplastic due to the low circulating levels of ACTH

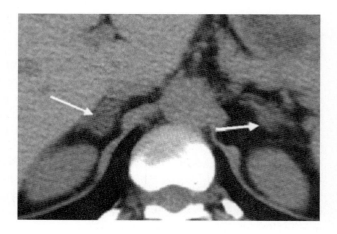

Histologically in addition to multiple pigmented nodules there is atrophy of the intervening cortex due to low circulating ACTH levels. On imaging, where nodules are 1–2 cm in size, atrophy of intervening cortex helps distinguish this from ACTH-dependent hyperplasia. In the absence of a central gradient on petrosal venous sampling and normal cross sectional imaging, a presumptive diagnosis of PPNAD may be assumed by bilateral uptake of ^{131}I-cholesterol scinitigraphy [15]. The adrenal uptake of ^{131}I-cholesterol analogues confirms an adrenal source of cortisol excess as opposed to ectopic adrenal rests.

ACTH-independent Macronodular Adrenal Hyperplasia (AIMAH)

ACTH-independent macronodular adrenal hyperplasia is a very rare cause of Cushing's syndrome.

Clinically the patients, usually male, present in their 40s, about 10 years older than the mean age of presentation for Cushing's syndrome and the clinical manifestations of the syndrome tend to be mild. The pathophysiology of AIMAH remains obscure. The imaging appearances of the adrenal glands are striking. They show massive bilateral adrenal enlargement, nodularity and distortion of adrenal contour. Nodules vary in size from 1 cm to 5.5 cm and on CT are of low attenuation in keeping with lipid rich adenomas (Fig. 6.7). Coronal imaging, either with MDCT reconstruction or MR imaging best demonstrate the cranio-caudal extent of the adrenal glands which frequently extend from the diaphragm to below the renal hila [16]. On MRI, nodules are hypointense relative to liver on T1-weighted images and hyperintense or isointense to

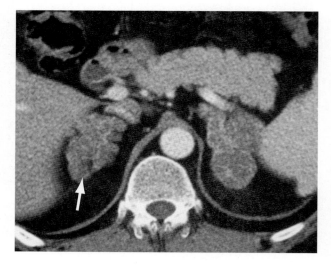

Fig. 6.7 Contrast enhanced CT of the adrenal glands in a patient with low plasma ACTH levels. Both adrenal glands demonstrate massive nodular hyperplasia (*arrows*) with retention of the adreniform shape in keeping with AIMAH

liver on T2-weighted images. In ACTH-dependent Cushing's syndrome nodules are isointense to liver on T2 images while in PPNAD nodules are hypointense on both T1 and T2 weighted images. On chemical shift imaging, nodules due to their high lipid content, lose signal intensity on out-of-phase images. Iodine-131-Iodomethylnor-cholesterol (NP-59) scintigraphy shows adrenal uptake. There is controversy regarding the inter-nodular adrenal cortex. This is usually histologically difficult to identify due to the gross nodular distortion of the adrenals. Hyperplastic, normal and atrophic changes have all been reported and because of this controversy, the morphology of the inter-nodular cortex is not a criteria for the pathological diagnosis of AIMAH [17]. In contrast, the inter-nodular cortex in ACTH-dependent macronodular hyperplasia is always hyperplastic.

Primary Hyperaldosteronism (Conn's Syndrome)

Primary hyperaldosteronism is characterised by low plasma renin and elevated serum and urinary aldosterone production. In 80% of cases, this is caused by an adrenocortical aldosterone producing adenoma (APA). In the remainder, bilateral adrenal hyperplasia is responsible; only rarely is it due to an adrenal carcinoma. The primary role of imaging is to distinguish between a solitary aldosteronoma which is best treated surgically and bilateral adrenal hyperplasia which is managed medically. Adenomas account for 80% and BAH for up to 20% of Conn's syndrome. CT or MRI are the mainstay of imaging in the investigation of these patients. Aldosteronomas tend to be low attenuation on CT, less than 10 HU. They are usually small, rarely calcify and demonstrate no significant contrast enhancement. The mean size of APAs is 1.6–2.2 cm, median size of 2 cm and range between 1 cm and 5 cm [18] (Fig. 6.8). Several studies have examined the performance of thin section CT (3 mm) in the detection of APA, with sensitivities and specificities varying between 88% and 100% and 33% and 100% respectively [18–20]. The diagnosis of BAH on imaging usually relies on failure to identify an APA. However the diagnosis is favoured by demonstrating enlargement of the adrenal limbs on CT (Fig. 6.9). On CT, if the adrenal limb width is 3 mm or greater, sensitivity for diagnosing BAH is 100% but the specificity is only 54%. The specificity is greatly improved if the limb width is 5 mm or greater approaching 100% [21].

In the detection of APA, MRI has been shown to have a sensitivity, specificity and accuracy of 70%, 100% and 85% respectively. As many as 86% of adenomas and 89% of glands with BAH have intracellular lipid and will demonstrate loss of signal intensity on chemical shift imaging on MRI (CSI) [22]. Few studies have directly

(a)

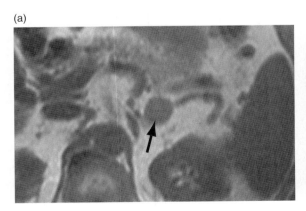

(b)

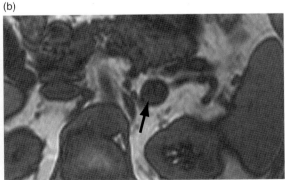

Fig. 6.8 A In-phase chemical shift imaging of the adrenals showing a left sided adrenal mass (*arrow*) in a patient with elevated aldosterone levels. **B** Out-of-phase chemical shift imaging shows loss of signal intensity in the mass (*arrow*) relative to splenic intensity indicating a lipid rich adenoma consistent with a functioning Conn's aldosteronism

Fig. 6.9 Contrast enhanced CT demonstrating bilateral thickened adrenal limbs and bilateral adrenal nodules (*arrows*) in keeping with bilateral adrenal hyperplasia causing Conn's syndrome

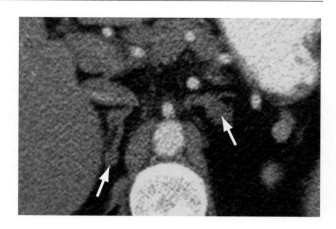

compared the diagnostic performance of CT and MRI in determining the cause of hyperaldosteronism. Nevertheless our data suggests CT and MRI have a comparable diagnostic performance in the detection of APAs with a sensitivity and specificity of 87%–93% and 82%–85% for CT and 83% and 92% for MRI respectively [18].

There are several reasons for the poor specificity in the detection of APA, including concomitant contralateral non-functioning nodules, presence of unilateral dominant nodules in BAH and the increasing bilateral nodularity with age and hypertension. The sensitivity is limited by the small size of APAs, although this may improve with the increasing use of thinner adrenal sections (1–2 mm) acquired by multidetector CT. In the overall management of Conn's syndrome a high specificity for the detection of APAs is desirable to avert unnecessary and unsuccessful surgery in patients with BAH.

Adrenal venous sampling (AVS) for aldosterone levels is very accurate in pre-operative assessment of Conn's syndrome. It is the most accurate method for distinguishing between unilateral and bilateral aldosterone production. Although now generally safe, it is technically difficult and even with modern techniques and per-procedural ACTH stimulation, bilateral adrenal vein catherization is only successful in 44%–50% of patients [23, 24]. Catherization of the right adrenal vein remains elusive with a cumulative failure rate of 26%. The accuracy of AVS in lateralising an APA exceeds 95% when the procedure is technically

successful [25, 26]. As AVS is not without risks, in our practice it is used selectively and reserved for patients with biochemically confirmed hyperaldosteronism and:

– Normal or equivocal adrenal glands or
– There are bilateral nodules, which may either be macronodules of adrenal hyperplasia or multiple adenomas or
– There is disagreement between CT and MRI findings or between imaging and biochemical findings.

AVS is essential in the above patients to avoid unnecessary and inappropriate adrenelectomy.

Nuclear medicine is not widely used in the evaluation of patients with hyperaldosteronism and appears to be routinely available in only a few institutions worldwide. Dexamethasone-suppression nor-cholesterol scintigraphy (NP-59) correctly distinguishes unilateral from bilateral adrenal disease in 92% of cases. Its strength lies in the demonstration of bilateral disease when the adrenal CT is normal or shows a dominant unilateral nodule in BAH thereby avoiding adrenelectomy. The diagnostic value of NP-59 in identifying adrenal adenomas is sensitivity 100%, specificity 71%, accuracy 95%, positive predictive value 94% and negative predictive value 100%. False positive cases may be due to phaeochromocytomas, adrenal carcinomas or myelolipomas. The overall combined sensitivity of CT and NP-59 has been reported as 100% and proposed as a non-invasive diagnostic alternative to adrenal venous sampling [27–29].

Virilization

Virilization is the development of exaggerated masculine characteristics, usually in women, often as a result of the adrenal glands overproducing androgens. Symptoms of virilization include excess facial and body hair (hirsutism), baldness, acne, deepening of the voice, increased muscularity, and an increased sex drive. In women, the uterus shrinks, the clitoris enlarges, the breasts become smaller, and normal menstruation stops. Virilization can occur in childhood in either boys or girls. Typical effects of virilization in children are pubic hair, accelerated growth and bone maturation, increased muscle strength, acne, adult body odour and sometimes growth of the penis. The most common cause is congenital adrenal hyperplasia (CAH) in both male and female children, adrenal androgen producing adenomas, adrenocortical carcinomas or extra-adrenal pathologies (polycystic ovaries and gonadal tumours) in adults. In boys, virilization may signal precocious puberty as part of CAH.

The role of imaging lies in detection or exclusion of surgically resectable sources of androgen excess in the adrenals, ovaries or testes. In children MRI or ultrasound are the modalities of choice to avoid ionising radiation from CT. In our experience, all adult patients presenting with elevated androgen levels where the suspicion of an androgen secreting tumour is high, should have an adrenal CT and ovarian transvaginal ultrasound to detect the tumour. Venous catherization and sampling should be reserved for patients in whom uncertainty remains as the presence of a small ovarian tumour cannot be excluded on biochemical and imaging studies alone [30].

Congenital Adrenal Hyperplasia (CAH)

Congenital adrenal hyperplasia refers to any of several autosomal recessive diseases resulting from defects in steps of the steroidogenesis of cortisol from cholesterol by the adrenal cortex. Most of these diseases involve excessive or deficient production of sex steroids and can alter or impair development of primary or secondary sex characteristics in affected infants, children, and adults. Congenital adrenal hyperplasia due to 21-hydroxylase deficiency accounts for about 95% of diagnosed cases of CAH. Severe 21-hydroxylase deficiency causes salt-wasting CAH, with life-threatening vomiting

and dehydration occurring within the first weeks of life. It is also the most common cause of ambiguous genitalia due to prenatal virilization of genetically female infants. Moderate 21-hydroxylase deficiency is referred to as simple virilizing CAH and typically causes virilization of prepubertal children. Still milder forms of 21-hydroxylase deficiency are referred to as non-classical CAH and can cause androgen effects and infertility in adolescent and adult women. CAH due to deficiencies of enzymes other than 21-hydroxylase present many of the same management challenges as 21-hydroxylase deficiency, but some involve mineralocorticoid excess or sex steroid deficiency. These include 17α-hydroxylase deficiency, 3β-hydroxysteroid dehydrogenase deficiency and 11β-hydroxylase deficiency.

In CAH there is a combination of precocious puberty and an androgen excess due to an increase in circulating ACTH with chronic adrenal hyperstimulation. This gross enlargement of the adrenal glands is seen on CT and MRI as diffuse or nodular enlargement of both adrenal glands with preservation of normal adreniform configuration [31] (Fig. 6.10). On CT and MRI the adrenal glands can enhance inhomogenously and can be mass-like, indistinguishable from carcinomas. Adrenocortical adenomas have been reported in children with longstanding untreated or under-treated CAH [32]. These adenomas are thought to be ACTH dependent and regress after adequate steroid replacement. However, some reports have suggested not all such adenomas regress and may even increase in size despite adequate treatment [33].

Adrenal Virilizing Tumours

Adrenal carcinomas and rarely adenomas may cause virilization. Approximately 80% of children with adrenal cortical carcinoma present with virilization. Both males and females present with precocious puberty and hypertension [34]. In contrast only 20%–30% of adults with adrenal carcinoma present with virilization syndromes [35]. The adrenal masses usually exceed 2 cm in diameter and have the same imaging characteristics for adenomas and carcinomas described previously (Fig. 6.11). The role of imaging is detecting or excluding surgically resectable tumours in the adrenal glands, ovaries or testes.

Fig. 6.10 Coronal T1-weighted image demonstrating bilateral massive adrenal hyperplasia with preservation of the adreniform contour (*arrows*) in a teenager with virilization

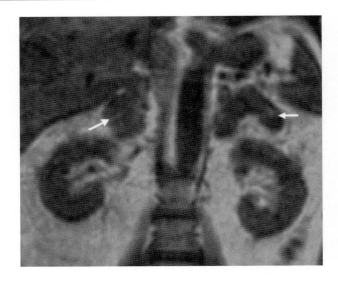

Fig. 6.11 Axial T2-weighted image demonstrating a large right sided high T2 signal intensity secretory adenoma in a patient with virilization

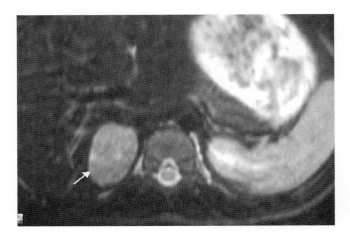

Functioning Adrenal Medullary Disorders

Adrenal Medullary Hyperplasia (AMH)

The normal adrenal gland weighs approximately 5 g, the medulla accounting for 1 g of its weight and is only found in the head and body of the gland. The diagnosis of medullary hyperplasia is made pathologically when there is extension of the medulla into the tail of the gland, an increase in the medullary/cortical ratio within the head and body and when morphometric weight calculations (estimated weight calculated from the volume of the medullary tissue) indicate the medulla exceeds 10% of the total weight

of the adrenal gland. The adrenal medulla shows a two-to three fold increase in the medullary volume and weight compared to age and sex matched controls [36]. It is associated with cystic fibrosis, non familial Beckwith-Wiedemann syndrome, MEN 2a or 2b and familial medullary thyroid carcinoma [37]. Adrenal medullary hyperplasia is a rare cause of clinical and biochemical findings identical to phaeochromocytomas. On imaging the adrenal glands may be normal, demonstrate unilateral or bilateral involvement and diffuse or nodular disease. The head and body of the adrenal glands are most frequently enlarged with relative preservation of the limbs [38–40] (Fig. 6.12). Several studies suggest AMH is

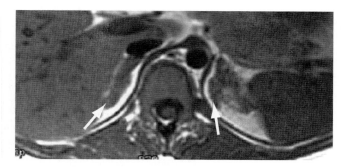

Fig. 6.12 Axial T1-weighted image demonstrating bilateral smooth adrenal enlargement (*arrows*) in a patient with markedly elevated plasma and urinary catecholamines. In the absence of a focal mass indicating a pheochromocytoma, this would be compatible with adrenal medullary hyperplasia which was confirmed pathologically in this patient

a precursor to pheochromocytomas [41, 42]. I-123 metaiodobenzylguanidine (MIBG) uptake has been demonstrated in all cases of adrenal hyperplasia and remains the most sensitive imaging modality [40, 42]. In patients with clinical and biochemical evidence of phaeochromocytoma, the absence of a focal mass on CT or MRI and adrenal MIBG uptake should raise the suspicion of adrenal medullary hyperplasia especially in the setting of an associated syndrome. The management of AMH is surgical. In unilateral disease, adrenelectomy is performed. In patients with bilateral disease or asynchronous recurrence of AMH in the contralateral adrenal, cortical-sparing surgery or resection of the largest gland has been proposed to preserve adrenal cortical function. Long term follow-up indicates patients thus treated retain normal clinical and biochemical function for up to 20 years [43].

Pheochromocytomas

Please refer to the Imaging Pheochromocytoma chapter.

Neuroblastoma and Ganglioneuroblastoma

Neuroblastomas and ganglioneuroblastomas are neuroendocrine tumours derived from neuroblastic and mature ganglion cells distributed along the sympathetic nervous system and the adrenal medulla. Both neuroblastomas and ganglioneuroblastomas produce abnormally high catecholamines that are detected by the measurement of urinary catecholamine metabolites; vanillylmandelic acid (VMA) and homovanillic acid (HVA).

Whereas pheochromocytomas secretes epinephrine, neuroblastomas and ganglioneuroblastomas secrete norepinephrine and gastrointestinal hormones particularly vaso-active intestinal peptide (VIP). Clinically the elevated catecholamines result in hypertension, palpitations and fever. The adrenal glands are the commonest primary site of involvement.

Neuroblastomas occur most frequently in infants and children. It is the most common extracranial, solid malignant tumours of childhood accounting for 8% of childhood malignancies, with 50%–80% arising in adrenal glands. 60% of patients have metastases in cortical bone, bone marrow, lymph nodes, liver and rarely to lung or brain. Assessment of disease status requires multiple imaging modalities. Plain films can identify lytic lesions. Ultrasound can detect the characteristically large supra-renal mass and liver involvement. CT is useful for defining the extent of primary tumour and for detecting contiguous retroperitoneal or distant lymph node and metastatic involvement [44, 45]. CT features of neuroblastoma are a large mass, often extending across the mid-line to engulf and displace the aorta anteriorly (Fig. 6.13). The majority are irregularly shaped, lobulated, and unencapsulated. They invade adjacent organs or encase adjacent vessels, tend to be inhomogeneous owing to tumor necrosis and hemorrhage. They contain coarse, amorphous, mottled peripheral calcification in approximately 85% of cases at CT [44]. Inhomogenous contrast enhancement is usual. CT and MRI are useful for defining morphological features and precisely assessing tumor extent for planning biopsies and surgical resection. Liver metastases may take two forms: diffuse infiltration, sometimes

Fig. 6.13 Axial T2-weighted image showing a large hetrogenous mass (*arrow*) extending into the retro-aortic space, encasing and displacing the aorta anteriorly. These features are characteristic of neuroblastomas

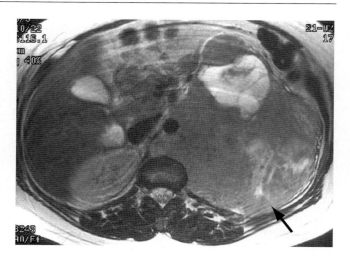

missed at CT because it may uniformly increase parenchymal attenuation or focal hypoenhancing masses. MRI has become the modality of choice for staging due to its multiplanar capabilities, lack of ionising radiation and good contrast between the very high signal tumour and surrounding tissues on T2-weighted images [44]. MRI is the preferred modality for investigating intraspinal extension of primary tumor (the so-called dumbbell tumours, seen in 10% of abdominal, 28% of thoracic, and occasionally in cervical neuroblastomas), for detection of diffuse hepatic metastases; these metastases manifest as areas of high signal intensity on T2-weighted images and intracranial metastases which are undetected by FDG PET and MIBG. Imaging with [131]I- or ^{123}I-labelled MIBG has gained increasing use as it has a high sensitivity and specificity for cortical bone, bone marrow and nodal metastases. The reported cumulative sensitivity and specificity of I-123-MIBG for detection of neuroblastoma is 69% and 85% respectively [45]. As approximately 30% of tumours are MIBG negative, normal results do not exclude the diagnosis. Routine use of MIBG is controversial; recent studies show MRI has the highest sensitivity (86%), MIBG the highest specificity (85%) and combined integrated imaging improves both sensitivity (99%) and specificity (95%) [45, 46]. Recently FDG PET CT has been shown to correlate well with MIBG, CT, MRI, clinical and biochemical findings. It is superior to MIBG in demonstrating liver metastases which are obscured by normal MIBG accumulation [45, 47].

On gross examination ganglioneuroblastomas are completely or partially encapsulated and have variable amounts of calcification (Fig. 6.14). The appearance depends upon degree of differentiation and primitive elements. Reported CT findings reflect this diversity and vary from predominantly solid to predominantly cystic masses with strands of solid tissue [47].

Adrenal Hypofunction (Addison's Disease)

Primary Adrenal Hypofunction

Adrenal hypofunction affects about 1 in 100,000 people [48]. This can result either from primary adrenal insufficiency or secondary to hypothalamic-pituitary ACTH deficiency. In primary adrenal hypofunction there is a reduction in aldosterone whilst in ACTH deficiency this remains unaffected as aldosterone production is controlled by the renin-angiotensin pathway rather than ACTH. The acquired causes of primary adrenal hypofunction include autoimmune disease, infection (Tuberculosis (TB), AIDS, cytomegalovirus, histoplasmosis),drugs, adrenal haemorrhage, Waterhouse-Friderichsen syndrome, metastatic disease, sarcoidosis, amyloidosis and haemochromatosis. The prevalence of primary adrenal insufficiency has increased threefold in the general population since the 1970 s [48]. Autoimmune disease is the most common cause in the

(a)

(b)

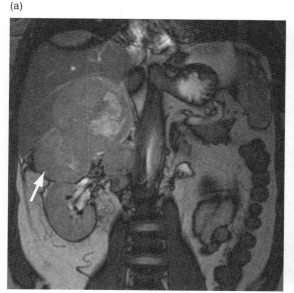

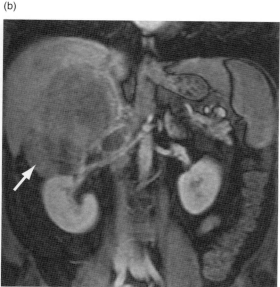

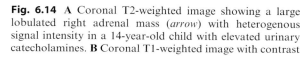

Fig. 6.14 **A** Coronal T2-weighted image showing a large lobulated right adrenal mass (*arrow*) with heterogenous signal intensity in a 14-year-old child with elevated urinary catecholamines. **B** Coronal T1-weighted image with contrast enhancement and fat saturation. The mass (*arrow*) is poorly enhancing and separate from the right kidney. Histologically this was a ganglioneuroblastoma

Western countries accounting for 68%–94% of primary adrenocortical failure. Worldwide, TB of the adrenal glands remains the commonest cause of adrenal insufficiency [49]. Congenital or hereditary causes of primary adrenal insufficiency include congenital adrenal hyperplasia, X-linked adrenoleukodystrophy, congenital familial glucocorticoid deficiency and triple A syndrome [49]. X-linked adrenoleukodystrophy is the most frequent genetic cause of primary adrenal insufficiency accounting for up to 20% of male cases.

The clinical symptoms and signs of Addison's disease manifest when more then 90% of the adrenal cortex is destroyed [50]. Addison's disease may be acute, subacute or chronic. Acute disease is rare and usually results from acute bilateral adrenal haemorrhage (Fig. 6.15). Chronic Addison's disease is most commonly due to autoimmune adrenal atrophy. The classical adrenal cortex autoantibody assay is the best marker for autoimmune adrenal disease. These antibodies are present in between 50%–90% of patients with autoimmune adrenal failure. Detection of circulating adrenal antibodies, particularly in low titres, does not always permit the unambiguous diagnosis because these have been detected in patients with TB adrenalitis [48, 49]. On imaging, autoimmune adrenal disease results in often barely discernable atrophic non-calcified adrenal glands (Fig. 6.16).

Bilateral adrenal haemorrhage may result from anticoagulant use or other bleeding diathesis and in the context of septicaemia in Waterhouse-Friderichsen syndrome. The commonest pathogens in Waterhouse-Friderichsen syndrome are meningococcus, *Haemophilus influenzae*, *Pseudomonas aeruginosa*, *Escherichia coli* and *Streptococcal pneumoniae*. Non traumatic acute adrenal haematomas characteristically appear as round or oval areas of high attenuation ranging between 50 HU and 90 HU and can be readily seen on non-contrast enhanced CT. As the haematoma organises it demonstrates mixed attenuation with increasing central low attenuation and cystic change. On MRI, in the acute stage (less than 7 days), the haematomas typically appear as iso or hypo-intense masses on T1-weighted images and markedly hypointense on T2-weighted images. Subacute haematomas (7 days–7 weeks) are hyperintense on both T1 and T2-weighted imaging. Chronic haematomas (>7 weeks) have a hypointense rim on T1 and

(b)

(a)

(c)

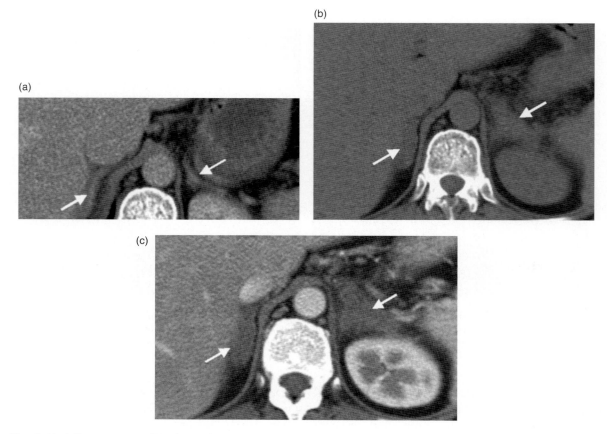

Fig. 6.15 A Post contrast CT of a patient undergoing a staging CT for a colo-rectal carcinoma demonstrating normal adrenal glands (*arrows*). **B** Non contrast enhanced post operative CT of the patient performed as the patient failed to recover from surgery with persistent hypotension. The CT demonstrates bilateral adrenal enlargement with preservation of the adreniform contour and high attenuation measurement of between 50 HU and 65 HU bilaterally. **C** Post contrast enhanced CT demonstrating no enhancement of the adrenal glands in keeping with bilateral adrenal haematomas

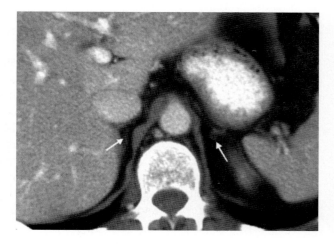

Fig. 6.16 Contrast enhanced CT demonstrating very small non-calcified adrenal glands bilaterally secondary to autoimmune adrenal atrophy (*arrows*)

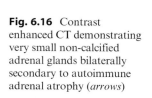

(a)

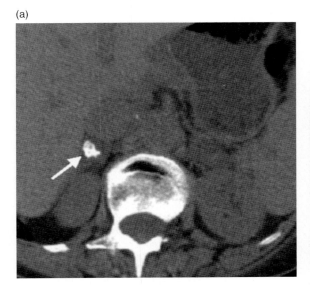

(b)

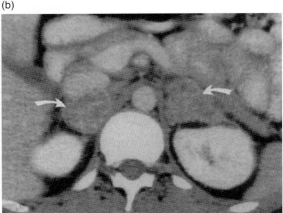

Fig. 6.17 **A** Non-contrast enhanced CT of the adrenal glands in untreated TB showing calcification in the right adrenal (*arrow*) and enlarged bilateral adrenal glands indicating adrenalitis. **B** Contrast enhanced CT demonstrating enhancement of the adrenal glands with scattered areas of non-enhancement which were histologically caseating granulomata in acute TB (*curved arrows*)

T2-weighted imaging [51]. Over time adrenal haematomas decrease in size, may calcify or organise appearing as adrenal pseudocysts which may contain areas of calcification.

In patients without discernable risk factors with unilateral or bilateral non-traumatic adrenal haemorrhage, careful imaging is essential to exclude an underlying adrenal mass. Underlying mass lesions including phaeochromocytomas, lymphoma and metastases from bronchogenic carcinoma and melanoma may cause bilateral adrenal haemorrhage and acute Addisonian crisis [52]. Contrast enhanced CT and MRI are of value to distinguish between an uncomplicated haemorrhage where non-enhancing blood products are the sole component and haemorrhage within an underlying mass lesion which demonstrates contrast enhancement.

Disease that is present for less than 2 years is defined as subacute Addison's disease and is usually a result of adrenalitis. CT plays an important role in evaluating these cases. Typically in untreated adrenalitis the adrenal glands are enlarged and may demonstrate central necrosis and rim enhancement. These features are not typical of any one pathogen and a CT guided biopsy may be required to distinguish between the causes of adrenalitis which include TB, histoplasmosis and other fungal infections (Fig. 6.17). In acute adrenal TB, bilateral adrenal enlargement is seen in 91% of cases. This can be mass like and calcification is seen in up to 59% [53]. Hypo-attenuating centres representing caseating granulomata with peripheral rim enhancement is seen in 47% of patients. After successful treatment 88% of enlarged glands decrease or return to normal size and configuration [54]. Calcification in atrophic adrenal glands is most often seen in granulomatous diseases (TB, histoplasmosis and sarcoidosis). However calcification in adrenal glands is not pathognomonic for granulomatous adrenalitis and is indistinguishable on CT from calcification due to previous haemorrhage. The adrenal glands return to normal size and may calcify after successful treatment of the adrenalitis.

Secondary Adrenal Hypofunction

Secondary adrenal insufficiency is much more common than primary adrenal insufficiency. In secondary adrenal insufficiency, the pituitary gland no longer triggers the adrenals to produce cortisol, and DHEA production also declines. Causes of pituitary hypofunction include tumors or infections of the pituitary, loss of blood flow and radiation or surgery for the treatment of pituitary or hypothalamic tumours. Hypopituitarism due to any cause results in ACTH and cortisol deficiency but not aldosterone deficiency.

Exogenous steroid administration by any route can also result in ACTH deficiency and the patient is at risk of Addisonian crisis if the steroids are stopped abruptly. Imaging of the hypothalamic-pituitary axis excludes pituitary apoplexy in acute onset of secondary adrenal failure and granulomatous diseases, macroadenomas and metastases in insidious secondary adrenal failure. The low circulating levels of ACTH results in normal or small adrenal glands on CT evaluation [55].

Summary

Imaging is an essential adjunct to the clinical and biochemical findings in the diagnosis of adrenal dysfunction. Close collaboration is required between the endocrinologists and radiologist to obtain the correct diagnosis and to select the most appropriate imaging strategy.

Key Points

1. Functional pathology of the adrenal gland usually presents as a clinical syndrome and imaging plays a critical role in localising and characterising the underlying pathology and to determine whether the pathology is unilateral or bilateral.
2. Thin section CT (3–5 mm) images obtained with and without intravenous contrast media are the mainstay of adrenal imaging.
3. MRI with T1- and T2-weighted axial images and chemical shift imaging is also used for the assessment of the adrenal glands particularly in children and patients with contrast media hypersensitivity.
4. 123-I-MIBG and other scintigraphy techniques supplement CT and MRI in the detection and localization of adenomas, primary and metastatic phaeochromocytomas, neuroblastomas and ganglioneuroblastomas. Adrenal venous sampling has a problem solving role. FDG-PET has a limited role in identifying an ectopic source of ACTH when CT is equivocal.
5. Imaging features are highly variable depending upon the nature of the adrenal disorder and must be interpreted along with clinical and biochemical findings.

References

1. Isidori AM, Kaltsas GA, Pozza C, Frajese V, Newell-Price J, Reznek RH et al. (2006) The ectopic adrenocorticotropin syndrome: clinical features, diagnosis, management, and long-term follow-up. J Clin Endocrinol Metab 91(2):371–377
2. Sohaib SA, Hanson JA, Newell-Price JD, Trainer PJ, Monson JP, Grossman AB et al. (1999) CT appearance of the adrenal glands in adrenocorticotrophic hormone-dependent Cushing's syndrome. AJR Am J Roentgenol 172(4):997–1002
3. Doppman JL, Miller DL, Dwyer AJ, Loughlin T, Nieman L, Cutler GB, Chrousos GP, Oldfield E, Loriaux DL (1988) Macronodular adrenal hyperplasia in Cushing disease. Radiology 166(2):347–352
4. Vincent JM, Trainer PJ, Reznek RH, Marcus AJ, Dacie JE, Armstrong P, Besser GM (1993) The radiological investigation of occult ectopic ACTH-dependent Cushing's syndrome. Clin Radiol 48(1):11–17
5. Ilias I, Torpy DJ, Pacak K, Mullen N, Wesley RA, Nieman LK (2005) Cushing's syndrome due to ectopic corticotropin secretion: twenty years' experience at the National Institutes of Health. J Clin Endocrinol Metab 90(8):4955–4962
6. Pacak K, Ilias I, Chen CC, Carrasquillo JA, Whatley M, Nieman LK (2004) The role of [(18)F]-fluorodeoxyglucose positron emission tomography and [(111)In]-diethylenetriaminepentaacetate-D-Phe-pentetreotide scintigraphy in the localization of ectopic adrenocorticotropin-secreting tumors causing Cushing's syndrome. J Clin Endocrinol Metab 89(5):2214–2221
7. Boscaro M, Fallo F, Barzon L, Daniele O, Sonino N (1995) Adrenocortical carcinoma: epidemiology and natural history. Minerva Endocrinol 20(1):89–94
8. Rockall AG, Babar SA, Sohaib SA, Isidori AM, Diaz-Cano S, Monson JP, Grossman AB, Reznek RH (2004) CT and MR imaging of the adrenal glands in ACTH-independent Cushing's syndrome. Radiographics 24(2):435–452
9. Dinneen SF, Carney JA, Carpenter PC, Grant CS, Young WF Jr (1995) Acth-independent Cushing's syndrome: bilateral cortisol-producing adrenal adenomas. Endocr Pract 1(2):77–81
10. Tung SC, Wang PW, Huang TL, Lee WC, Chen WJ (2004) Bilateral adrenocortical adenomas causing ACTH-independent Cushing's syndrome at different periods: a case report and discussion of corticosteroid replacement therapy following bilateral adrenalectomy. J Endocrinol Invest 27(4):375–379
11. Nomura K, Saito H, Aiba M, Iihara M, Obara T, Takano K (2003) Cushing's syndrome due to bilateral adrenocortical adenomas with unique histological features. Endocr J 50(2):155–162
12. Ayala AR, Basaria S, Udelsman R, Westra WH, Wand GS (2000) Corticotropin-independent Cushing's syndrome caused by an ectopic adrenal adenoma. J Clin Endocrinol Metab 85(8):2903–2906
13. Szolar DH, Korobkin M, Reittner P, Berghold A, Bauernhofer T, Trummer H, Schoellnast H, Preidler KW, Samonigg H (2005) Adrenocortical carcinomas and

adrenal pheochromocytomas: mass and enhancement loss evaluation at delayed contrast-enhanced CT. Radiology 234(2):479–485

14. Slattery JM, Blake MA, Kalra MK, Misdraji J, Sweeney AT, Copeland PM, Mueller PR, Boland GW (2006) Adrenocortical carcinoma: contrast washout characteristics on CT. AJR Am J Roentgenol 187(1):W21–W24

15. Doppman JL, Travis WD, Nieman L, Miller DL, Chrousos GP, Gomez MT, Cutler GB Jr, Loriaux DL, Norton JA (1989) Cushing syndrome due to primary pigmented nodular adrenocortical disease: findings at CT and MR imaging. Radiology 172(2):415–420

16. Doppman JL, Chrousos GP, Papanicolaou DA, Stratakis CA, Alexander HR, Nieman LK (2000) Adrenocorticotropin-independent macronodular adrenal hyperplasia: an uncommon cause of primary adrenal hypercortisolism. Radiology 216(3):797–802

17. Lieberman SA, Eccleshall TR, Feldman D (1994) ACTH-independent massive bilateral adrenal disease (AIMBAD): a subtype of Cushing's syndrome with major diagnostic and therapeutic implications. Eur J Endocrinol 131(1):67–73

18. Lingam RK, Sohaib SA, Rockall AG, Isidori AM, Chew S, Monson JP et al. (2004) Diagnostic performance of CT versus MR in detecting aldosterone-producing adenoma in primary hyperaldosteronism (Conn's syndrome). Eur Radiol 14(10):1787–1792

19. Ikeda DM, Francis IR, Glazer GM, Amendola MA, Gross MD, Aisen AM (1989) The detection of adrenal tumors and hyperplasia in patients with primary aldosteronism: comparison of scintigraphy, CT, and MR imaging. AJR Am J Roentgenol 153(2):301–306

20. Geisinger MA, Zelch MG, Bravo EL, Risius BF, O'Donovan PB, Borkowski GP (1983) Primary hyperaldosteronism: comparison of CT, adrenal venography, and venous sampling. AJR Am J Roentgenol 141(2):299–302

21. Lingam RK, Sohaib SA, Vlahos I, Rockall AG, Isidori AM, Monson JP et al. (2003) CT of primary hyperaldosteronism (Conn's syndrome): the value of measuring the adrenal gland. AJR Am J Roentgenol 181(3):843–849

22. Sohaib SA, Peppercorn PD, Allan C, Monson JP, Grossman AB, Besser GM et al. (2000) Primary hyperaldosteronism (Conn syndrome): MR imaging findings. Radiology 214(2):527–531

23. Harvey A, Kline G, Pasieka JL (2006) Adrenal venous sampling in primary hyperaldosteronism: comparison of radiographic with biochemical success and the clinical decision-making with "less than ideal" testing. Surgery 140(6):847–853; discussion 853–855

24. Espiner EA, Ross DG, Yandle TG, Richards AM, Hunt PJ (2003) Predicting surgically remedial primary aldosteronism: role of adrenal scanning, posture testing, and adrenal vein sampling. J Clin Endocrinol Metab 88(8):3637–3644

25. Young WF, Stanson AW, Thompson GB, Grant CS, Farley DR, van Heerden JA (2004) Role for adrenal venous sampling in primary aldosteronism. Surgery 136(6):1227–1235

26. Tan YY, Ogilvie JB, Triponez F, Caron NR, Kebebew EK, Clark OH et al. (2006) Selective use of adrenal venous sampling in the lateralization of aldosterone-producing adenomas. World J Surg 30(5):879–885; discussion 886–887

27. Nocaudie-Calzada M, Huglo D, Lambert M, Ernst O, Proye C, Wemeau JL et al. (1999) Efficacy of iodine-131 6-beta-methyl-iodo-19-norcholesterol scintigraphy and computed tomography in patients with primary aldosteronism. Eur J Nucl Med 26(10):1326–1332

28. Maurea S, Klain M, Caraco C, Ziviello M, Salvatore M (2002) Diagnostic accuracy of radionuclide imaging using 131I nor-cholesterol or meta-iodobenzylguanidine in patients with hypersecreting or non-hypersecreting adrenal tumours. Nucl Med Commun 23(10):951–960

29. Lumachi F, Marzola MC, Zucchetta P, Tregnaghi A, Cecchin D, Favia G et al. (2003) Non-invasive adrenal imaging in primary aldosteronism. Sensitivity and positive predictive value of radiocholesterol scintigraphy, CT scan and MRI. Nucl Med Commun 24(6): 683–688

30. Kaltsas GA, Mukherjee JJ, Kola B, Isidori AM, Hanson JA, Dacie JE, Reznek R, Monson JP, Grossman AB (2003) Is ovarian and adrenal venous catheterization and sampling helpful in the investigation of hyperandrogenic women? Clin Endocrinol (Oxf) 59(1):34–43

31. Harinarayana CV, Renu G, Ammini AC, Khurana ML, Ved P, Karmarkar MG, Ahuja MM, Berry M (1991) Computed tomography in untreated congenital adrenal hyperplasia. Pediatr Radiol 21(2):103–105

32. Falke TH, van Seters AP, Schaberg A, Moolenaar AJ (1986) Computed tomography in untreated adults with virilizing congenital adrenal cortical hyperplasia. Clin Radiol 37(2):155–160

33. Bhatia V, Shukla R, Mishra SK, Gupta RK (1993) Adrenal tumor complicating untreated 21-hydroxylase deficiency in a 5 1/2-year-old boy. Am J Dis Child 147(12):1321–1323

34. Bonfig W, Bittmann I, Bechtold S, Kammer B, Noelle V, Arleth S et al. (2003) Virilising adrenocortical tumours in children. Eur J Pediatr 162(9):623–628

35. Allolio B, Fassnacht M (2006) Clinical review: adrenocortical carcinoma: clinical update. J Clin Endocrinol Metab 91(6):2027–2037

36. DeLellis RA, Wolfe HJ, Gagel RF, Feldman ZT, Miller HH, Gang DL, Reichlin S (1976) Adrenal medullary hyperplasia. A morphometric analysis in patients with familial medullary thyroid carcinoma. Am J Pathol 83(1):177–196

37. Lack EE (1997) Tumours of the adrenal gland and extra-adrenal paraganglia. Third series ed. Armed Forces Institute of Pathology, Washington DC

38. Chen M, Lu G, Zhang Q (2002) Adrenal cortical and medullar hyperplasia–a retrospective analysis of 6 cases. J Huazhong Univ Sci Technolog Med Sci 22(4): 367–368, 374

39. Rudy FR, Bates RD, Cimorelli AJ, Hill GS, Engelman K (1980) Adrenal medullary hyperplasia: a clinicopathologic study of four cases. Hum Pathol 11(6):650–657

40. Yung BC, Loke TK, Tse TW, Tsang MW, Chan JC (2000) Sporadic bilateral adrenal medullary hyperplasia: apparent false positive MIBG scan and expected MRI findings. Eur J Radiol 36(1):28–31

41. Qupty G, Ishay A, Peretz H, Dharan M, Kaufman N, Luboshitzky R (1997) Pheochromocytoma due to

unilateral adrenal medullary hyperplasia. Clin Endocrinol (Oxf) 47(5):613–617

42. Carney JA, Sizemore GW, Tyce GM (1975) Bilateral adrenal medullary hyperplasia in multiple endocrine neoplasia, type 2: the precursor of bilateral pheochromocytoma. Mayo Clin Proc 50(1):3–10

43. Jansson S, Khorram-Manesh A, Nilsson O, Kolby L, Tisell LE, Wangberg B, Ahlman H (2006) Treatment of bilateral pheochromocytoma and adrenal medullary hyperplasia. Ann N Y Acad Sci 1073:429–435

44. Kushner BH (2004) Neuroblastoma: a disease requiring a multitude of imaging studies. J Nucl Med 45(7):1172–1188

45. Pfluger T, Schmied C, Porn U, Leinsinger G, Vollmar C, Dresel S, Schmid I, Hahn K (2003) Integrated imaging using MRI and 123I metaiodobenzylguanidine scintigraphy to improve sensitivity and specificity in the diagnosis of pediatric neuroblastoma. AJR Am J Roentgenol 181(4):1115–1124

46. Ilias I, Shulkin B, Pacak K (2005) New functional imaging modalities for chromaffin tumors, neuroblastomas and ganglioneuromas. Trends Endocrinol Metab 16(2):66–72

47. Mehta N, Tripathi RP, Popli MB, Nijhawan VS (1997) Bilateral intraabdominal ganglioneuroblastoma in an adult. Br J Radiol 70:96–98

48. Lovas K, Husebye ES (2002) High prevalence and increasing incidence of Addison's disease in western Norway. Clin Endocrinol (Oxf) 56(6):787–791

49. Falorni A, Laureti S, De Bellis A, Zanchetta R, Tiberti C, Arnaldi G et al. (2004) SIE Addison Study Group. Italian Addison network study: update of diagnostic criteria for the etiological classification of primary adrenal insufficiency. J Clin Endocrinol Metab 89(4):1598–1604

50. Chin R (1991) Adrenal crisis. Crit Care Clin 7:23–42

51. Itoh K, Yamashita K, Satoh Y, Sawada H (1988) MR imaging of bilateral adrenal hemorrhage. J Comput Assist Tomogr 12(6):1054–1056

52. Kawashima A, Sandler CM, Ernst RD, Takahashi N, Roubidoux MA, Goldman SM, Fishman EK, Dunnick NR (1999) Imaging of nontraumatic hemorrhage of the adrenal gland. Radiographics 19(4):949–963

53. Yang ZG, Guo YK, Li Y, Min PQ, Yu JQ, Ma ES (2006) Differentiation between tuberculosis and primary tumors in the adrenal gland: evaluation with contrast-enhanced CT. Eur Radiol 16(9):2031–2036. Epub 2006 Jan 25

54. Betterle C, Dal Pra C, Mantero F, Zanchetta R (2002) Autoimmune adrenal insufficiency and autoimmune polyendocrine syndromes: autoantibodies, autoantigens, and their applicability in diagnosis and disease prediction. Endocr Rev 23(3):327–364. Review. Erratum in: Endocr Rev 23(4):579

55. Trainer PJ, Besser GM (2002) Addison's Disease. In: Besser GM, Thorner MO (eds) Clinical endocrinology, 3rd edn, Mosby, London, pp 203–212

Imaging of Pheochromocytomas

7

Erick M. Remer and Frank H. Miller

Contents

E.M. Remer (✉)
Associate Professor of Radiology, Director, Abdominal Imaging Fellowship Program, Section of Abdominal Imaging, Division of Diagnostic Radiology, Cleveland Clinic, 9500 Euclid Ave. A21, Cleveland, OH 44195
E-mail: remere1@ccf.org

Clinical Features

Pheochromocytomas are rare, hormonally active tumors that arise from the paraganglia of the sympathetic nervous system and secrete epinephrine and norepinephrine. The paraganglia are collections of specialized neural crest cells that arise in association with autonomic ganglia throughout the body [1], including the adrenal medulla and other widely dispersed sites. Frankel first described the pheochromocytoma in 1886 when he reported a patient with hypertension and subsequent sudden death due to an adrenal tumor [2]. Since that time, pheochromocytoma has become better understood, but it remains elusive clinically [3, 4] and has such varied imaging manifestations that it has been termed an "Imaging Chameleon." [5].

Tumors of the paraganglia are considered differently if they occur in the adrenal or outside of it. Tumors arising from the adrenal medulla are termed pheochromocytomas and comprise 80%–90% of these tumors [1]. Approximately 98% occur below the diaphragm [1]. Sporadic pheochromocytomas occur equally in males and females and typically present in the fourth to fifth decades of life and have a slight female predominance [1]. While the true prevalence of pheochromocytomas is unknown, it is estimated to be the cause of 0.1–0.5% of newly diagnosed cases of hypertension [6].

Although usually sporadic, pheochromocytomas are associated with many different syndromes. Multiple endocrine neoplasia syndromes (MEN) 2a and 2b include pheochromocytomas. MEN syndromes

M.A. Blake, G. Boland (eds.), *Adrenal Imaging*, DOI 10.1007/978-1-59745-560-2_7,
© 2009 Humana Press, a part of Springer Science+Business Media, LLC

are caused by rare, autosomal dominant mutations in genes regulating cell growth. In MEN 2A, pheochromocytomas are small, multifocal, bilateral in 70% and develop on the background of adrenomedullary hyperplasia secondary to an *RET* germline mutation. Biochemical and/or imaging manifestations occur in about 50% of patients. Other syndromes that include pheochromocytomas are neurofibromatosis, von Hippel-Lindau disease, tuberous sclerosis, and Sturge-Weber syndrome [6–8]. Pheochromocytomas occur in 1% of patients with neurofibromatosis type-1 and are most commonly solitary adrenal tumors. In one study, 84% were solitary adrenal masses, 9.6% were bilateral adrenal masses, and 6.1% were ectopic in location [6]. One caveat is that up to 25% of apparently sporadic pheochromocytomas may herald germline mutations, indicating hereditary disease and, therefore, a predisposition for extra-adrenal, often multifocal, tumors [9].

Approximately 10% of pheochromocytomas occur in children. In children, 50% of pheochromocytomas are solitary and intra-adrenal, 25% are bilateral, and 25% are extra-adrenal. In children, multifocal and extraadrenal tumors are found in up to 30%–43% of cases of tumors of the paraganglia [10].

Sporadic pheochromocytoma is malignant about 2%–11% of the time [1]. Malignancy is seen more frequently in patients with hereditary syndromes at a rate than has been estimated at 26%–35% [10]. Unfortunately, there are no clinical findings, imaging features, or histopathological appearances that can exclude malignant behavior [10]. Typical histological markers of malignancy, such as nuclear atypia, number of mitoses, and capsular or vascular invasion, do not consistently predict malignant behavior [10]. Conversely, benign features at histopathology do not ensure benign clinical behavior in the future. However, distant metastases to sites without paraganglion tissue, such as bone, lungs, lymph nodes and liver, are reliable indicators of malignancy and, thus, the diagnosis of malignancy is often made by radiologists.

Tumors arising outside the adrenal, in the sympathetic ganglia, are called extra-adrenal pheochromocytomas or paragangliomas. Some authors reserve the term extraadrenal pheochromocytomas only for functioning tumors. They occur with greatest frequency in the second and third decades, without gender predominance [1], and comprise 10%–20% of all pheochromocytomas. They are less commonly hormonally active than adrenal pheochromocytomas [11].

Extraadrenal tumors occur anywhere along the sympathetic chain from the base of the skull to the bladder. At least 85% of extraadrenal tumors occur below the diaphragm, with the most common site being in the superior paraaortic region (46%), especially at the level of the renal hila (46%) [1] (Fig. 7.1). The second most common site is the inferior paraaortic region (29%). The most common location in this region is at the organ of Zuckerkandl, a paraganglion that contains small groups of chromaphil cells connected with the ganglia of the sympathetic trunk and is located at the aortic bifurcation near the inferior mesenteric artery origin [12]. The next most common sites are along the sympathetic nerve chain in the intrathoracic region (10%) and in the urinary bladder (10%) (Fig. 7.2). Rare sites include the anus, vagina, sacrococcygeal region, pelvis (Fig. 7.3), mediastinum, pericardium, and in the neck (carotid body), middle ear (glomus jugulare and glomus tympanicum) (Fig. 7.4), and vagus nerve.

Extra-adrenal pheochromocytomas are multifocal 15%–24% of the time [13, 14]. It has been more common to identify multiple tumors at extraadrenal sites than to find coexistent adrenal and extra-adrenal tumors. Extra-adrenal tumors are more likely to be malignant than those in the adrenal, with malignancy rates ranging from 29%–40% (Fig. 7.5).

Patients with pheochromocytomas present with a variety of symptoms that include headaches, palpitations, excessive sweating, tremor, vomiting, chest or abdominal pain, constipation, and visual disturbances. The classic clinical findings are hypertension (often episodic or refractory to therapy) associated with headaches, diaphoresis, and palpitations. Hypertension is characteristically labile or sustained. These symptoms are typically paroxysmal. The symptomatic episodes may vary in occurrence from monthly to several times per day, and the duration may vary from seconds to hours.

The pattern of symptoms relates to the relative amounts of epinephrine and norepinephrine secreted by a particular tumor [15]. Tumors in the adrenal and organ of Zuckerkandl tend to produce more epinephrine than those in the

(a)

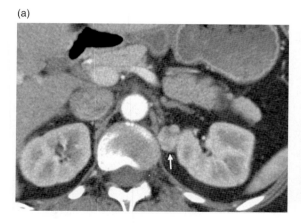

(b)

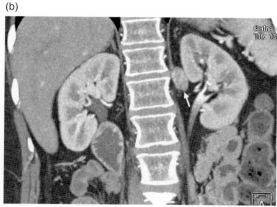

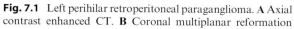

Fig. 7.1 Left perihilar retroperitoneal paraganglioma. **A** Axial contrast enhanced CT. **B** Coronal multiplanar reformation show ovoid mass that is isoattenuating with renal parenchyma (*arrow*). A normal left adrenal gland is visualized

Fig. 7.2 A 16-year-old girl with history of micturition symptoms. Sagittal gadolinium-enhanced T1-weighted spin echo image shows enhancing bladder-base mass (*arrow*)

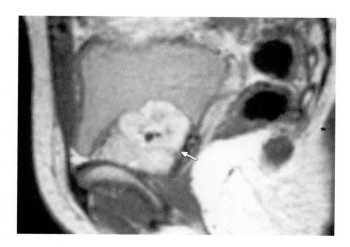

other paraganglia which tend to produce norepinephrine. Symptoms of epinephrine-predominant tumors include hypotension, tachyarrhythmia and palpitations.

Patients with nonfunctional retroperitoneal paragangliomas present with symptoms from compression of other structures by the tumor. Because of "attention-getting" symptoms, functional tumors are usually small when detected, but nonfunctional tumors may be large. Tumors of the bladder may present with micturitional symptoms, including micturition syncope. Tumors arising near the renal hilus have been associated with renal artery stenosis [16, 17]. In some patients, this association may represent a "pseudostenosis"

due to catecholamine-induced arterial constriction, resulting from local leakage of vasoactive catecholamines from an adjacent pheochromocytoma into the renal hilum or from mass effect of the tumor itself [18].

Some patients may also be asymptomatic and have tumors found by serendipitous imaging. Pheochromocytomas have increasingly been identified in patients imaged for unrelated symptoms and conditions [19]. In recent series, 23%–59% of pheochromocytomas were found incidentally [19–23]. This is considerably higher than the typically quoted 10% asymptomatic rate. One explanation for this discrepancy relates to an increasing number of all types of adrenal masses that are

(a)

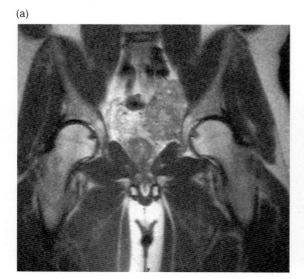

(b)

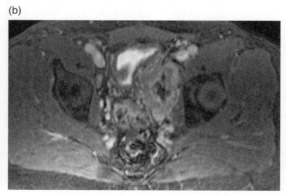

Fig. 7.3 Left pelvic paraganglioma. **A** Coronal T2-weighted MRI shows large mass in the left pelvis adjacent to external iliac vessels that is intermediate signal intensity. **B** Axial gadolinium-enhanced T1-weighted image shows enhancing tumor with central nonenhancing region

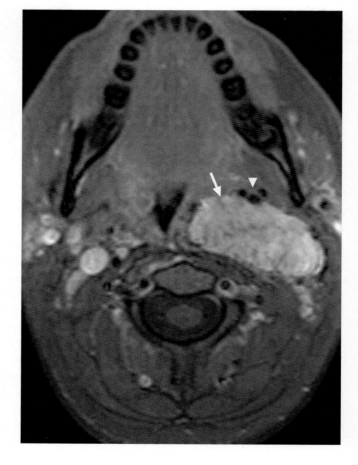

Fig. 7.4 Left parapharyngeal space vagal paraganglioma (Glomus vagale). Gadolinium-enhanced axial T1-weighted image shows large uniformly enhancing parapharyngeal space mass (*arrow*) that displaces the internal carotid artery anteriorly and medially (*arrowhead*)

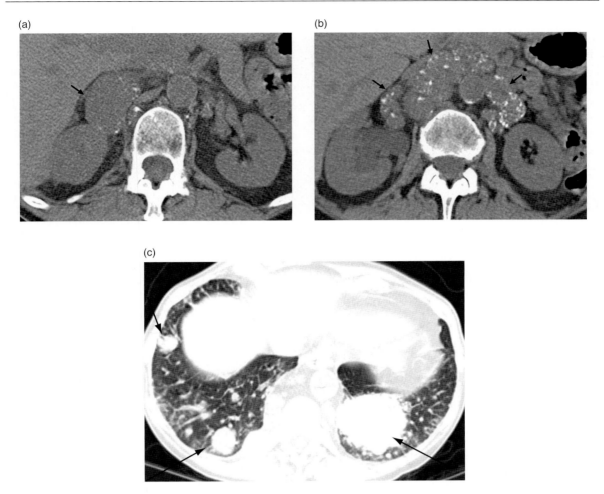

Fig. 7.5 Metastatic pheochromocytoma. Unenhanced CT images show a peripherally calcified right adrenal pheochromocytoma (*arrow*) (**A**), metastatic lymphadenopathy with multifocal punctate calcifications (*arrows*) (**B**), and metastatic pulmonary nodules (*arrows*) (**C**)

being discovered incidentally because of the common use of imaging to evaluate abdominal symptoms and diseases. With increased imaging, pheochromocytomas may be detected earlier, before they are symptomatic. Because pheochromocytomas are elusive clinically, the prevalence of incidental pheochromocytomas in any series relates in part to how attuned the physician ordering the imaging study was to the symptoms and signs of pheochromocytoma. One could speculate that the physicians were not attuned to the patients' symptoms in these earlier series. However, considering the indications for the CT examinations in one study [19] included pancreatitis, diverticulitis, pelvic pain, ulcerative colitis, and abdominal aortic aneurysm, it was likely that incidental pheochromocytomas in this series were merely discovered during an evaluation of unrelated problems. It, therefore, behooves the radiologist to be circumspect of any incidental adrenal mass. The measurement of fractionated metanephrines and catecholamines in a 24-h urine specimen has been recommended for all patients with adrenal incidentalomas by one author [24].

There is varying information in the literature regarding the size of asymptomatic vs symptomatic tumors. Some studies suggest that asymptomatic patients tend to have larger tumors [20]. The size difference has been attributed to secreted catecholamines being metabolized within large tumors

[25]. Smaller tumors, in contrast, have slower turnover rates and release free catecholamines into the circulation that lead to hyperadrenergic symptoms [26]. Other, larger series found no statistically significant size difference (maximum diameter or volume) between incidental and symptomatic masses. This result is similar to that of an autopsy series of 54 pheochromocytomas that found no size difference between pheochromocytomas diagnosed before death and those detected after death [27].

Laboratory Tests

Screening laboratory tests should be considered in patients presenting with classic symptoms or those with a family history of the tumor or associated syndromes. The most common screening examination is a urinary measurement of unconjugated catecholamines, namely epinephrine and norepinephrine, or their metabolites, metanephrine and vanillylmandelic acid. Ninety percent of patients with pheochromocytomas have elevated urinary metanephrine or vanillylmandelic acid [28, 29].

The combination of plasma catecholamines and urinary metanephrines measurements has an accuracy of close to 98% in both sporadic and hereditary pheochromocytoma [4]. If available, plasma free metanephrines should be performed, especially if hereditary pheochromoctyoma is suspected. It has a reported sensitivity of 97% and specificity of 96% for hereditary pheochromocytoma and a sensitivity of 99% and specificity of 82% in sporadic pheochromocytoma [4]. The particular screening tests used vary from institution to institution based on the expertise of the particular laboratory. Further, because pheochromocytomas are such a heterogeneous group of tumors with variable metabolism, in order to achieve 100% diagnostic accuracy, multiple tests should be performed [4].

While biopsy can definitively confirm the diagnosis of pheochromocytoma, it is uncommonly warranted. The combination of positive biochemical studies and an imaging localized mass mandate surgical resection. One scenario to avoid, however, is the inadvertent biopsy of a pheochromocytoma. This most typically occurs when the diagnosis has not been previously entertained and no biochemical evaluation has been performed. Indiscriminant biopsy of pheochromocytoma can lead to disastrous

consequences from the hypertensive crisis that can be provoked by manipulation of the mass [30]. Hypertension is thought to be less common from the biopsy of a paraganglioma than a pheochromocytoma, but there have been rare reports of the former [31]. Pharmacological adrenergic blockade is recommended before biopsy of a mass that may potentially be a pheochromocytoma with inconclusive biochemical studies.

Pathology

The main cellular feature of normal paraganglia is chief (type 1) cells that are oval or round and contain neurosecretory granules that store catecholamines [1]. Spindle-shaped sustentacular (type 2) cells are a minor cell population on the periphery of the chief cells. This dual cell population is present in all paraganglia and in the adrenal medulla, but the organization varies in paraganglia from different regions.

The histological appearance of tumors is similar to the paraganglion of origin; thus, tumors occurring in different paraganglia have differing histological appearances [1]. Adrenal pheochromocytomas usually have cells arranged in large trabeculae, interspersed with thin-walled sinusoids. Head and neck vagal paraganglion tumors are typically comprised of cells in small clusters or nests (zellballen) [5] or cords, containing eosinophilic cytoplasm, separated by prominent fibrovascular stroma. Paraganglion tumors may have either the trabecular or zellballen pattern or both.

A range of different patterns, however, may be seen. In general, smaller tumors tend to be solid, while larger tumors tend to have more areas of hemorrhage [5]. Some tumors have features that include calcification, cystic change, and fibrosis.

Imaging Examinations

While elevated levels of urinary and plasma catecholamines and clinical history are used to diagnose pheochromocytomas, imaging studies are used to preoperatively localize the tumors, to determine multifocality or bilaterality, and to aid in determining surgical approach. The main imaging modalities utilized to localize pheochromocytomas are CT, MRI, and nuclear medicine studies.

Computed Tomography

Whether intravenous iodinated contrast can be used safely in patients with pheochromocytoma has been the subject of some debate. The risk of inducing a hypertensive crisis has been reported with ionic contrast [32–34]. In a small series, however, intravenous injection of nonionic contrast has been shown to cause no increase in plasma catecholamine levels [35]. Some authors suggest that current accepted practice would avoid the use of iodinated contrast in patients with known pheochromocytoma [5]. However, no patient in a recent study of 25 patients with pheochromocytoma or paraganglioma (21 functionally active) had an adverse advent after the intravenous administration of nonionic contrast media [36]. Contrast issues aside, the role of CT in studying a pheochromocytoma in any particular patient is directly related to the clinical situation for which the examination is performed. If a patient presents with clinical symptoms suggesting pheochromocytoma and has positive biochemistries, the goal of imaging is not characterization, but is localization of the hormone-secreting tumor. When clinically suspected, some authors suggest that CT is the study of choice to confirm the diagnosis of pheochromocytomas [37]. An unenhanced CT of the adrenals and retroperitoneum will achieve this goal in the majority of patients. Pheochromocytomas are most typically relatively large (averaging 3 cm or more) and localize to the adrenals or, if extraadrenal, in the retroperitoneum from the renal hila to the organ of Zuckerkandl. On unenhanced CT, adrenal pheochromocytoma is typically a soft-tissue attenuation mass [19] that is 3 cm or greater [38] (Fig. 7.6). Calcifications are present in 10%–20% [19, 38] (Fig. 7.7). Most have areas of low attenuation, thought to be from necrosis (Fig. 7.8). In a recent series, only 1 of 33 pheochromocytomas had no focal areas of diminished attenuation in comparison to the remainder of the mass [19]. Cystic changes can also occur and are the result of intratumoral hemorrhage with subsequent liquefaction and fibrous capsule formation [39] (Fig. 7.9). Fluid-fluid levels may be present within the cystic components (Fig. 7.10).

Should the tumor go undetected in evaluation of the abdomen, then an evaluation of the pelvis, followed by the chest and neck, if necessary, should be performed to exclude the possible 2% of extraadrenal pheochromocytomas that are not below the diaphragm.

The reported sensitivity of CT for detection for adrenal pheochromocytomas ranges from 93% to 100% [40, 41]. For extra-adrenal tumors, sensitivity decreases to approximately 90% [42].

A second scenario involves a patient with a known adrenal mass, but no symptoms of pheochromocytoma or available biochemistries at the time of the CT examination. In this scenario, the goal of imaging is to characterize the adrenal mass. CT densitometry and post contrast washout, have been used to characterize adrenal masses. The goal of these tests is to rule in the common benign adrenal mass, the adenoma. Noncontrast CT densitometry has been used to distinguish adenomas from metastases [43, 44] based on the amount of intracellular lipid content in adenomas. There is incomplete information about the use of CT densitometry in pheochromocytoma identification. In general, excluding areas of necrosis, pheochromocytoma has been shown to have noncontrast attenuation above 10 Hounsfield units (H) [19, 45] (Fig. 7.6). One study [19] of 33 pheochromocytomas showed none to be lower than 10 H (median 35 H, range 17–59 H). There have been case reports, however, of adrenal pheochromocytomas and medullary hyperplasia (a suspected pheochromocytoma precursor) with an attenuation <10 H [46] because of fat in either medullary cells or intermingled cortical cells. Also, macroscopic fat has been rarely identified in pheochromocytomas, confounding the key diagnostic feature of adrenal myelolipoma [5].

Often, when an unenhanced CT attenuation measurement is greater than 10 H, which should be expected of almost all pheochromocytomas, a contrast-enhanced CT followed by washout phase CT is performed. The aim of this technique is to identify adenomas, in this case by detecting rapid contrast loss. If this technique is applied in a patient with a previously uncharacterized pheochromocytoma, the best outcome for which one could hope is to identify the mass as a nonadenoma. If the mass were correctly identified as a nonadenoma, then additional workup, including biochemistries would be performed. That said, there is only preliminary information about the washout characteristics of pheochromocytomas. Pheochromocytomas characteristically enhance briskly (Fig. 7.6.), but non- or minimally-enhancing areas from necrosis or cystic change are common (Figs. 7.7 and 7.8).

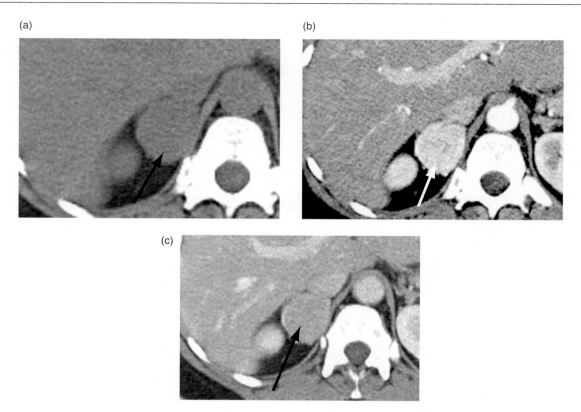

Fig. 7.6 "Typical" CT findings in pheochromocytoma (*arrows*). **A** Unenhanced axial CT shows soft tissue attenuation right adrenal mass (*arrow*). **B** Arterial phase contrast-enhanced CT shows avid homogeneous enhancement. **C** Portal venous phase contrast-enhanced CT shows rapid contrast loss. Reprinted with permission from the American Journal of Roentgenology

The only series studying the washout characteristics of pheochromocytoma showed washout compatible with a nonadenoma (>60% washout) in all 17 pheochromocytomas that were evaluated [45]. There have several been reports, however, of pheochromocytoma with washout greater than 60%; thus a pheochromocytoma could be mistaken for adenoma using enhancement characteristics. Caoili et al. [47] reported a pheochromocytoma with 68% washout. Blake et al. [48] reported a

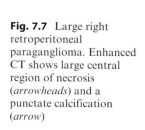

Fig. 7.7 Large right retroperitoneal paraganglioma. Enhanced CT shows large central region of necrosis (*arrowheads*) and a punctate calcification (*arrow*)

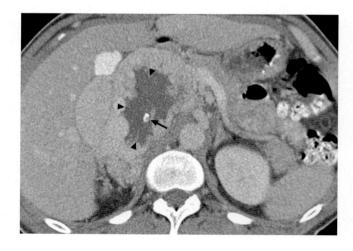

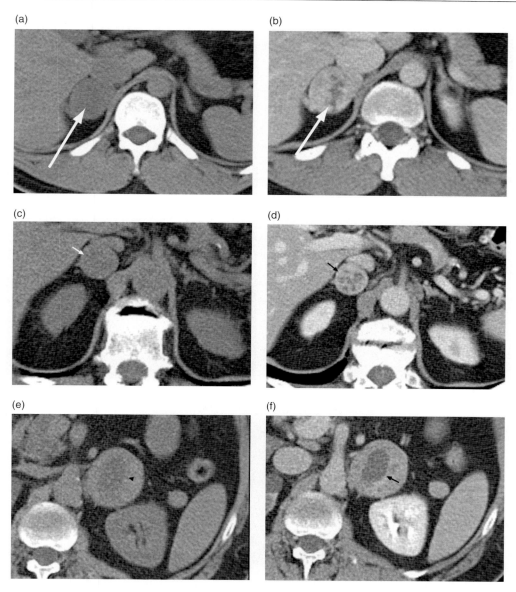

Fig. 7.8 Pheochromocytoma with necrosis. Unenhanced (**A,C,E**) and contrast-enhanced CT (**B,D,F**) images show areas of several patterns and degrees of low attenuation, nonenhancing necrosis (*arrowhead* and *arrow* in e,f) within pheochromocytomas (*arrows*) in three different patients

symptomatic patient with pheochromocytoma and another with medullary hyperplasia, each measuring less than 10 H on unenhanced CT and showing washout >60%. Yoon and colleagues [49] reported an incidental pheochromocytoma in a patient with an esophageal carcinoma with an unenhanced attenuation of 37 H and washout of 72%. Szolar et al. [45] compared a series of 23 adenomas with 17 pheochromocytomas and found that CT washout at 10 minutes was 100% sensitive.

Another clinical and specific for adenoma scenario involves a routine diagnostic study performed with intravenous contrast for an issue unrelated to pheochromocytoma. While there are findings commonly seen in pheochromocytoma, it has a variable appearance on CT. Pheochromocytomas are varied in attenuation and can be either homogeneous or heterogeneous. Contrast-enhanced images often demonstrate brisk enhancement secondary to the tumor's hypervascularity (Fig. 7.11). Calcifications and areas

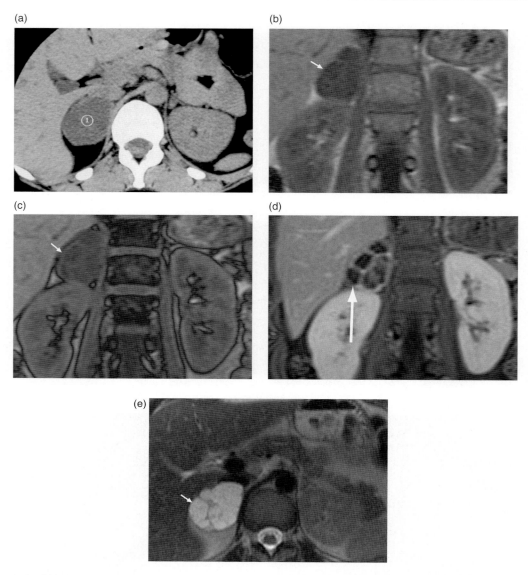

Fig. 7.9 **A** Ovoid homogeneous right adrenal pheochromo-cytoma measures 14 Hounsfield units on unenhanced CT scan. **B,C** Coronal in- (**B**) and opposed-phase (**C**) gradient echo T1-weighted images show low signal intensity lesion without signal loss on opposed phase image. **D** Coronal contrast-enhanced three-dimensional gradient echo MR image shows enhancing septa (*arrow*) within the mass. **E** Axial T2-weighted image shows uniformly high signal intensity except for regions of septa

of low attenuation from necrosis are common [19] (Fig. 7.7). Upon discovering a previously unknown adrenal mass, it is incumbent upon the radiologist to suggest biochemical evaluation.

Finally, pheochromocytoma may be the cause of nontraumatic adrenal hemorrhage. In a patient who presents without a discernable risk for adrenal hemorrhage, it is necessary to determine whether the hemorrhage occurred in a preexisting tumor [50] (Fig. 7.12). Pheochromocytoma is the most common cause of massive bleeding from a primary adrenal tumor [50]. CT can be helpful for this determination, assessing enhancement and serial imaging can document resolution of the hematoma. In some patients, biopsy or surgery may be required.

Fig. 7.10 Left adrenal pheochromocytoma. Axial turbo spin echo T2 weighted image shows fluid-fluid level (*arrow*) and septation (*arrowhead*) in central cystic component of the mass

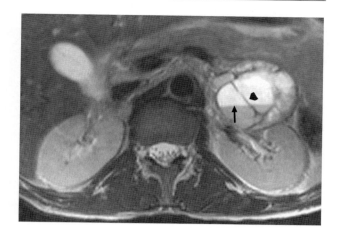

(a)

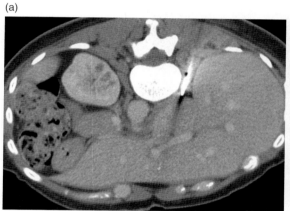

(b)

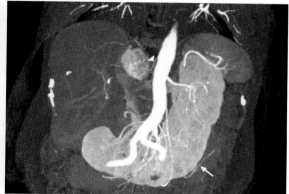

Fig. 7.11 Retroperitoneal mass was discovered during a work-up for back pain. Imaging-guided biopsy was requested. **A** Enhanced CT image, with patient in prone position, shows biopsy needle placed to margin of retrocaval mass. **B** Thin slab coronal maximal intensity projection of CT obtained for surgical planning after histopathology found pheochromocytoma. Note marked tumor vascularity, arterial supply from aorta (*arrowhead*) and horseshoe kidney (*arrow*)

CT can be used to evaluate for metastases. Direct extension of the tumor into the inferior vena cava or adjacent organs can occur. Metastases occur most commonly in the axial skeleton, lymph nodes, liver and lungs (Fig. 7.5).

Magnetic Resonance Imaging

MRI can be utilized to both localize pheochromocytoma and paraganglioma in patients with clinical symptoms and positive biochemistries and to characterize an adrenal mass as a pheochromocytoma in patients with suspected pheochromocytoma, but with equivocal biochemical values or clinical findings. Some authors believe that MR imaging should be the initial modality when a functioning paraganglioma is suspected [14]. In 1 series of 282 patients with pheochromocytoma, MRI provided higher sensitivity than CT or metaiodobenzylguanidine (MIBG) scintigraphy [51]. The advantages of MRI when compared to CT are its primary multiplanar capability and lack of ionizing radiation.

Generally, the signal intensity of a pheochromocytoma on T1-weighted sequences is equivalent to or lower than that of liver, kidney, or muscle. If hemorrhage is present, then a higher signal may be seen [52] (Fig. 7.12). Unlike adrenal

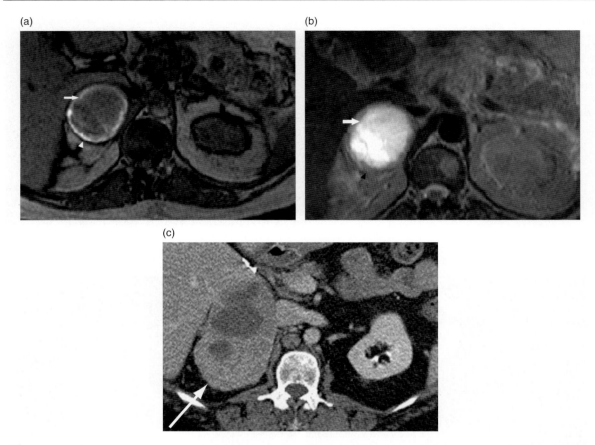

Fig. 7.12 A 56-year-old woman who had incidental left adrenal lesion detected during episode of severe acute pancreatitis. **A** T1-weighted axial spin echo MRI shows majority of 6 cm mass is isointense to liver (*arrow*) with a peripheral hyperintense rim (*arrowhead*). **B** T2-weighted spin echo MRI shows majority of mass to be markedly hyperintense (*arrow*) with peripheral rim of lower signal intensity (*arrowhead*). Signal intensities are consistent with hemorrhage. Biochemistries were normal and a follow-up CT 9 months later showed reduction of mass to 2 cm. **C**. Enhanced CT six years later shows 11 cm right adrenal pheochromocytoma (*arrow*) with areas of unenhancing necrosis

adenomas, pheochromocytomas typically do not show phase cancellation on out-of-phase gradient-echo sequences in comparison to in phase sequences [53] (Fig. 7.9B,C). However, they can occasionally be erroneously characterized as adenomas if they contain fat [5].

On T2-weighted sequences, pheochromocytomas typically have long T2 relaxation times and are, therefore, markedly hyperintense [52, 54]. Classically, they were described as "light bulb" bright. Currently, however, this description is not considered accurate. In one series, only 60% of lesions demonstrated the characteristic marked hyperintensity [55] (Fig. 7.13). Another study showed that 35% of the pheochromocytomas had atypically short T2 relaxation times [56]. Others have shown that the majority of lesions have heterogeneous and moderate hyperintensity on T2 imaging [57]. Therefore, a pheochromocytoma cannot be excluded based on a lack of high signal intensity on T2-weighted images. Further, when high T2 signal intensity is seen, it is not completely specific for pheochromocytoma. Gadolinium-enhanced images demonstrate rapid and prolonged enhancement secondary to the marked vascularity of the tumor. Areas of necrosis or cystic change do not enhance and are typically high signal intensity on T2-weighted images (Fig. 7.9).

Fig. 7.13 Left adrenal pheochromocytoma. Coronal T2-weighted image shows intermediate signal intensity left adrenal mass (*arrow*)

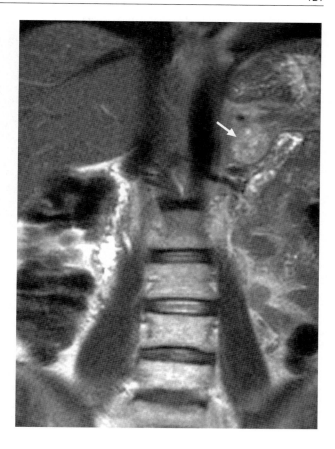

The MR signal intensities of paragangliomas are similar to those of adrenal pheochromocytomas. Like CT, MRI may also be used to search for metastases and direct extension into the inferior vena cava or adjacent organs, such as the liver or kidney.

MRI is an appropriate first choice to image children and pregnant women in search of pheochromocytoma since no ionizing radiation is delivered during the study.

They may be homogeneous or heterogeneous and anechoic to echogenic depending on the degree of necrosis, hemorrhage, cystic change or calcification (Fig. 7.14). Hemorrhage is typically hyperechoic, while necrosis appears hypoechoic [59]. Factors that can help distinguish cystic pheochromocytomas from simple adrenal or renal cysts include the presence of a relatively thick capsule, solid components, and internal low-level echoes [60].

Ultrasound

Ultrasound is rarely recommended as a test to diagnose pheochromocytoma except in children and pregnant patients. But, as a noninvasive, rapid, and inexpensive test, ultrasound may be used in localizing adrenal pheochromocytomas with a reported sensitivity of 89%–97% [58]. Pheochromocytomas have a variable appearance.

Nuclear Scintigraphy

Functional imaging is typically not used as a primary localizing modality for pheochromocytomas [10]. It is recommended in patients in whom pheochromocytoma is suspected but CT or MRI is negative [37]. Also, functional imaging is used to confirm that a tumor identified on CT or MRI is a pheochromocytoma when biochemical studies are

Fig. 7.14 Sagittal ultrasound shows left suprarenal mass that it isoechoic to spleen and more echogenic than kidney

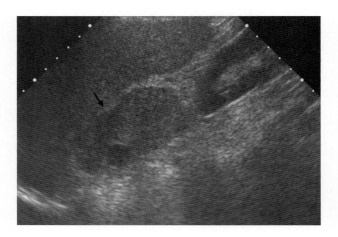

equivocal, or it may be used to guide further workup [10]. Some authors suggest that even when CT or MRI localizes a suspected tumor, functional imaging is required to confirm that a tumor is a pheochromocytoma and to exclude metastatic disease [10]. Others have found that in the setting of a unilateral adrenal mass in a patient with biochemically-proven pheochromocytoma, that ^{123}I-MIBG did not alter management [61].

In most cases, functional studies can exclude metastases or search for multifocal disease by imaging the entire body – a difficult task with MRI or CT.

Metaiodobenzylguanidine (MIBG) is an aralkyl derivative of guanethidine, a structural analog of norepinephrine, and is capable of imaging adrenergic tissue and detecting pheochromocytomas. Both ^{131}I and ^{123}I are used for imaging, but ^{123}I is preferable due to its higher sensitivity, lower radiation dose, and better image quality [62]. Due to its lower cost and the possibility of obtaining delayed scans, as well as difficulty obtaining ^{123}I-MIBG in the U.S. [10], [121]I-MIBG is still used at some centers [63]. The recommended dose is 185–370 MBq of ^{123}I-MIBG (30–37 MBq ^{131}I-MIBG) for adults [62]. Thyroid blockade is needed and some medications that reduce MIBG uptake should be stopped. Imaging is performed with a large field of view gamma camera with low energy (^{123}I) or high energy ([121]I) parallel hole collimators. Planar images of the whole body are obtained at 24 and 48 h and, with ^{123}I-MIBG, SPECT images at 24 h after injection are usually carried out. ^{123}I-MIBG is

especially useful in detecting recurrent or metastatic pheochromocytoma, tumors with fibrosis, or tumors in unusual locations or areas with distorted anatomy [64]. Normal uptake is seen in the heart, salivary glands, liver, spleen and urinary tract [62] (Fig. 7.15). Therefore, if a paraganglioma near the urinary bladder is suspected, then bladder catheterization may be necessary.

Pheochromocytomas have increased uptake on MIBG studies (Fig. 7.15). The specificity of ^{131}I-MIBG ranges from 88% to 100% [65, 66]. However, occasional false-negative studies occur, resulting in a sensitivity between 80% and 90% [64, 65]. A meta-analysis of ^{123}I-MIBG found overall sensitivity of 96% and specificity of 100%, with a sensitivity of 79% for malignant tumors [67]. While not widely used currently, fusion of ^{123}I scintigraphic images with CT or MRI hold much potential in evaluation for pheochromocytoma (Fig. 7.15) [68].

Practically, for most patients, a negative MIBG study excludes the diagnosis of pheochromocytoma and abnormal uptake confirms it. Rare false positive results have been seen in adrenocortical carcinoma and infection [10]. False negative results can occur with necrotic tumors or when medications that block agent uptake are not stopped before the study.

[111]Indium-octreotide (IN), a second agent that can be used to detect pheochromocytomas, is a synthetic octapeptide analog of somatostatin that shows uptake in a variety of tumors that contain

(a) 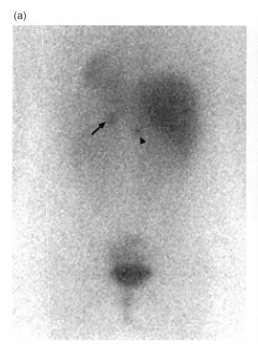 (b)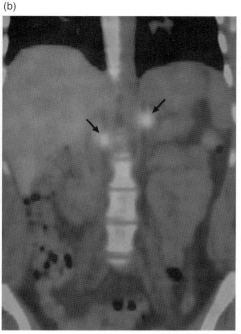

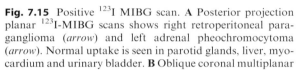

Fig. 7.15 Positive ^{123}I MIBG scan. **A** Posterior projection planar ^{123}I-MIBG scans shows right retroperitoneal paraganglioma (*arrow*) and left adrenal pheochromocytoma (*arrow*). Normal uptake is seen in parotid glands, liver, myocardium and urinary bladder. **B** Oblique coronal multiplanar reformation of fused ^{123}I-MIBG SPECT and CT scan provides improved spatial resolution and anatomic cues. Note that the combination of an adrenal pheochromocytoma and a paraganglioma is unusual

somatostatin receptors. A total of 5 mCi (185 MBq) of ^{111}In octreotide is administered intravenously, and whole-body imaging is performed at 4 and 24 h after injection. ^{111}In octreotide has a sensitivity of 75%–90% for detection of pheochromocytomas [37]. Only a few studies have compared MIBG and octreotide in the same patients [10]. They have not found octreotide to be helpful in localization of primary pheochromocytomas [69], with octreotide negative in up to 75% of benign tumors, even in tumors with positive MIBG scans. However, malignant or metastatic pheochromocytoma is detected more frequently with octreotide than with ^{123}I-MIBG (87% vs 57% of lesions) [68]. Therefore, a more appropriate role for octreotide is in patients with malignant or metastatic disease.

Studies have evaluated the use of positron emission tomography (PET) in pheochromocytoma, but this test has not yet achieved widespread use. PET is performed in minutes to hours after injecting a positron-emitting agent with a short half-life. Low radiation dose and superior spatial resolution are two advantages of PET compared to other functional studies (Fig. 7.16).

A number of agents have been studied including ^{18}F-FDG, ^{11}C hydroxyephedrine or ^{11}C epinephrine, ^{18}F DOPA and ^{18}F Dopamine. ^{18}F FDG PET has been shown to identify more metastases than MIBG [70]. However, all rapidly metabolizing cells take up glucose, so imaging with ^{18}F FDG PET is nonspecific for pheochromocytoma and should not be performed as an initial study [10]. ^{18}F DA, developed at the National Institutes of Health, has been shown to provide more accurate information about the number and location of metastatic disease compared to ^{131}I-MIBG [71]. It is a more specific substrate for the norepinephrine transporter than other amines and should be a better agent than others [10]. While promising, it is currently only available at a few centers [10] and needs further study.

Fig. 7.16 Positive ^{18}F-FDG PET. Axial ^{18}F-FDG PET/CT image shows focal, marked uptake in right adrenal pheochromocytoma

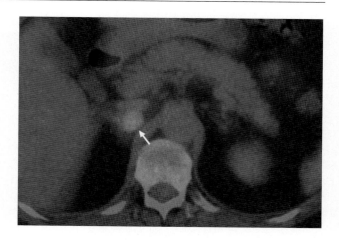

Summary Points

- Pheochromocytoma and paragangliomas are elusive clinically and have widely variable imaging features.
- The radiologist should be circumspect of adrenal masses and remain vigilant that even incidentally discovered adrenal masses may be a pheochromocytoma.
- The role of CT in pheochromocytoma depends highly on the clinical circumstances in which it is used.
- As much as 35%–40% of pheochromocytomas are not markedly hyperintense on MRI.
- Functional imaging can help confirm pheochromocytoma or paraganglioma when CT or MRI is negative. Also, it is used to identify a pheochromocytoma or paragangliomas when CT or MRI is negative or if biochemical studies are equivocal.

References

1. Whalen RK, Althausen AF, Daniels GH (1992) Extra-adrenal pheochromocytoma. J Urol 147:1–10
2. Miles RM (1960) Pheochromocytoma. Arch Surg 80:283
3. Manger WM (2002) In search of pheochromocytoma. J Clin Endocrinol Metab 88:4080–4082
4. Bravo EL, Tagle R (2003) Pheochromocytoma: state of the art and future prospects. Endocr Rev 24:539–553
5. Blake M, Kalra MK, Maher MM et al. (2004) Pheochromocytoma: an imaging chameleon. Radiographics 24(Suppl 1)S87–99
6. Goldfien A (1994) Adrenal gland endocrinology. In: Greenspan FS, Baxter TD (eds) Basic and clinical endocrinology, edn 4. Appleton and Lange, Norwalk, CT, p 370
7. Thomas JL, Bernardino ME, Samaan NA, Hickey RC (1980) CT of pheochromocytoma. AJR Am J Roentgenol 135:477–483
8. Korobkin M, Francis IR (1995) Adrenal imaging. Semin Ultrasound CT MR 16:317
9. Neumann HPH, Bausch B, McWhinney SR et al. (2002) Germ-line mutations in nonsyndromic pheochromocytomas N Engl J Med 346:1459–1466
10. Ilias I, Pacak K (2004) Current approaches and recommended algorithm for the diagnostic localization of pheochromocytoma. J Clin Endocrinol Metab 89:479–491
11. Sahdev A, Sohaib A, Monson JP, Grossman AB, Chew SL, Reznek RH (2005) CT and MR imaging of unusual locations of extra-adrenal paragangliomas (pheochromocytomas). Eur Radiol 15:85–92
12. Cirillo RL, Bennett WF, Vitellas KM, Poulos AG, Bova JG (1998) Pathology of the adrenal gland. AJR Am J Roentgenol 170:429–435
13. Goldfarb DA, Novick AC, Bravo EL, Straffon RA, Montie JE, Kay RE (1989) Experience with extra-adrenal pheochromocytoma. J Urol 142:931
14. Melicow MM (1987) One hundred cases of pheochromocytoma at the Columbia-Presbyterian Medical Center. Cancer 40:1977
15. Bravo EL (1983) Pheochromocytoma. Current concepts in diagnosis, localization, and mangement. Prim Care 10:75–86
16. Del Gaudio A (1985) Pheochromocytoma and renal artery stenosis. Int Surg 70:153
17. Gill IS, Meraney AM, Bravo EL, Novick AC (2000) Pheochromocytoma coexisting with renal artery lesions J Urol 164:296–301
18. Walther WM, Choyke PL (2001) Re: pheochromoctyoma coexisting with renal artery lesions. J Urol 165:2005–2006
19. Motta-Ramirez GA, Remer EM, Herts BR, Gill IS, Hamrahian AH (2005) Comparison of CT findings in symptomatic and incidentally discovered pheochromocytomas. AJR Am J Roentgenol 185:684–688
20. Miyajima A, Nakashima J, Baba S, Tachibana M, Nakamura K, Murai M (1997) Clinical experience with incidentally discovered pheochromocytoma. J Urol 157:1566–1568

21. Aso Y, Homma Y (1992) A survey on incidental adrenal tumors in Japan. J Urol 147:1478–1481

22. Cheah WK, Clark OH, Horn JK, Siperstein AE, Duh Q-Y (2002) Laparoscopic adrenalectomy for pheochromocytoma. World J Surg 26:1048–1051

23. Baguet JP, Hammer L, Mazzuco TL et al. (2004) Circumstances of discovery of phaeochromocytoma: a retrospective study of 41 consecutive patients. Eur J Endocrinol 150:681–686

24. Young WF (2007) The incidentally discovered adrenal mass. N Engl J Med 356:601–610

25. Crout JR, Sjoerdsma A (1964) Turnover and metabolism of catecholamine in patients with pheochromocytoma. J Clin Invest 43:94–102

26. Bravo EL (1991) Pheochromocytoma: new concepts and future trends. Kidney Int 40:544–556

27. Lucon AM, Pereira MA, Mendonca BB, Halpern A, Wajchenberg BL, Arap S (1997) Pheochromocytoma: study of 50 cases. J Urol 157:1208–1212

28. Kawashima A, Sandler CM, Fishman EK et al. (1998) Spectrum of CT findings in nonmalignant disease of the adrenal gland. RadioGraphics 18:393–412

29. Lenders JW, Pacak K, Walther MM et al. (2002) Biochemical diagnosis of pheochromocytoma: which test is best? JAMA 287:1427–1434

30. Casola G, Nicolet V, vanSonnenberg E et al. (1986) Unsuspected pheochromocytoma: Risk of blood-pressure alterations during percutaneous adrenal biopsy. Radiology 159:733–735

31. Dalal T, Maher MM, Kalra MK, Mueller PR (2005) Extraadrenal pheochromoctyoma: a rare cause of tachycarida and hpertension during percutaneous biopsy. AJR Am J Roentgenol 185:554–555

32. Gold RE, Wisinger BM, Geraci AR, Heinz LM (1972) Hypertensive crisis as a result of adrenal venography in a patient with pheochromocytoma. Radiology 102:579–580.

33. Christenson R, Smith CW, Burko H (1976) Arteriographic manifestations of pheochromocytoma. AJR Am J Roentgenol 126:567–575

34. Raisanen J, Shapiro B, Glazer GM et al. (1984) Plasma catecholamines in pheochromocytoma: Effect of urographic contrast media. AJR Am J Roentgenol 143:43–46

35. Mukherjee JJ, Peppercorn PD, Reznek RH et al. (1997) Pheochromocytoma: effect of nonionic contrast medium in CT on circulating catecholamine levels. Radiology 202:227–231

36. Bessell-Browne R, O'Malley ME (2007) CT of pheochromocytoma and paraganglioma: risk of adverse events with IV administration of nonionic contrast material. AJR Am J Roentgenol 188: 970–974

37. Mayo-Smith WW, Boland GW, Noto RB, Lee MJ (2001) State-of-the-art adrenal imaging. RadioGraphics 21:995–1012

38. Kawashima A, Sandler CM, Fishman EK et al. (1998) Spectrum of CT findings in nonmalignant disease of the adrenal gland. RadioGraphics 18:393–412

39. Bush WH, Elder JS, Crane RE, Wales LR (1985) Cystic pheochromocytoma. Urology 25:332–334

40. Francis IR, Korobkin M (1996) Pheochromocytoma. Radiol Clin North Am 34:1101–1112

41. Quint LE, Glazer GM, Francis IR, Shapiro B, Chenevert TL (1987) Pheochromocytoma and paraganglioma: comparison of MR imaging with CT and I-131 MIBG scintigraphy. Radiology 165:89–93

42. Mannelli M, Ianni L, Cilotti A, Conti A (1999) Pheochromocytoma in Italy: a multicentric retrospective study. Eur J Endocrinol 141:619–624

43. Korobkin M, Giordano TJ, Borduer FJ et al. (1996) Adrenal adenomas: relationship between histologic lipid and CT and MR findings. Radiology 200:743–747

44. Boland GW, Lee MJ, Gazelle SG et al. (1998) Characterization of adrenal masses using unenhanced CT: an analysis of the CT literature. AJR Am J Roentgenol 171:201–204

45. Szolar DH, Korobkin M, Reittner P et al. (2005) Radiology Adrenocortical Carcinomas and adrenal pheochromocytoma: mass and enhancement loss evolution at delayed contrast-enhanced CT. 234:479–485

46. Blake MA, Krishnamoorthy SK, Boland GW et al. (2003) Low-density pheochromocytoma on CT: a mimicker of adrenal adenoma. AJR Am J Roentgenol 181:1663–1668

47. Caoili EM, Korobkin M, Francis IR et al. (2002) Adrenal masses: characterization with combined unenhanced and delayed enhanced CT. Radiology 222:629–633

48. Blake MA, Krishnamoorthy SK, Boland GW et al. (2003) Low-density pheochromocytoma on CT: a mimicker of adrenal adenoma. AJR Am J Roentgenol 181:1663–1668

49. Yoon JK, Remer EM, Herts BR (2006) Incidental pheochromocytoma mimicking adrenal adenoma because of rapid contrast enhancement loss. AJR Am J Roentgenol 187:1309–1311

50. Kawashima A, Sandler CM, Ernst RD et al. (1999) Imaging of nontraumatic hemorrhage of the adrenal gland. Radiographics 19:949–963

51. Jalil ND, Pattou FN, Combemale F et al. (1998) Effectiveness and limits of preoperative imaging studies for the localization of pheochromocytomas and paragangliomas: a review of 282 cases—French Association of Surgery (AFC) and the French Association of Endocrine Surgeons (AFCE). Eur J Surg 164:23–28

52. van Gils APG, Falke THM, van Erkel AR et al. (1991) MR imaging and MIBG scintigraphy of pheochromocytomas and extra adrenal functioning paragangliomas. RadioGraphics 11:37–57

53. Namimoto T, Yamashita Y, Mitsuzaki K et al. (2001) Adrenal masses: quantification of fat content with double-echo chemical shift in-phase and opposed-phase FLASH MR images for differentiation of adrenal adenomas. Radiology 218:642–646

54. Glazer GM, Woolsey EJ, Borrello J et al. (1986) Adrenal tissue characterization using MR imaging. Radiology 158:73–79

55. Krebs TL, Wagner BJ, Penney PJ (1997) MR appearances of pheochromocytoma of the adrenal gland with pathologic correlation (abstr.) Radiology 205:342

56. Varghese JC, Hahn PF, Papanicolaou N, Mayo-Smith WW, Gaa JA, Lee MJ (1997) MR differentiation of phaeochromocytoma from other adrenal lesions based on

qualitative analysis of T2 relaxation times. Clin Radiol 52:603–606

57. Brown ED, Semelka RC (1995) Magnetic resonance imaging of the adrenal gland and kidney. J Magn Reson 7:90–101

58. Yeh HC (1980) Sonography of the adrenal glands: normal glands and small masses. AJR Am J Roentgenol 135:1167–1177

59. Bowerman RA, Silver TM, Jaffe MH, Stuck KJ, Hinerman DL (1981) Sonography of adrenal pheochromocytomas. AJR Am J Roentgenol 137:1227–1231

60. Schwerk WB, Gorg C, Gorg K, Restrepo IK (1994) Adrenal pheochromocytomas: a broad spectrum of sonographic presentation. J Ultrasound Med 13:517–521

61. Miskulin J, Shulkin BL, Doherty GM, Sisson JC, Burney RE, Gauger PG (2003) Is preoperative iodine 123 meta-iodobenzylguanidine scintigraphy routinely necessary before initial adrenalectomy for pheochromocytoma? Surgery 134(6):918–922

62. Mozley PD (1994) The efficacy of iodine = 123 = MIBG as a screening test for pheochromocytoma. J Nucl Med 35:1138–1144

63. Brink I, Hoegerle S, Klisch J, Bley TA (2005) Imaging of pheochromocytoma and paraganglioma. Famil Cancer 4:61–68

64. Shulkin BL, Shapiro B, Francis IR, Dorr R, Shen SW, Sisson JC (1986) Primary extra-adrenal pheochromoytomas: positive I-123 MIBG imaging with negative I-131 MIBG imaging. Clin Nucl Med 11:851–854

65. van Gils APG, Falke THM, van Erkel AR et al. (1991) MR imaging and MIBG scintigraphy of pheochromocytomas and extra adrenal functioning paragangliomas. Radio-Graphics 11:37–57

66. Berglund AS, Hulthen UL, Manhem P, Thorrson O, Wollmer P, Tornquist C (2001) Metaiodobenzylguanidine (MIBG) scintigraphy and computed tomography (CT) in clinical practice. Primary and secondary evaluation for localization of pheochromocytomas. J Int Med 249:247–251

67. Van Der Horst-Schrivers ANA, Jager PL, Boezen HM, Schouten JP, Kema IP, Links TP (2006) Iodine-123 metaiodobenzylguanidine scintigraphy in localising phaeochromocytomas–experience and meta-analysis. Anticancer Res 26:1599–1604

68. Fujita A, Hyodoh H, Kawamura Y, Kanegae K, Furuse M, Kanazawa K (2000) Use of fusion images of I-131 metaiodobenzylguanidine, SPECT, and magnetic resonance studies to identify malignant pheochromocytoma. Clin Nucl Med 24:440–442

69. van der Harst E, de Herder WW, Bruining HA et al. (2001) [123I]Metaiodoenzylguandine and [111In]octreotide uptake in benign and malignant pheochromocytomas. J Clin Endorinol Metab 86:685–693

70. Shulkin BL, Thompson NW, Shapiro B, Francis IR, Sisson JC (1999) Pheochromocytomas: imaging with 2-[fluorine-18]fluoro-2-deoxy-D-glucose PET. Radiology 212:35–41

71. Pacak K, Eisenhofer G, Carasquillo JA, Chen CC, Li ST, Goldstein DS (2001) 6-[18F]Fluorodopamine positron emission tomographic (PET) scanning for diagnostic localization of pheochromoctyomas. Hypertension 38:6–8

Contents

Introduction

Adrenal mass characterization using non invasive diagnostic imaging has gained more interest in recent years due to the prevalence of adrenal pathology detected on routine CT examinations performed for clinical conditions that are not related to suspicion of adrenal diseases, as well as adrenal masses detected at the time of staging CT exams performed for various extra-adrenal malignancies. The clinically silent adrenal masses incidentally detected by these imaging studies are commonly referred to as adrenal "incidentalomas" and were first described more than 20 years ago [1]. Their prevalence approaches 3% in middle age, and increases to as much as 10% in the elderly. Up to 5% of abdominal CT scans obtained for reasons other than suspected functioning adrenal mass will demonstrate an adrenal mass [2]. Differentiating benign adrenal adenomas from malignant masses using noninvasive imaging methods can reduce the need both for percutaneous adrenal biopsy in patients with cancer and the follow-up imaging of incidental adrenal masses.

Adrenal masses found on imaging studies can be benign or malignant. These include adenomas, adrenal cysts (Fig. 8.1), hematomas, myelolipomas (Fig. 8.2), ganglioneuromas, pheochromocytomas, adrenal cortical carcinomas, metastases from other cancers, and other rare entities [4]. Clinical diagnostic evaluation is used to further subdivide adrenal adenomas into (a) functional or

M.M. Al-Hawary (✉)
Department of Radiology, University of Michigan Hospitals, 1500 E. Medical Center Drive, Ann Arbor, Michigan 48109-0030
E-mail: alhawary@umich.edu

M.A. Blake, G. Boland (eds.), *Adrenal Imaging*, DOI 10.1007/978-1-59745-560-2_8,
© 2009 Humana Press, a part of Springer Science+Business Media, LLC

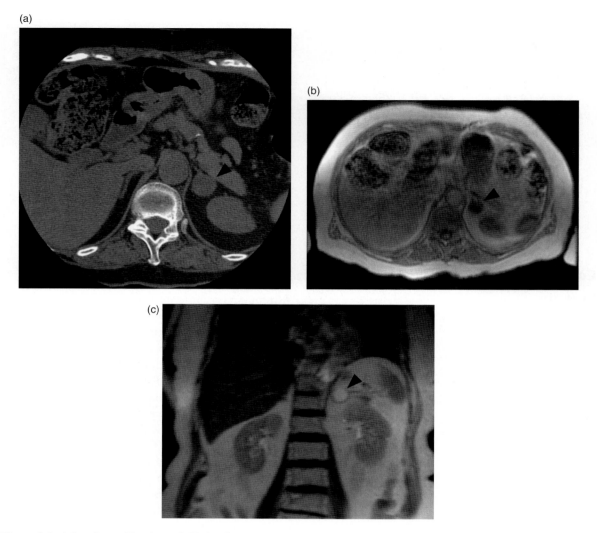

Figure 8.1 Adrenal cyst. Unenhanced CT (**a**) showing a well defined hypodense mass (*arrowhead*) in the left adrenal gland with −3 HU density. Axial T1-weighted (**b**) and coronal T2-weighted (**c**) MR images show fluid intensity signal in the lesion

hypersecreting and (b) non-functional depending on whether or not they elaborate adrenal hormones such as aldosterone, cortisol or androgens [5]. Complete history and physical examination in addition to biochemical evaluation of all pertinent hormones will help confirm the diagnosis in cases of functional (clinical or sub clinical) adrenal masses [6]. Radiological evaluation in these instances will be performed mainly for tumor detection and localization, prior to surgical removal. In non-functioning masses, additional testing, primarily using imaging studies, will be required for further evaluation and characterization. The focus of our chapter addresses the role of CT in the characterization for guiding management of adrenal masses, with emphasis on distinguishing between adenomas and non-adenomas.

CT

CT is the most commonly used diagnostic imaging modality for the detection and in many centers (including our own) for the characterization of adrenal masses. Care should be first taken to exclude extraadrenal normal variants or other

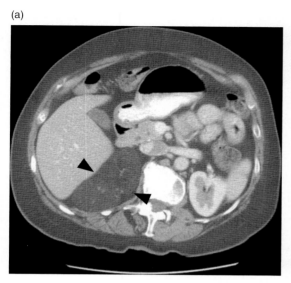

(a)

(b)

Figure 8.2 Adrenal myelolipoma. Right adrenal myelolipoma (**a**) with predominant fat attenuation and minimal soft tissue (*arrowheads*). Left adrenal myelolipoma (*arrowhead*) with predominant soft tissue attenuation and small focus of macroscopic fat (*arrow*)

conditions that may masquerade as adrenal tumors on CT including exophytic upper pole renal masses, tortuous splenic vessels, periadrenal and adrenal portosystemic collaterals, pancreatic tail masses, splenic lobulation / accessory spleen (Fig. 8.3), gastric diverticulum, prominent lobation of the hepatic lobe, exophytic hepatic tumors, fluid-filled colon and retroperitoneal tumors.

Once an adrenal lesion is detected, the important initial imaging characteristics that are evaluated include lesion size, homogeneity, and presence of fat, hemorrhage or calcifications. Additional characterization includes CT density evaluation on both unenhanced and enhanced CT studies.

Nodule/mass Size

It is generally considered that the risk of malignancy in an adrenal mass increases with increasing size. Most masses smaller than 4 cm are likely to be benign; however most studies have shown that size alone cannot be used to exclude malignancy [6]. Autopsy series show that less than 2% of adrenal adenomas are greater than 4 cm in diameter and less than 0.03% are greater than 6 cm, whereas 92% of adrenal cortical carcinomas are greater than 6 cm [7]. Another review reported that adrenal

cortical carcinoma accounts for 2% of tumors that are 4 cm or less, 6% of tumors that are 4.1–6 cm, and 25% of tumors that are >6 cm [4]. Since 25% of adrenal masses >6 cm are adrenocortical carcinomas, this size is usually considered a threshold for surgical resection [4].

Nodule/mass Homogeneity

Most adrenal adenomas are relatively homogeneous, and rarely undergo hemorrhagic degeneration, necrosis, or calcifications. The homogeneous nature of most adrenal adenomas is helpful in distinguishing them from malignant lesions. However adrenal adenomas, especially larger ones, may occasionally undergo intratumoral hemorrhagic degeneration with development of avascular and cystic internal regions and subsequent fibrosis and ultimate calcification [8]. These uncommon adenomas may show variable CT attenuation and enhancement pattern and can be confused with adrenal malignancy and biopsy or resection may be necessary for ultimate diagnosis (Fig. 8.4). Large adenomas may also undergo internal hemorrhage and ultimately evolve to become a "pseudocyst." Therefore the differential diagnosis for calcified cystic lesions includes adrenocortical carcinoma, hydatid

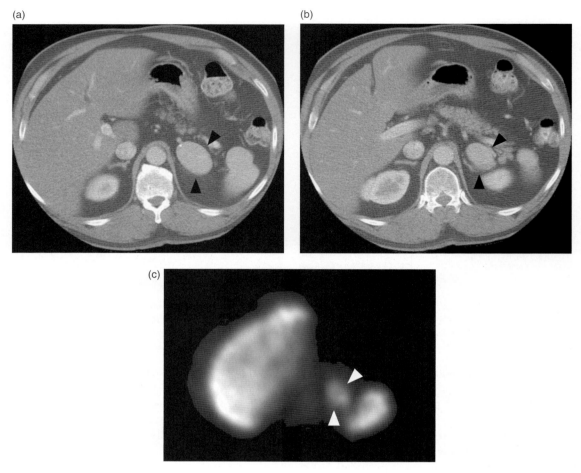

Figure 8.3 Adrenal pseudotumor. Accessory spleen simulating an adrenal mass. Enhanced CT (**a,b**) showing a soft tissue lesion in the region of the left adrenal gland (*arrowheads*). Sulfur colloid SPECT/CT examination (**c**) shows radiocolloid localization to the same lesion in the left juxta-adrenal position (*white arrowheads*), consistent with an accessory spleen

disease, hemorrhage, metastases, myelolipomas, hemangiomas, pheochromocytomas, neuroblastomas (mainly seen in children), granulomatous disease and epithelial cysts [3, 8, 9]. Imaging findings such as presence of fat which suggest a diagnosis of myelolipoma or high density in patients with adrenal hemorrhage can at times be helpful in making a specific diagnosis, but this is true in only a small percentage of adrenal masses. Occasionally adrenal adenomas may calcify or may undergo myelolipomatous metaplasia appearing as macroscopic fat (Fig. 8.5). The heterogeneous appearance of adrenal lesions alone is not helpful in distinguishing between benign and malignant adrenal masses. In addition to the imaging appearance, knowledge of

the biochemical abnormalities in suspected cases of hyper-secreting tumors and presence or absence of extra-adrenal primary neoplasm should also be taken into account when attempting to characterize adrenal masses [10].

Nodule/mass Density

Many studies have shown the usefulness of attenuation measurements or CT densitometry using unenhanced CT in the differentiation of benign from malignant adrenal masses [11, 12]. This is based on the premise that unenhanced CT can detect intracytoplasmic lipid (composed mainly of cholesterol, fatty acids, and neutral fat), which is often

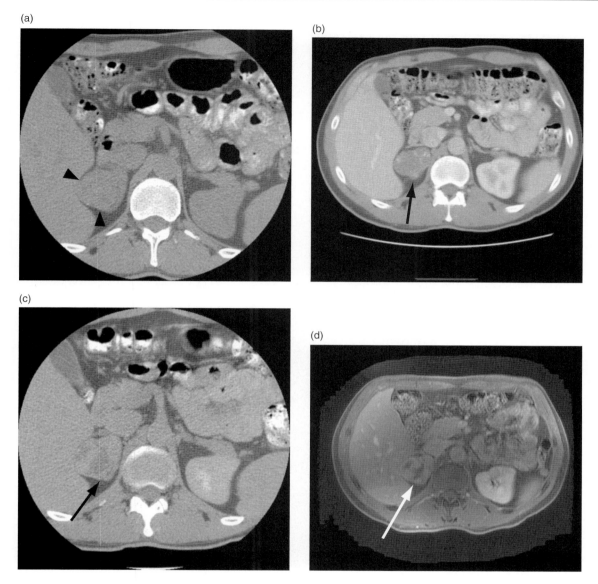

Figure 8.4 Heterogeneous adrenal adenoma mimicking adrenal carcinoma. Pathology proven adrenal cortical adenoma with organizing hematoma (*arrowheads*) on: **a** unenhanced; **b** enhanced; **c** 15-min-delayed CT; **d** axial delayed post contrast T1-weighted 3D SPGR MRI images. There is a heterogeneous right adrenal mass (*arrows*) showing several thin peripheral areas of enhancement on the early enhanced images with central lower attenuation areas demonstrating progressive increased enhancement on the delayed enhanced images on CT and MRI

abundantly present within most adenomas but rarely present within malignant lesions [11]. Korobkin et al. [11] showed an inverse linear relationship between the percentage of lipid-rich cortical cells in resected adrenal adenomas and the unenhanced CT attenuation number and concluded that the presence and amount of histologic lipid in many adrenal adenomas accounts for their

low attenuation on the unenhanced CT scans. Meta-analysis of a number of studies by Boland et al. [12] that evaluated attenuation values at unenhanced CT, found that sensitivity for characterizing a lesion as benign ranged from 47% at a threshold of 2 HU to 88% at a threshold of 20 HU. Similarly, specificity varied from 100% at a threshold of 2 HU to 84% at a threshold of

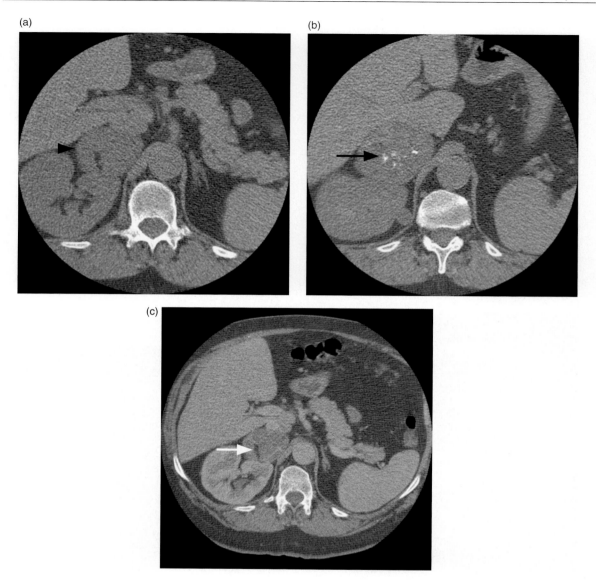

Figure 8.5 Heterogeneous adrenal adenoma with macroscopic fat and calcifications. Pathology proven right adrenal cortical adenoma with myelolipomatous metaplasia and secondary degenerative changes and hemorrhage. Unenhanced (**a,b**) and enhanced (**c**) CT examinations showing a heterogeneous right adrenal gland mass (*arrowhead*) containing low attenuation areas with high attenuation areas consistent with calcification (*black arrow*) and areas of fat density (*white arrow*)

20 HU. They suggested that 10 HU was most optimal, with sensitivity of 71% and specificity of 98%. Another study by Korobkin et al. [13], which compared their results to other prior reported studies [14–16] on the value of unenhanced CT, found that a threshold value of 10 HU gave the most optimal overall ratio of 73% sensitivity and 96% specificity for the diagnosis of adenoma.

Adenomas containing relatively small amounts of lipid, or "lipid poor" adenomas, account for 10%–40% of all adenomas. They have an attenuation value of more than 10 HU on unenhanced CT and therefore cannot be distinguished from non adenomas (metastases or primary adrenocortical carcinomas and most pheochromocytomas). Unlike unenhanced attenuation values, those

(a)

(b)

(c)

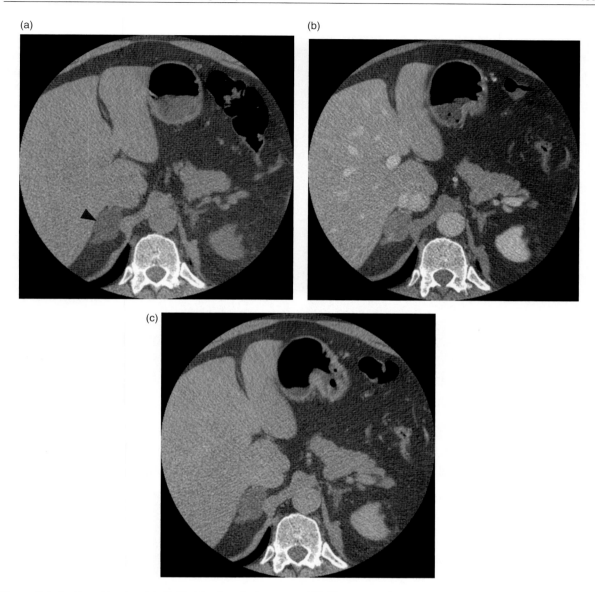

Figure 8.6 Incidental benign right lipid-rich adrenal adenoma (arrow head) on: **a** unenhanced; **b** enhanced; **c** 15-min-delayed CT. The attenuation values were −3, 52 and 14 HU respectively giving an absolute contrast washout value of 69%

obtained on adrenal masses following intravenous contrast-enhancement on routine abdominal CT scans show overlap between adenomas and metastases to a degree that does not allow reliable differentiation between them [13, 17–19]. In one study the mean enhanced attenuations of adrenal adenomas and non adenomas were nearly identical (64 HU vs 62 HU), confirming the inability of CT attenuation values on routine enhanced abdominal CT scans to differentiate adenomas from non adenomas [17]. However, it has been shown in several studies performed to evaluate the enhancement features of adrenal masses that adenomas, in contrast to malignant masses, tend to have a rapid loss of attenuation value or rapid washout soon after enhancement with intravenous contrast (IV) material on delayed scans (Fig. 8.6) [13, 17, 18, 20, 21]. The washout features were also shown to be independent of the lipid content of an adenoma, as lipid-poor adenomas, (those with attenuation values greater than 10 H on unenhanced CT) demonstrate enhancement washout features nearly identical to lipid-rich adenomas [22, 23] (Fig. 8.7).

Depending on whether an unenhanced scan is obtained or not, two types of percentage washout,

(1) absolute and (2) relative to the initial enhancement of adrenal masses can be calculated. The absolute percent enhancement washout is obtained using the enhanced attenuation value, the delayed enhanced value, and the unenhanced value using the following formula:

$$\text{Absolute enhancement washout} = \frac{\text{Enhanced attenuation value} - \text{Delayed enhanced value}}{\text{Enhanced attenuation value} - \text{Unenhanced attenuation value}}$$

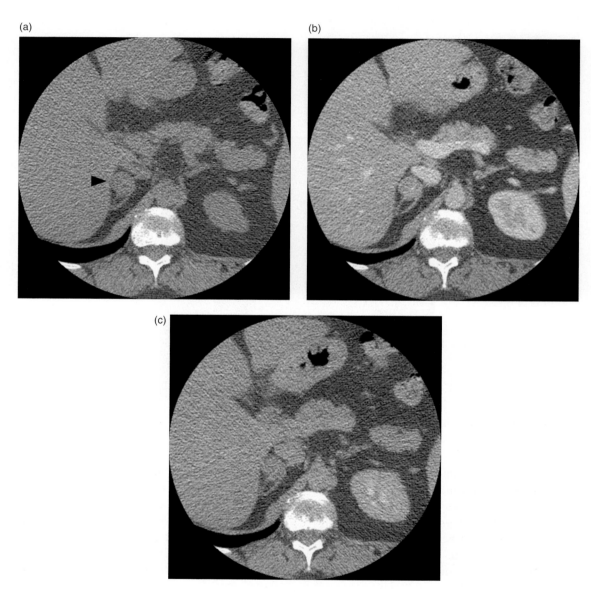

(a)

(b)

(c)

Figure 8.7 Incidental right adrenal lipid-poor adenoma (*arrowhead*) on: **a** unenhanced; **b** enhanced; **c** 15-min-delayed CT. The attenuation values were 25, 90 and 45 HU respectively giving an absolute contrast washout value of 69%

If an incidental adrenal mass is detected on routine contrast-enhanced CT, delayed images through the adrenal mass can be performed at 15 min following the initial scan to calculate the relative percent enhancement washout. The relative percent enhancement washout is obtained using the enhanced attenuation value and the delayed enhanced using the following formula:

$$\text{Relative enhancement washout} = \frac{\text{Enhanced attenuation value} - \text{Delayed enhanced value}}{\text{Enhanced attenuation value}}$$

Several studies have attempted to systematically assess the shortest time delay required after contrast enhancement to accurately differentiate adenomas from nonadenomas.

Szolar and Kammerhuber [20] showed that the mean absolute percentage loss of enhancement on 10-min-delayed scans was 62% for adenomas and 31% for metastases. Using a threshold of 60% for the diagnosis of adenoma, a sensitivity of 97% and specificity of 100% was achieved. Korobkin et al. [18] analyzed a group of patients with adrenal masses who had undergone delayed CT scans at 5, 10, 15, 30 and 45 min after enhancement. A much greater washout of initial enhancement occurred at each delay time for the adenomas than for the nonadenomas. The mean washout at 5 and 15 min after enhancement was 51% and 70% for the adenomas and only 8% and 19% for the nonadenomas (Fig. 8.8). The optimal combination of sensitivity and specificity for the diagnosis of adrenal adenoma occurred on the 15-min-delayed images, with sensitivity: specificity ratio of 88% and 96% at a threshold of 60% washout. Using a relative percentage washout threshold of 40% at the 15 min delay, the sensitivity: specificity ratio was 96% and 100% respectively. Using a 10 min enhancement delay, Blake et al. [24] showed that a threshold of 52% absolute enhancement washout yielded a sensitivity and specificity of 100% and 98%, but only if masses less than 0 HU or higher than 43 HU on unenhanced CT were excluded. For the calculation of relative enhancement washout, a threshold of 37.5% resulted in a sensitivity and specificity of 100% and 95% respectively.

Our adrenal mass CT protocol is mostly based on the study published by Caoili et al. [25] assessing the adrenal mass characterization with combined unenhanced and delayed enhanced CT. Use of this protocol resulted in a sensitivity: specificity ratio for the diagnosis of adenoma of 98% and 92%, respectively. Our protocol for characterizing adrenal masses using CT densitometry can be summarized as follows.

For an adrenal mass detected on prior contrast-enhanced CT that is referred for CT characterization, we start by performing an unenhanced CT. If the attenuation value is <10 HU, then the mass is characterized as a likely lipid rich adenoma and no further workup is done. If the attenuation value is >10 HU, then intravenous contrast is administered (our current protocol includes the use of 125 cc of Ultravist-300, Bayer HealthCare pharmaceuticals, administered at a rate of 3 cc/s) and images obtained during the portal venous phase of hepatic enhancement with a 65-s scan delay, and then 15-min-delayed images are acquired. Absolute enhancement washout calculations are performed using the above-described equation. If absolute enhancement values are = or >60%, the mass is characterized as a lipid poor adenoma and no further evaluation is recommended. If the absolute enhancement washout is less than 60%, further evaluation is usually necessary, such as with chemical shift MRI, FDG-PET, percutaneous biopsy, surgical resection or clinical follow up (Table 8.1).

CT Histogram Analysis

One recently described method using a different approach to the CT density evaluation of the adrenal nodule/mass is based on histogram analysis of the pixels contained within the adrenal mass [26, 27]. The rationale of the histogram analysis in trying to differentiate adrenal adenoma from nonadenoma is based on the distribution of tissue attenuation inside the lesion which might be more sensitive than one based on the calculation of the overall mean attenuation value. The histogram analysis

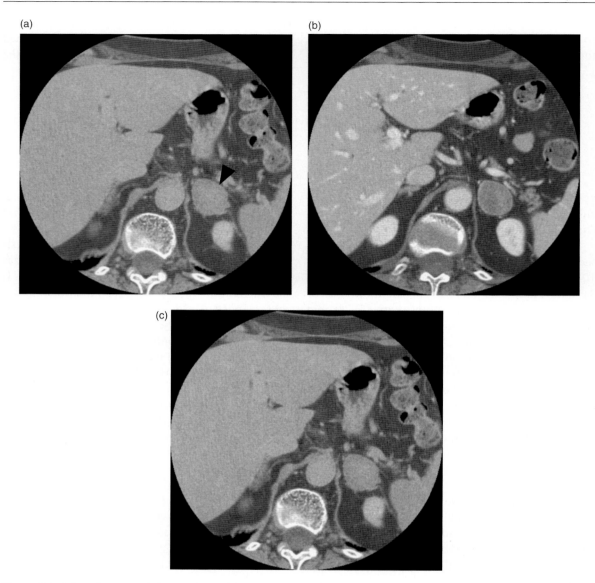

Figure 8.8 Adrenal metastasis in a patient with history of lung and breast carcinoma. Left adrenal gland mass (*arrowhead*) on: **a** unenhanced; **b** enhanced; **c** 15-min- delayed CT. The attenuation values were 25, 75 and 71 HU respectively giving an absolute contrast washout value of 8%

would allow detection of negative pixels (fat) < 0 HU and probably more accurately characterize adenomas since they usually contain intracytoplasmic lipid. On enhanced CT obtained after contrast administration, there is overall increase in the mean attenuation value in an adenoma even though lipid tissue is present, leading to too much overlap in mean attenuation between the adenomas and non adenomas.

The study conducted by Bae et al. [26] showed that the sensitivity of diagnosis of adrenal adenoma at contrast-enhanced CT was higher with the histogram method than with the mean attenuation method. Whereas only 10.9% (20 of 184) of adrenal adenomas had a mean attenuation of 10 HU or less, 52.7% (97 of 184) of them contained negative pixels. Out of the 31 metastases, none demonstrated negative pixels (excluding obvious necrotic or fatty

Table 8.1. CT evaluation algorithm for distinguishing adenomas from non-adenomas

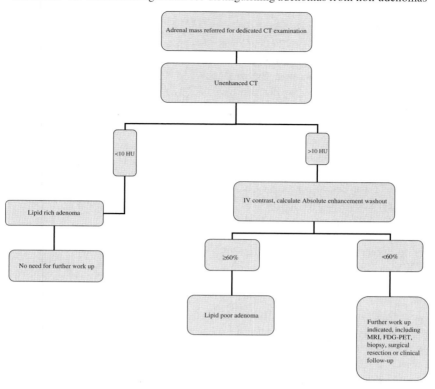

masses), but it was uncertain if the presence of just a single pixel with a negative attenuation provides 100% specific evidence for the diagnosis of adrenal adenoma. If more conservative criteria were used—for example, diagnosis of adenomas for masses with more than 5% or more than 10% negative pixels, sensitivity decreased to 35.9% (66 of 184) or 27.7% (51 of 184). A threshold of at least 10% negative pixels was suggested as an appropriate criterion for diagnosis of an adenoma because the lowest percentage negative pixels in masses with mean attenuation of 10 HU or less was 9.8%.

Another series published by Remer et al. [27] performed a study of pixel analysis and found that there were metastases, pheochromocytomas, and adrenocortical carcinomas that contained negative pixels. This decreased the specificity of the histogram technique on enhanced scans to between 64.4% and 88.5%. Comparing adenomas and metastases only improved specificity to 93.2%–95.5% on enhanced CT. Although using a 10% negative pixel threshold maintained high specificity of 98.9%, sensitivity dropped to unacceptably low levels of between 11.3% and

12.9% on enhanced studies. In conclusion, this study showed that using a 10% negative pixel threshold to discriminate adenomas from nonadenomas on enhanced scans had a high specificity of 98.9% but suffered from poor sensitivity, limiting its clinical application. Further modifications of this technique may be necessary before it is clinically useful.

CT Density Measurement Accuracy

The use of a universal, scanner-independent threshold inherently assumes that different scanner types and different scanning protocols lead to constant density measurements. Stadler et al. [28] assessed the variability in CT density measurements of adrenal tumors using a range of different scanning protocols and different CT scanners. The authors found a wide range of CT attenuation for a particular tissue type, depending on the tube voltage (peak kilovoltage), scanner type, reconstruction algorithm, and tissue surrounding the lesion. Slice thickness did not affect the CT density measurements significantly in their study. They showed a protocol-dependent variation (different kilovoltage) in mean densities of up to 6.4 HU. After varying both scanner and protocol, they also observed a maximum intraindividual variation in CT attenuation measurements of 12 HU. This finding raised questions on the accuracy of lesion classification with CT attenuation around the suggested threshold level of 10 HU. In another study, Hahn et al. [29] compared the unenhanced density of the same adrenal lesion on two different manufacturers' scanners and showed only very slight differences. Despite the variations discussed above, both studies confirmed the benefit of using attenuation values of unenhanced CT for discrimination of adrenal adenomas from non adenomatous lesions. More recently Birnbaum et al. [30] have also shown that CT attenuation values vary significantly between different manufacturers' multi-detector row scanners, different generations of multi-detector row scanners, and combination of scanners and convolution kernels. This was especially true for densities in the lower range of CT number scales, thus affecting the reliability of density measurements of cysts and adrenal adenomas. These observations raised doubt about the recommendation of a universal scanner- and protocol-independent threshold. Therefore quantitative methods relying on absolute CT attenuation values should be always be used with calibration phantoms to ensure that accurate CT numbers are obtained that are specific for a specific scanner.

Summary

1. Incidental adrenal lesions are commonly detected on CT scans.
2. Characterization needs to determine if the mass if functioning or non-functioning, benign or malignant.
3. Malignancy is rare in patients without a history of malignant disease.
4. The liklihood of malignancy increases with lesion size.
5. Non-contrast CT can differentiate those adenomas that are lipid-rich adenomas from lipid poor malignant disease.
6. Up to 40% of adenomas are lipid poor and cannot be characterized by non-contrast CT.
7. Contrast enhanced washout CT is the imaging test of choice and effectively differentiates benign from malignant masses in most patients.

References

1. Geelhoed GW, Druy EM (1982) Management of the adrenal "incidentaloma". Surgery 92:866–874
2. Kloos RT, Gross MD, Francis IR, Korobkin M, Shapiro B (1995) Incidentally discovered adrenal masses. Endocr Rev 16:460–484
3. Dunnick NR, Korobkin M (2002) Imaging of adrenal incidentalomas: current status. AJR Am J Roentgenol 179:559–568
4. Grumbach MM, Biller BM, Braunstein GD, Campbell KK, Carney JA, Godley PA, Harris EL, Lee JK, Oertel YC, Posner MC, Schlechte JA, Wieand HS (2003) Management of the clinically inapparent adrenal mass ("incidentaloma"). Ann Intern Med 138:424–429
5. Mayo-Smith WW, Boland GW, Noto RB, Lee MJ (2001) State-of-the-art adrenal imaging. Radiographics 21(4):995–1012
6. Mansmann G, Lau J, Balk E, Rothberg M, Miyachi Y, Bornstein SR (2004) The clinically inapparent adrenal mass: update in diagnosis and management. Endocr Rev 25(2):309–340
7. Copeland PM (1999) The incidentally discovered adrenal mass: an update. Endocrinologist 9:415–423
8. Newhouse JH, Heffess CS, Wagner BJ, Imray TJ, Adair CF, Davidson AJ (1999) Large degenerated adrenal adenomas: radiologic-pathologic correlation. Radiology 210(2):385–391
9. Kenney PJ, Stanley RJ (1987) Calcified adrenal masses. Urol Radiol 9:9–15
10. Korobkin M (2000) CT characterization of adrenal masses: the time has come. Radiology 217:629–632
11. Korobkin M, Giordano TJ, Bordeur FJ et al. (1996) Adrenal adenomas: relationship between histologic lipid and CT and MR findings. Radiology 200:743–747
12. Boland GW, Lee MJ, Gazelle GS, Halpern EF, McNicholas MM, Mueller PR (1998) Characterization of adrenal masses using unenhanced CT: an analysis of the CT literature. AJR Am J Roentgenol 171:201–204
13. Korobkin M, Brodeur FJ, Yutzy GG et al. (1996) Differentiation of adrenal adenomas from nonadenomas using CT attenuation values. AJR Am J Roentgenol 166:531–536
14. Lee MJ, Hahn PF, Papanicolaou N et al. (1991) Benign and malignant adrenal masses: CT distinction with attenuation coefficients, size, and observer analysis. Radiology 179:415–418
15. Van Erkel AR, Van Gils APG, Lequin M, Kruitwagen C, Bloem JL, Falke THM (1994) CT and MR distinction of adenomas and nonadenomas of the adrenal glands. J Comput Assist Tomogr 18:432–438
16. Singer AA, Obuchowski NA, Einstein DM, Paushter DM (1994) Metastasis or adenoma?: computed tomographic evaluation of the adrenal mass. Cleve Clin J Med 61:200–205
17. Korobkin M, Brodeur FJ, Francis IR et al. (1998) CT time-attenuation washout curves of adrenal adenomas and non-adenomas. AJR Am J Roentgenol 170:747–752
18. Korobkin M, Brodeur FJ, Francis IR, Quint LE, Dunnick NR, Goodsitt M (1996) Delayed enhanced CT

for differentiation of benign from malignant adrenal masses. Radiology 200:737–742

19. Boland GW, Hahn PF, Pena C, Mueller PR (1997) Adrenal masses: characterization with delayed contrast-enhanced CT. Radiology 202:693–696

20. Szolar DH, Kammerhuber FH (1998) Adrenal adenomas and nonadenomas: assessment of washout at delayed contrast-enhanced CT. Radiology 207:369–375

21. Szolar DH, Kammerhuber F (1997) Quantitative CT evaluation of adrenal gland masses: a step forward in the differentiation between adenomas and nonadenomas? Radiology 202:517–522

22. Caoili EM, Korobkin M, Francis IR, Cohan RH, Dunnick NR (2000) Delayed enhanced CT of lipid-poor adrenal adenomas. AJR Am J Roentgenol 175:1411–1415

23. Pena CS, Boland GW, Hahn PF, Lee MJ, Mueller PR (2000) Characterization of indeterminate (lipid-poor) adrenal masses: use of washout characteristics at contrast-enhanced CT. Radiology 217:798–802

24. Blake MA, Kaira MK, Sweeney AT et al. (2006) Distinguishing benign from malignant adrenal masses: multi-detector row CT protocol with 10-minute delay. Radiology 238:578–585

25. Caoili EM, Korobkin M, Isaac R. Francis IR et al. (2002) Adrenal masses: characterization with combined unenhanced and delayed enhanced CT. Radiology 222:629–633

26. Bae KT, Fuangtharnthip P, Prasad SR, Joe BN, Heiken JP (2003) Adrenal masses: CT characterization with histogram analysis method. Radiology 228:735–742

27. Remer EM, Motta-Ramirez GA, Shepardson LB, Hamrahian AH, Herts BR (2006) CT Histogram analysis in pathologically proven adrenal masses. AJR Am J Roentgenol 187:191–196

28. Stadler A, Schima W, Prager G et al. (2004) CT Density measurements for characterization of adrenal tumors ex vivo: variability among three CT scanners. AJR Am J Roentgenol 182:671–675

29. Hahn PF, Blake MA, Boland GW (2006) Adrenal lesions: attenuation measurement differences between CT scanners. Radiology 240:458–463

30. Birnbaum BA, Hindman N, Lee J, Babb JS (2007) Multi-detector row CT attenuation measurements: assessment of intra and interscanner variability with an anthropomorphic body CT phantom. Radiology 242:109–119

MRI of the Adrenal Glands

9

Philip J. Kenney

Contents

P.J. Kenney (✉)
Department of Diagnostic Radiology, University of
Alabama at Birmingham, JT N370, 619 19th Street South,
Birmingham, AL 35249-6830, USA
E-mail: pkenney@uabmc.edu

Introduction

Early in the history of abdominal Magnetic Resonance Imaging (MRI) publications on its ability to image adrenal glands and adrenal disorders appeared [1, 2]. Despite limits of the MRI technology of the time, these studies showed MRI could depict normal and pathologic adrenals, and provided new features for analysis. Initial diagnostic criteria rested largely on signal intensity characteristics on T1 and T2 weighted sequences. Later, with release of intravenous gadolinium based contrast agents, the varying enhancement patterns of different masses was reported [3, 4] to be discriminatory. The recognition that MRI techniques could document the presence of lipid in adrenal masses [5] was the last key piece in classic MRI methods for adrenal evaluation.

Despite high statistical accuracy for MRI diagnosis of adrenal disease, the role of MRI in practice has been persistently limited. This is due to continued high expense of MRI compared to computed tomography (CT), as well as limited availability and expertise in adrenal imaging. In addition, both technical advances (helical, then multislice CT, Positron Emission Tomography (PET)) as well as increased knowledge (CT attenuation, CT assessment of washout, histogram analysis) in other methodologies has continued to limit the utility of MRI. In no area except perhaps suspected pheochromocytoma, is MRI clearly the first and preferred imaging method. For most other uses, MRI is considered equivalent, and used either in patients for whom

M.A. Blake, G. Boland (eds.), *Adrenal Imaging*, DOI 10.1007/978-1-59745-560-2_9,
© 2009 Humana Press, a part of Springer Science+Business Media, LLC

iodinated contrast is contraindicated, in pregnant patients or others for whom avoidance of radiation is desired, or in whom preceding studies have not been conclusive.

Technique for MRI of the Adrenals

A typical MRI protocol for adrenal imaging includes: three plane localizer to make certain of proper coverage. High quality axial T1 and T2 weighted images (3–5-mm sections preferably with suspended respiration) are standard. Chemical shift imaging with Gradient Echo T1 weighted images done with suspended respiration using same TR (repetition time) and different TE (echo time) to obtain images with fat and water protons in-phase on one set of images, and opposed-phase on another are now standard; again usually axial plane. Typically a standard dose of intravenous gadolinium contrast is also given and breath-hold T1 weighted images repeated.

Details of the imaging sequences have varied over time, with individual preference, and specific MR instruments. Axial images are obtained due to their similarity to CT images, and familiarity of most radiologists with that orientation. Coronal T1, T2, and T1 weighted images after contrast are very useful when a large mass is present, as differentiation of adrenal origin (vs renal hepatic or other) is commonly more clear on coronal (or sagittal plane). Radiofrequency fat suppression on T2 weighted images markedly improves visualization of normal adrenals and small masses. Without fat suppression, chemical shift edge artifact on heavily T2 weighted images can make visualization of the normal adrenal problematic (as the chemical shift can be as much as the thickness of normal adrenal limbs) and obscure small lesions. We prefer fat suppressed T1 weighted images for gadolinium enhanced series.

Because of the location of the adrenal glands near both the diaphragm and large blood vessels (aorta, vena cava), and the small size of the normal glands, certain technical factors are key, including high spatial resolution and limiting artifact due to respiratory motion and blood flow. Higher field strength, stronger gradients, and more sensitive specialized coils have evolved over the years to help improve these goals, and likely improvements

will continue. Phased array or multichannel coils with higher field strength (1.0–3.0 Tesla) combined with short sequences that can collect adequate anatomic coverage with thin slice technique (5 mm or less) in a single breath hold are necessary for adequate imaging. Use of dual echo in- and opposed phase sequences allows for comparable images for chemical shift images without misregistration or other technical issue (altered TR or flip angle).

Normal Anatomy

The morphology of the adrenal glands on transverse MRI images is the same as on transverse CT. While no definitive study has been performed with MRI, the same size criteria can be applied as with CT, since adrenal volume correlates well with CT volume—smooth thin limbs no thicker than 3–4 mm. On coronal images the normal adrenals can be seen as small "tricorn hat" shaped structures superomedial to the kidneys. With use of multiplanar imaging, and T1 and T2 weighted images and signal void in blood vessels, MRI is less prone than CT to pseudotumors from adjacent structures such as the spleen, gastric diverticulum, other bowel, or vascular structures.

Early studies described the normal adrenal glands as hypointense on both T1 and T2. When fat suppression is used, the adrenal tissue in fact is mildly more intense on T1 than liver, and clearly more intense on T2. It has not been clearly shown that differentiation between adrenal cortex and medullary tissue is possible with MRI, although high resolution T2 weighted scans of surgical adrenal specimens have shown differentiation between cortex and medulla [6].

MRI of Pheochromocytoma

Pheochromocytoma is a unique neuroendocrine tumor that arises from the adrenal medulla or paraganglia (see Chap. 7). It can present in a variety of ways, and represents a surprising percentage of incidentalomas. While pheochromocytoma can be detected by other noninvasive imaging methods, even early studies showed promise that MRI may be more specific [1, 2]. These early studies concentrated on the very high signal seen on heavily T2 weighted spin echo images, and the term "lamp bulb bright" became associated with pheochromocytoma. This became overemphasized, as about one-third of pheochromocytomas are only moderately hyperintense on T2 [7]. In fact, in one of the early reports, while 74% of the 19 pheochromocytomas reported were "superintense", 26% were only moderately hyperintense, and thus overlapped with adrenocortical carcinoma and metastatic disease [8].

Nevertheless, MRI is an excellent method for imaging detection of pheochromocytoma. The pathology of this tumor, which arises from medullary tissue, is that of cells with usually no lipid but a high amount of water protons. These tumors are of a size that are readily detected using current MRI technology. When small, pheochromocytomas typically are round, homogeneous masses with medium signal intensity (greater than muscle, near that of liver or kidney) and either hyperintense (greater than liver but less than water/CSF) or very hyperintense (similar to water/CSF). Even if benign, when these tumors exceed a certain size, hemorrhage and necrosis are common, and they may become predominantly cystic [9]. If so, the hemorrhagic and necrotic areas are typically hyperintense on T1 weighted images resulting in marked heterogeneity. On T2 weighted images cystic areas may be very hyperintense, while some hemorrhagic components may be hypointense, again resulting in marked heterogeneity.

The solid component of pheochromocytoma is quite vascular and tends to enhance considerably. Some studies [3] reported that pheochromocytoma on MRI after intravenous gadolinium contrast typically showed high early peak enhancement and prolonged washout. However, in Ichikawa's study[4], one of the seven pheochromocytomas had washout overlapping with adenoma. A study using CT washout reported high sensitivity and specificity for distinguishing adrenal adenomas from carcinoma or pheochromocytoma using threshold of 50% absolute percent washout [10]. Whether washout of MR contrast matches of that of CT contrast has or has not been proven, one report based on MRI contrast washout [11] indicated that as many as 50% of pheochromocytomas may have rapid washout.

Since pheochromocytomas may become large, MRI with its multiplanar imaging capability is often useful to demonstrate clearly the adrenal origin, although this advantage is less with the availability of very thin slice multidetector CT. MRI retains some advantage over CT regarding evaluation of paragangliomas, as they have the same MR characteristics as adrenal pheochromocyomas, and thus MR is somewhat more sensitive and specific than CT [12]. Paragangliomas, whatever their location, have the same MRI features as adrenal pheochromocytoma, and are readily detected with MRI (Fig. 9.1). Aside from the presence of metastasis or local invasion, there are no MRI features that indicate malignancy.

While scintigraphic procedures such as radiolabelled meta-iodo-benzyl-guanidine (MIGB) has some advantage in specificity as well as whole body imaging, several reports show MRI has some sensitivity advantage, and MRI is more readily available [12]. While there have been reports that some pheochromocytomas are FDG-PET avid, that is not a specific test, and does not separate pheochromocytoma from malignancy, and PET is neither more readily available nor cheaper than MRI [13].

MRI of Adrenocortical Carcinoma

Primary malignant tumors arising from adrenal cortex are rare tumors that are highly aggressive, with poor prognosis (see Chaps. 4 and 6). About half produce an endocrine disorder due to secretion of excess hormones, with cortisol production being most frequent. Thus these tumors must be suspected in a variety of clinical settings, that of an endocrine disorder of adrenal type, or in a patient with nonspecific symptoms of an upper abdominal mass due to a nonfunctional tumor, and also in a patient with incidental discovery of an adrenal mass.

Since these tumors typically are large at presentation, 5–15 cm, they are readily detected with MRI. Functional tumors can present with smaller sizes, 4–5 cm, and may be relatively homogeneous with medium signal intensity on T1 and moderately hyperintense on T2 weighted images (Fig. 9.2). These small tumors may overlap in appearance with benign adenoma; even histologic evaluation may be nonspecific and only biological behavior is definitive—that is development of metastasis or recurrence indicates malignancy [26]. However, they are usually quite large and heterogeneous due to central necrosis; although there may be

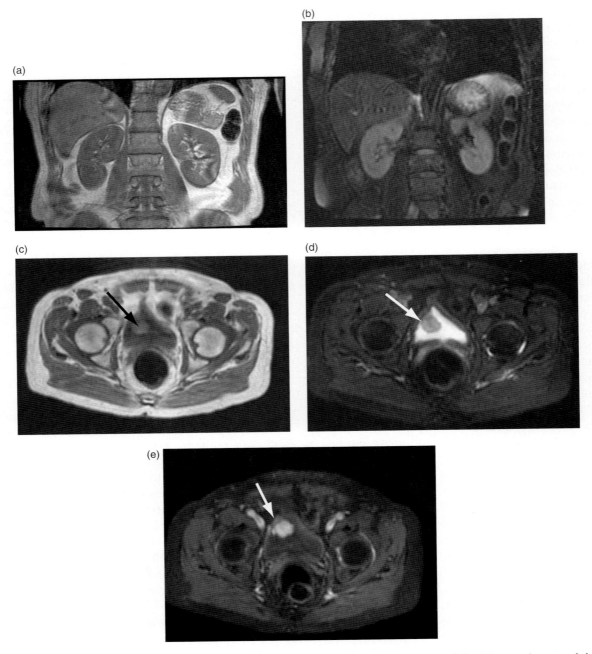

Fig. 9.1 MRI of pheochromocytoma. **A** MRI of abdomen requested due to uncontrolled hypertension with headaches stimulated by urination in this 43-year-old male. Coronal T1 weighted images of the upper abdomen show normal adrenal glands. **B** Coronal T2 weighted images showed no hyperintense mass in upper abdomen or adrenals. **C** Axial T1 weighted image shows nodular lesion (*arrow*) of bladder wall. **D** On axial fat suppressed T2 image the mass (*arrow*) is hyperintense although less so that urine. **E** After intravenous gadolinium contrast injection, marked enhancement (*arrow*) is noted; a paraganglioma of bladder wall was resected

hemorrhagic necrosis this is less common that with pheochromocytoma. Typically the necrotic component is very low signal on T1 and very high signal on T2 images [14]. The solid component will enhance, and the pattern typically described is somewhat less avid enhancement than seen with pheochromocytoma, but prolonged washout [3, 15]. Although many of these malignancies are poorly differentiated and contain no lipid, some (especially the smaller ones that may present earlier due to endocrine function) may be well differentiated and have areas that do contain lipid [14, 16]. The large size, marked heterogeneity and heterogenous enhancement will indicate that adrenal carcinoma is the diagnosis even if opposed phase images show some area of signal drop. However some small lesions may overlap with adenoma and their true nature only discovered on follow up [17]. Calcification, a common finding on CT, is not readily recognizable on MRI.

MRI may be quite useful in staging evaluation of adrenal carcinoma, since staging has marked impact on prognosis. A study of 34 patients with adrenocortical carcinoma showed that accurate determination of IVC extension was achieved in 50% with US, 66% with CT but 100% with MRI – only one-third of those with IVC invasion were alive 2 years after resection [18].

MRI of Adrenal Functional Disorders

A patient presenting with an endocrine disorder of adrenal origin may be evaluated with MRI. Hypertensive patients with elevated catecholamines may have pheocrhromocytoma, previously discussed. A patient with hypercortisolism, hyperaldosteronism, virilization or feminization may have an adrenocortical carcinoma, a benign autonomously hyperfunctioning adenoma, or cortical hyperplasia. The MRI

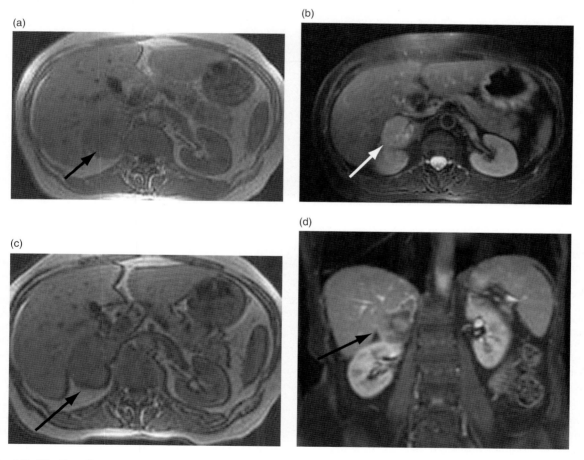

Fig. 9.2 (Continued)

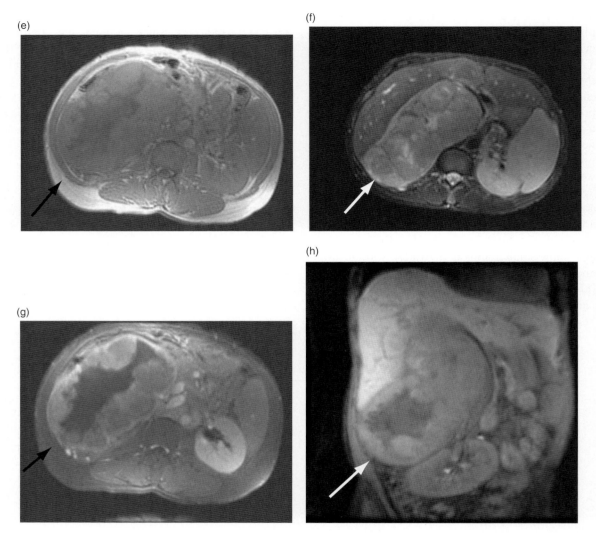

Fig. 9.2 MRI of adrenocortical carcinoma. **A** Sonogram for right upper quadrant pain detected a mass in this 54-year-old female. Axial T1 weighted image shows a non-round intermediate signal intensity 5 cm mass (*arrow*). **B** The mass (*arrow*) is heterogeneous with high signal areas on fat suppressed T2 weighted image. **C** There is no appreciable drop in signal of the mass (*arrow*) on opposed phase image. **D** After intravenous injection Gadolinium contrast, heterogenous enhancement noted, with clear separation of mass (*arrow*) from kidney on coronal image. After biochemical evaluation was negative, surgical resection was performed revealing adrenocortical carcinoma. **E** In another middle aged male with no endocrine disorder presenting with abdominal pain, CT had shown a very large upper abdominal mass thought to be renal carcinoma. An extremely large mass (*arrow*) with central necrosis is evident on axial T1 weighted image. **F** Hyperintensity with central necrosis is noted in the mass (*arrow*) on fat suppressed T2 weighted axial image. **G** There was marked, heterogeneous and sustained enhancement of the mass (*arrow*) after intravenous gadolinium contrast, with central necrosis. **H** Coronal image shows clearly the mass (*arrow*) does not arise from liver or kidney; adrenal carcinoma was successfully resected

features of adrenal carcinoma have been discussed; the features of benign adenoma are distinctly different (and will be discussed below) allowing clear distinction by MRI. Both present as a unilateral mass, one large and heterogeneous the other small and homogeneous. Adrenal cortical hyperplasia may be diagnosed in the absence of a focal mass with a proven endocrine disorder; the glands may or

(a)

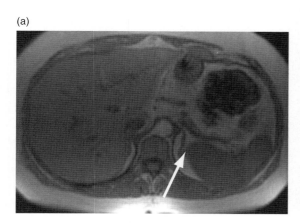

(b)

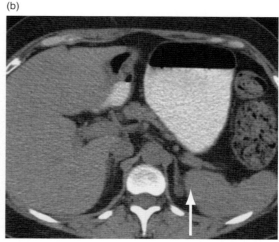

Fig. 9.3 MRI of functional disease. **A** This 41-year-old female with poorly controlled hypertension developed palpitations. Serum catecholamines were mildly elevated. Octreatide nuclear scan was negative. Axial T1 weighted MR image show normal right adrenal with tiny nodule (*arrow*) arising from posterior edge of left adrenal, which dropped in signal on opposed phase; overall findings consistent with adenoma, not pheochromocytoma. **B** Unenhanced CT image confirms the MRI finding of a nodule (*arrow*) with attenuation 4 HU. Surgical resection confirmed diagnosis of 0.7 cm aldosteronoma

may not appear abnormally thick (>5 mm). There have been few reports on the MRI appearance of cortical hyperplasia; however there is likely to be high lipid content so drop in signal on opposed phase can be expected.

Imaging evaluation of a patient with an adrenal endocrine disorder can be done either with CT or MRI [19]. Aside perhaps from pheochromocytoma, there is no particular advantage for MRI aside from avoidance of radiation. While MRI can detect aldosteronomas, some concern has persisted since aldosteronomas tend to be small in size (1.0–1.5 cm is common) at presentation, thus CT with its higher spatial resolution should be more accurate. However, studies with current state of the art MRI show it is capable of accurate diagnosis in this area (Fig. 9.3). In a study of 20 patients, MRI had sensitivity of 70% and specificity of 100% for evaluating hyperaldosteronism [20].

Adrenal insufficiency (Addison's disease) can occur from a variety of causes. MRI is probably equivalent to CT for imaging evaluation. Bilateral adrenal hematoma, or bilateral metastases including lymphoma may be detected with MRI. Bilateral granulomatous disease is a not infrequent finding; while MRI may show bilateral masses, distinct diagnostic features have not been reported. In contrast, autoimmune Addison's disease or acute pituitary apoplexy [21] or adrenal infarction without hematoma will show normal or atrophic adrenal glands without a mass. Primary antiphospholipid antibody syndrome usually presents with bilateral hemorrhage [22] but may result in adrenal atrophy without detectable hematomas [23], both resulting in adrenal insufficiency.

MRI of Adrenal Adenoma vs Nonadenoma

Incidentalomas

Over the past few decades, the seemingly ever increasing use of noninvasive imaging of the abdomen has led to the now commonplace finding of an adrenal "incidentaloma" defined as an adrenal mass detected incidentally on imaging done for some other reason in a patient with no signs or symptoms of adrenal disease, and without a known malignancy. Early on, such masses raised great concerns for incidental malignancy including primary adrenal carcinoma, however only a small minority of such lesions have been found to be malignant. In fact most such masses are benign with adenoma the single most common lesion, up to 57% [24]. Incidentalomas not diagnosable with CT are commonly followed as a single follow up of 6 months or greater showing lack of growth effectively excludes malignancy. However MRI has been shown to be particularly accurate in evaluation [24] – a study on oncologic patients with incidental adrenal mass in which all lesions were resected after imaging evaluation reported sensitivity for diagnosis of malignancy of 66%, 81% and 100% for US, CT and MRI respectively, and sensitivity for diagnosis of adenoma of 46%, 39% and 100% [25].

Adenoma Characteristics on MRI

The potential accuracy of MRI in evaluating incidentalomas largely comes from the fairly specific MRI features of benign cortical adenomas. Early studies which concentrated on T1 and T2 characteristics showed that the majority of adenomas are small (< 3–4 cm) smooth, round or oval and homogenous

with signal intensity little different from that of liver on both T1 and T2 weighted images, which often distinguished them from malignancies which typically have higher signal on T2 weighted images [26] (Fig. 9.4).

In addition, when intravenous gadolinium contrast was investigated, the relatively low level of enhancement with rapid washout was typical of adenomas whereas malignancies tended to display longer retention of contrast [3, 4]. Strict washout criteria, interestingly, have never been developed and promulgated for use in MRI, probably because of the limitations and variability in the way MRI signal intensities are derived.

A major breakthrough was the reporting of the ability of MRI to reliably detect [5] (and even

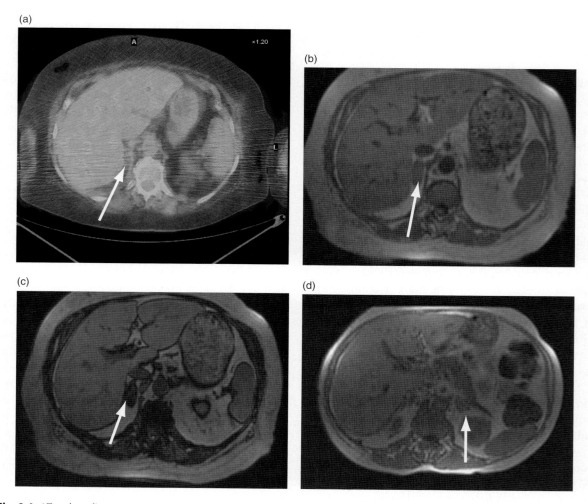

(a) (b) (c) (d)

Fig. 9.4 (Continued)

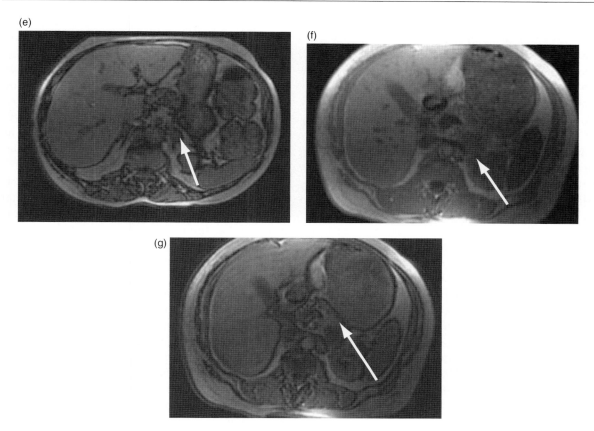

Fig. 9.4 MRI of adrenal adenomas. **A** This 72-year-old female had PET done because of pulmonary nodule on chest radiography. A right adrenal nodule (*arrow*) with abnormal uptake (SUV 4.3) was identified. **B** MRI for definitive evaluation shows right adrenal ovoid mass (*arrow*) on in phase T1 weighted gradient echo image. **C** Opposed phase image shows incontrovertible visual drop in signal of the mass (*arrow*). The nodule remained stable in size on 1 year follow up. (Note dark outline of liver, spleen kidney-the "India ink artifact". **D** In another patient, a 60-year-old female with thyroid cancer, routine postcontrast staging CT showed a left adrenal nodule (*arrow*). The nodule is of intermediate signal intensity on in-phase T1 weighted imaged. **E** There is no appreciable signal intensity drop on opposed phase image of the mass (*arrow*). Dedicated adrenal CT showed precontrast attenuation of 34 HU, early postcontrast 110 HU and 15 min delay of 50, consistent with lipid poor adenoma. **F** In a third patient, a nonhypertensive 43-year-old female had a 3.0-cm. indeterminate left adrenal mass detected on CT done for abdominal pain with routine enhanced technique. The mass (*arrow*) is of intermediate signal intensity on in-phase T1 weighted image. **G** Although minimal visual difference is evident on opposed phase image, calculated adrenal/spleen ratio was indicative of benign adenoma (*arrow*), confirmed on follow up

quantify [27]) the presence of intracellular lipid, a common histologic feature of benign cortical adenomas. This can be demonstrated by the decrease in signal intensity when comparing images initially performed with standard spin echo technique, then repeating the same sequence with radiofrequency fat suppression (this remains the more reliable method for documentation of macroscopic fat such as may be seen in myelolipoma, or angiomyolipoma). However, chemical shift imaging techniques quickly became the standard due to high sensitivity to small amounts of lipid, as well as speed [28–31]. A single short sequence done during a single breath-hold became the critical set of images (Fig. 9.4B,C).

Chemical Shift Principle

In MRI, the signal is produced from spinning protons, with the two major types being free water protons and fat protons. The magnetic field experienced by any proton is a combination of the externally applied magnetic field plus local effects; the local effects will be different between bound fat protons and free water protons; therefore they will precess (spin) at different rates. This is indicated by the Larmor equation which states the resonant frequency of a proton is proportional to the magnetic field it experiences. Because of the slight difference in resonant frequency, over time the fat and water protons vary between spinning in phase or in opposing phase. Because the signal comes from the sum of the protons, if in phase, the signal intensity in voxels with a near-equal mixture of fat and water protons will have an additive and thus higher signal; in contrast, when out of phase there will be some cancellation and thus a lower signal generated—seen as "signal drop" when comparing two images with the only difference being slight difference in echo time (TE) (Fig. 9.4B,C). This signal drop produces the "India ink artifact", a black line at the interface between a soft tissue structure like the spleen and adjacent fat, since the boundary voxels contain both fat and water (Fig. 9.4C). Intracellular lipid as in adrenal adenomas or fatty infiltration of the liver will reduce the signal. However, regions that are pure fat (subcutaneous fat) or pure water protons (kidney) do not reduce the signal on opposed phase images.

Metastasis Characteristics

Although metastases, like malignancies such as adrenocortical carcinoma, may be recognized due to large size, marked heterogeneity, central necrosis and heterogenous enhancement and poor washout, smaller lesions tend to be homogeneous and T1 and T2 intensities may overlap with benign adenomas. However, except for a few unusual exceptions—the aforementioned adrenal carcinoma [16], and metastases from hepatocellular carcinoma [32] and clear cell renal carcinoma [33], metastases do not contain appreciable fat so will not show signal drop on opposed phase (chemical shift) imaging (Fig. 9.5).

MRI: Benign vs Malignant

In a typical adenoma, with considerable intracellular lipid, a clearly visible drop in signal indicates benign diagnosis. There have been several proposals for more quantitative means for specific diagnosis, although in one study the visual qualitative assessment was equivalent in accuracy to quantitative analysis [30]. Ratio of the signal intensity change of the adrenal mass correlated with a reference standard (another organ on same images) has been proposed, with the spleen probably most reliable as fatty infiltration makes the liver unsuitable and muscle has very low inherent signal (Fig. 9.4F,G). Various studies report sensitivity and specificity as high as 100% for the ASR [29, 30]. The cutoff for ASR of 0.71 is relatively well established [34, 35]. The signal intensity index (signal intensity on inphase image minus signal intensity on opposed phase image divided by signal intensity on in-phase image) has also been proposed [36], with better results in some studies [37] and less good in others [29, 30]. Some have also advocated subtraction as a nonmathematical method to document signal drop [38]. In the preponderance of clinical cases, visual inspection is acceptable; the ASR is probably more widely used if visual assessment is not clear, but one must be wary of artifactual variation in signal intensity across a field of view.

Using the combination of features described above, MRI has shown considerable accuracy for diagnosis of adenoma, and distinction from other processes including malignancy. In a study of 229 adrenal masses with pathologic proof of diagnosis in all, MRI showed 96% sensitivity 90% specificity and 94% accuracy for adenoma [39]. A few unavoidable factors limit the accuracy of MRI. While drop in signal on chemical shift imaging is highly indicative of benign adenoma, there is variability in the lipid content with some adenomas being lipid poor. Also problematic are those adenomas with heterogenous composition, with some lipid rich and other lipid poor areas, which results in a disturbing heterogenous appearance on MRI [40]. Metastases that contain lipid (adrenal carcinoma [16], hepatocellular carcinoma [32] and renal carcinoma [33] may be falsely interpreted by chemical shift imaging. Particularly challenging are "collision tumors" in which a metastasis seeds a pre-existing adenoma, potentially resulting in a mass with drop in signal of most but not all of the lesion—thus indistinguishable from an adenoma with nonuniform lipid distribution [41, 42].

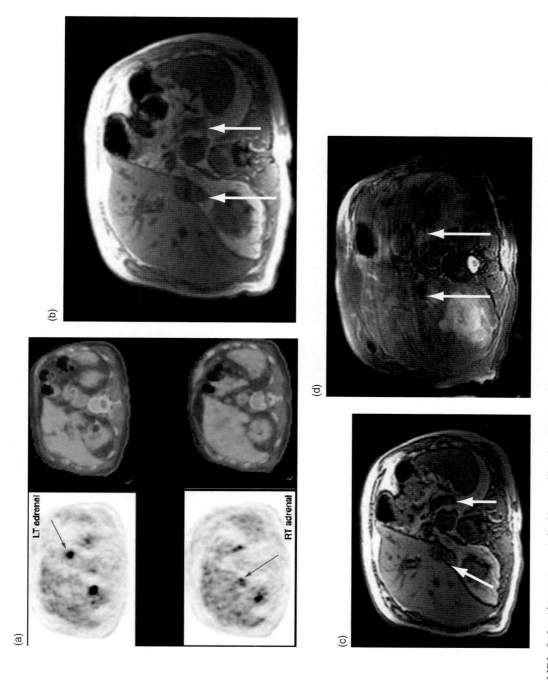

Fig. 9.5 MRI of adrenal metastases. **A** An 81 year old male with 60 pack/year smoking history presented with a lung mass. PET scan done for staging revealed abnormal uptake (*arrows*) in both adrenal glands (SUV 4.3-4.7). **B** On T1 weighted images from MRI done for further investigation, both lesions (*arrows*) are seen to have intermediate signal intensity. **C** There is no signal drop of the nodules (*arrows*) on opposed phase T1 image. **D** The lesions (*arrow*) are moderately hyperintense on fat suppressed T2 weighted images. The lesions showed moderate enhancement after gadolinium. Diagnosis of metastases to both adrenal glands was confirmed by follow up

Role of MRI for Incidentalomas

Following the popularization of chemical shift MRI, investigators published numerous reports indicating that the presence of lipid could be detected using CT, and statistical evaluation of criteria based on unenhanced CT attenuation were proposed [40] which were easy to apply and have good accuracy. Subsequently some of the limitations of the CT attenuation were addressed with CT contrast washout criteria [43].

These CT developments led to some loss of interest in MRI, questioning whether there was any value in using the more expensive modality to detect the same histologic feature. One study showed the evaluation of adrenal masses by CT attenuation and chemical shift MRI directly correlated with lipid content, and several lesions were misdiagnosed by both [34]; however, in that study the CT attenuation cutoff used was 17 HU, not the now more currently accepted 10 HU. Investigations on the results of MRI compared with CT attenuation including use of histogram analysis have shown MRI may add value [44]. One study showed a threshold of over 20% signal drop aided additional diagnoses to CT evaluation even using histogram analysis on CT [45]. Thus if a lesion is not diagnosable as adenoma by CT, MRI may still be worth performing.

MRI of Miscellaneous Pathology

Quite a wide variety of pathologic processes can occur in the adrenal infrequently to rarely. MRI features of several have been described although often nonspecific.

MRI of Myelolipoma

Myelolipoma is an uncommon but not rare benign mass-like process most commonly seen within the adrenal gland. The lesion is a variable composition of mature adipose cells mixed with bone marrow elements (although not true extramedullary hematopoiesis). Many are small, predominantly fatty lesions. Larger lesions can occur, and there may be moderate to high percentage of solid component which can enhance after either iodinated or gadolinium based contrast. The key diagnostic feature is demonstration of fat within the lesion. While opposed phase imaging may show this (including phase shift artifact within the lesion), since the fat is macroscopic and not intracellular lipid, radiofrequency fat suppression may be more definitive (Fig. 9.6). T1 and T2 characteristics can be quite variable and may be confusing as they depend on the mixture of fat and soft tissue components, but typically are quite heterogeneous. The marrow elements are moderately hyperintense on T2 weighted images.

MRI of Adrenal Hematomas

Adrenal hematomas can be demonstrated on MRI. The characteristics depend on the age of the hemorrhage and will evolve over time; this and the usual decrease in size is most discriminatory between hematoma and malignancy. Acute hemorrhage will have intermediate or high signal on T1. Chronic hematoma may have nonspecific low T1 high T2 signal or more suggestive low T1 low T2 pattern. In addition, a thick very low signal hemosiderin rim is typical of old hematomas.

MRI of Adrenal Cysts

A cystic mass in the adrenal may arise from necrosis of an originally solid mass, as mentioned from pheochromocytoma, possibly from adrenocortical carcinoma or metastasis. An adrenal pseudocyst may result from prior trauma and an organized hematoma. All of these lesions often have a thick enhancing rim, and complex contents. Calcification with the wall of a complex cyst is common, and may cause signal void on MR, but is difficult to recognize as calcification. It is thus not possible to distinguish absolutely the benign from the malignant [46]. More simple adrenal cysts may also occur, with thin rim, low signal on T1 and high signal on T2 weighted images. Although these can be predicted to be benign, they may be large and symptomatic [47]. Endothelial cysts can occur and tend to be multilocular, but may be complex [46].

MRI of Rare Adrenal Tumors

Lymphoproliferative lesions can rarely be found in the adrenal such as plasmacytoma and lymphoma [48, 49]. These can present as masses with relatively homogeneous medium intensity on T1 and hyperintensity on T2. MRI is rarely used for evaluation of lymphoma as CT is more effective for whole body evaluations. Neural sheath tumors including ganglioneuromas and schwannomas can occur in the adrenal or nearby in

(a)

(b)

(c)

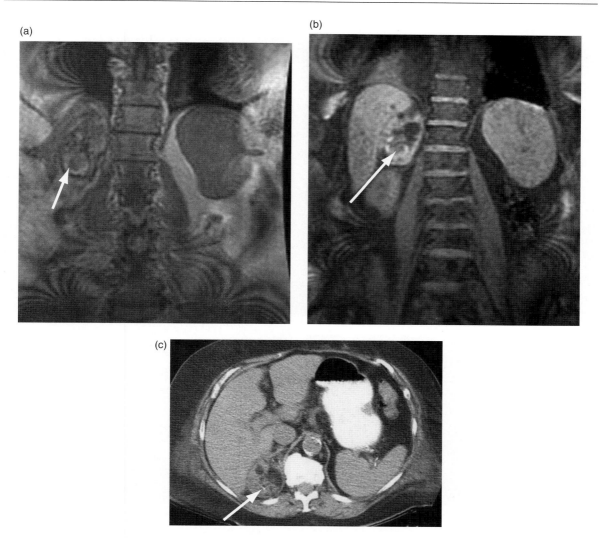

Fig. 9.6 MRI of myelolipoma. **A** A 79-year-old female with hypertension underwent magnetic resonance angiogram. Localizer image revealed a large heterogeneous right adrenal mass (*arrow*) with high signal regions on T1 weighted image, as shown. **B** Repeat T1 weighted image done with radiofrequency fat suppression shows focal areas of signal loss in the mass (*arrow*), with some remaining hyperintense areas consistent with hemorrhage. **C** Unenhanced CT confirms presence of macroscopic fat regions in this benign myelolipoma (*arrow*) of the adrenal

the retroperitoneum [50, 51]. These also have the rather nonspecific appearance of sizeable masses with medium T1 signal and T2 hyperintensity with enhancement, and thus cannot clearly be distinguished from malignancy and are usually only diagnosed from pathologic examination of a specimen (Fig. 9.7). Oncocytomas can very rarely arise in the adrenal; as with renal oncocytoma their MRI appearance is not distinguishable from malignancy, and the stellate scar seen in larger renal oncocytomas has not been reported in the adrenal [52] (Fig. 9.8).

MRI of Inflammatory Adrenal Disease

Inflammatory processes also rarely occur in the adrenal gland, including tuberculosis, histoplasmosis, paracoccidiodomycosis and adrenal abscess. Few reports exist on the MRI appearance of these entities, but they could be misconstrued as malignant processes since they will not show loss of signal on opposed phase, may be hyperintense on T2 weighted images, and in acute phase may show peripheral enhancement.

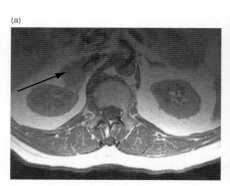

Fig. 9.7 MRI of ganglioneuroma. **A** MRI done for back pain (with lumbar coil) shows right adrenal mass (*arrow*) with irregular margins, intermediate signal intensity on the T1 weighted image. **B** The mass (*arrow*) is hyperintense on T2 weighted image, and showed enhancement. Because of nonspecific nature, after nondiagnostic percutaneous biopsy the mass was resected with histologic diagnosis of ganglioneuroma

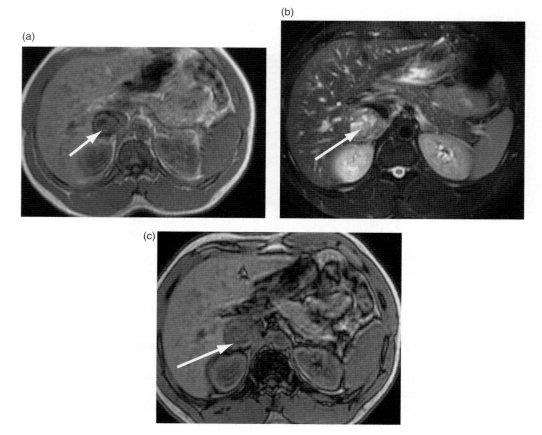

Fig. 9.8 MRI of adrenal oncocytoma. **A** MRI was done for further investigation of incidental finding on US in this asymptomatic 31-year-old male after CT showed 5-cm indeterminate mass. T1 weighted axial image shows slightly heterogenous medium signal intensity mass (*arrow*). **B** On T2 weighted image, the lesion (*arrow*) shows fairly marked heterogeneity with markedly hyperintense areas. **C** No appreciable drop in signal of the mass (*arrow*) is evident on the opposed phase image; the mass did enhance. Because of nonspecific, possibly malignant nature, the mass was resected with final pathology: adrenal oncocytoma

Summary and Future Directions

With increased technical capability and voluminous published experience, MRI offers great utility in diagnosis of adrenal disorders. Despite the inherent capabilities however, alternate methods limit the use of MRI. CT, although less specific, is less expensive and more widely available, will likely remain the first line imaging tool, with MRI more of a problem solving tool. Another limiting factor on the impact of MRI is that, due to the variation in characteristics of common lesions (such as atypical adenomas that can simulate malignancy or pheochromocytoma that may be purely cystic) and also due to the occurrence of rare nonspecific lesions (ganglioneuroma, oncocytoma) the diagnostic accuracy of MRI will never be 100%.

It had been expected some years ago that MRI of the adrenal would benefit from development of specific contrast agents, using biochemical probes tagged with an MR detectable molecule (whether gadolinium or some other), to allow specific diagnosis of lesions such as pheochromocytoma, adrenal cortical tumors etc. However, that development now seems very unlikely, not due to any inability to create such agents, but because the development and approval process is so long cumbersome and expensive that such niche market diagnostic agents are unlikely to be profitable enough to stimulate commitment from pharmaceutical industry. In addition, the previous use of MRI in patients in end stage renal disease is currently limited by concerns for development of nephrogenic systemic fibrosis if exposed to intravenous gadolinium agents.

Spectroscopy may hold the best offer for more specific diagnoses of adrenal masses as a large proportion of MR devices in use or being bought have this capability.

References

1. Moon KL, Hricak H, Crooks LE et al. (1983) Nuclear magnetic resonance imaging of the adrenal gland: a preliminary report. Radiology 147:155–160
2. Glazer GM, Woolsey EJ, Borello J et al. (1986) Adrenal tissue characterization using MR imaging. Radiology 158:73–79
3. Krestin GP, Steinbrich W, Friedman G (1989) Adrenal masses: evaluation with fast gradient echo MR imaging and Gd-DTPA-enhanced dynamic studies. Radiology 171:675–680
4. Ichikawa T, Ohtoma K, Uchiyama G et al. (1995) Contrast enhanced dynamic MRI of adrenal masses: classification of characteristic enhancement patterns. Clin Radiol 50:295–300
5. Mitchell DG, Crovello M, Matteucci T et al. (1992) Benign adrenocortical masses: diagnosis with chemical shift MR imaging. Radiology 185:345–351
6. Mitchell DG, Nasciemento AB, Alam F et al. (2002) Normal adrenal gland: in vivo observations and high resolution in vitro chemical shift MR imaging-histologic correlation. Acad Radiol 9:430–426
7. Krebs TL, Wagner BJ, Kenney PJ (1998) Unpublished data from Armed Forces Institute of Pathology, presented at annual meeting of RSNA 1998. Appearances of pheochromocytoma with pathologic correlation
8. Falke THM, Strake LT, Sandler MP et al. (1987) Magnetic resonance imaging of the adrenal glands. Radiographics 7:343–370
9. Belden CJ, Powers C, Ros PR (1995) MR demonstration of a cystic pheochromocytoma. JMRI 5:778–780
10. Szolar DH, Korobkin M, Reitner P et al. (2005) Adrenocortical carcinomas and adrenal pheochromocytomas: mass and enhancement loss evaluation at delayed contrast-enhanced CT. Radiology 234:479–485.
11. Happel B, Heinz-Peer G (2006) Enhancement characteristics of pheochromocytoma. Radiology 238:373–374
12. Quint LE, Glazer GM, Francis IR et al. (1987) Pheochromocytoma and paraganglioma: comparison. of MR imaging with CT and I-131 MIBG scintigraphy. Radiology 165:89–93
13. Shulkin BL, Thompson NW, Shapiro B et al. (1999) Pheochromocytomas: imaging with 2-Fluorine-18 fluoro-2-deoxy-D-glucose PET. Radiology 212:35–41
14. Schlund JF, Kenney PJ, Brown ED et al. (1995) Adrenocortical carcinoma: MR imaging appearance with current techniques. JMRI 5:171–174
15. Slattery JMA, Blake MA, Kalra MK et al. (2006) Adrenocortical carcinoma: contrast washout characteristics on CT. AJR Am J Roentgenol 187:197
16. Ferozzi F, Bova D (1995) CT and MR demonstration of fat within an adrenal cortical carcinoma. Abdom Imag 20:272–274
17. Outwater EK, Mitchell DM, Rubenfeld IG (1997) Correction to a previously published case: recurrence of invasive adrenocortical tumor after excision of atypical adenoma. Radiology 202:531-532
18. Tucci S, Martins ACP, Suaid HJ et al. (2005) The impact of tumor stage on prognosis in children with adrenocortical carcinoma. J Urol 174:2338–2442
19. Rockall AG, Babar SA, Sohaib AA et al. (2004) CT and MR imaging of the adrenal glands in ACTH-independent Cushing syndrome. Radiographics 24:435–452
20. Sohaib SA, Peppercorn P, Allan C et al. (2000) Primary hyperaldosteronism (Conn syndrome): MR imaging findings. Radiology 214:527–531
21. Scully RE, Mark EJ, McNeely WF et al. (2001) Case records of the Massachusetts General Hospital. NEJM 344:1536–1542
22. Provenzale JM, Ortel TL, Nelson R (1995) Adrenal hemorrhage in patients with primary antiphospholipid

syndrome: imaging findings.AJR Am J Roentgenol 165:361–364

23. Riddel AM, Khalili K (2004) Sequential adrenal infarction without MRI detectable hemorrhage in primary antiphospholipid-antibody syndrome. AJR Am J Roentgenol 183:220–222

24. Favia G, Lumachi F, Basso S et al. (2000) Management of incidentally discovered adrenal masses and risk of malignancy. Surgery 128:918–924

25. Frilling A, Tecklenborg K, Weber F et al. (2004) Importance of incidentaloma in patients with a history of malignancy. Surgery 136:1289–1296

26. Schwartz LH, Panicek DM, Koutcher JA et al. (1995) Adrenal masses in patients with malignancy: prospective comparison of echo-planar, fast spin echo and chemical shift MRI. Radiology 197:421–425

27. Namimoto T, Yamashita Y, Mitsuzaki K et al. (2001) Adrenal masses: quantification of fat content with double echo chemical shift in-phase and opposed-phase FLASH MR images for differentiation of adrenal adenomas. Radiology 218:642–646

28. Korobkin M, Lombardi TJ, Aisen AM et al. (1995) Characterization of adrena masses with chemical shift and gadolinium-enhanced MR imaging. Radiology 197:411–418

29. Bilbey JH, McLoughlin RF, Kurkijian PS et al. (1995) MR imaging of adrenal masses: value of chemical-shift imaging for distinguishing adenomas from other tumors. AJR Am J Roentgenol 164:637–642

30. Mayo-Smith WW, Lee MJ, McNicholas MMJ et al. (1995) Characterization of adrenal masses (<5 cm) by use of chemical shift MR imaging: observe performance versus quantitative measures. AJR Am J Roentgenol 165:91–95

31. Outwater EK, Siegelman ES, Radecki PD et al. (1995) Distinction between benign and malignant adrenal masses: value of T1-weighted chemical shift MR imaging. AJR Am J Roentgenol 165:579–583

32. Sydow BD, Rosen MA, Siegelman ES (2006) Intracellular lipid within metastatic hepatocellular carcinoma of the adrenal gland: a potential diagnostic pitfall of chemical shift imaging of the adrenal gland. AJR Am J Roentgenol 187:W550–551

33. Shinozaki K, Yoshimitsu K, Honda H et al. (2001) Metastatic adrenal tumor from clear-cell renal cell carcinoma: a pitfall of chemical shift MR imaging. Abdom Imag 26:439–442

34. Outwater EK, Siegelman ES, Huang AB et al. (1996) Adrenal masses: correlation between CT attenuation value and chemical shift ratio at MR imaging with in-phase and opposed-phase sequences. Radiology 200:749–752

35. McNicholas MM, Lee MJ, Mayo-Smith WW et al. (1995) An imaging algorithm for the differential diagnosis of adrenal adenomas and metastases. AJR Am J Roentgenol 165:1453–1459

36. Tsushima Y, Ishizaka H, Matsumoto M (1993) Adrenal masses: differentiation with chemical shift, fast low angle shot MR imaging. Radiology 186:705–709

37. Fujiyoshi F, Nakajo M, Fukukura Y et al. (2003) Characterization of adrenal tumors by chemical shift fast low-angle shot MR imaging: comparison of four methods of quantitative evaluation. AJR Am J Roentgenol 180:1649–1657

38. Savci G, Yazici Z, Sahin N et al. (2006) Value of chemical shift subtraction MRI in characterization of adrenal masses. AJR Am J Roentgenol 186:130–135

39. Honigschnabl S, Gallo S, Niederle B et al. (2002) How accurate is MR imaging in characterization of adrenal masses: update of a long-term study. Eur J Radiol 41:113–122

40. Korobkin M, Giordano TJ, Brodeur FJ et al. (1996) Adrenal adenomas: relationship between histologic lipid and CT and MR findings. Radiology 200:743–747

41. Schwartz LH, Macari M, Huvos AG et al. (1996) Collision tumors of the adrenal gland: demonstration and characterization at MR imaging. Radiology 201:757–760

42. Thorin-Savoure A, Tissier-Ribble F, Guignat L et al. (1005) Collision/composite tumors of the adrenal gland: a pitfall of scintigraphy imaging and hormone assays in the detection of adrenal metastasis. J Clin Endocrinol Metabo 90:4924–2572

43. Korobkin M, Brodeur FJ, Francis IR et al. (1998) CT time-attenuation washout curves of adrenal adenomas and non-adenomas. AJR Am J Roentgenol 170:747–752

44. Haider MA, Ghai S, Jhaveri K et al. (2004) Chemical shift MR imaging of hyperattenuating (>10 HU) adrenal masses: does it still have a role? Radiology 231:711–716

45. Jhaveri KS, Wong F, Ghai et al. (2006) Comparison of CT histogram analysis and chemical shift MRI in the characterization of indeterminate adrenal nodules. AJR Am J Roentgenol 187:1303–1308

46. Rozenblitt A, Morehouse HT, Amis ES (1996) Cystic adrenal lesions. Radiology 201:541–548

47. Habra MA, Feig BW, Waguespack SG (2005) Adrenal pseudocyst. J Clin Endocrinol Metab 90:3067–3068

48. Roger CG, Pinto PA, Weir EG (2004) Extraosseous (extramedullary) plasmacytoma of the adrenal gland. Arch Pathol Lab Med 128:e86–88

49. Kato J, Itami J, Shiina T et al. (1995) MR imaging of primary adrenal lymphoma. Clin Imag 20:126–128

50. Radin R, David CL, Goldfarb H et al. (1997) Adrenal and extra-adrenal retroperitoneal ganglioneuroma: imaging findings in 13 adults. Radiology 202:703–707

51. Goh BKP, Tan Y-M, Chung Y-FA et al. (2006) Retroperitoneal schwannoma. Am J Surg 192:14–18

52. Gandras EJ, Schwartz LH, Panicek DM et al. (1996) Adrenocortical oncocytoma: CT and MRI findings. JCAT 407–409

Single Photon Imaging of the Adrenal Gland

10

James A. Scott and Edwin L. Palmer

Contents

J.A. Scott (✉)
Division of Nuclear Medicine, Department
of Radiology, Massachusetts General Hospital, Boston,
Massachusetts 02114
E-mail: jscott2@partners.org

Introduction

The clinical niche inhabited by single photon radionuclide imaging in the evaluation of the adrenal has been progressively restricted by advances in CT, MRI and, more recently, PET imaging. The traditional advantages of single photon techniques have been high sensitivity, the ability to perform whole body imaging and to evaluate specific aspects of biochemistry and physiology. As is often the case, however, this more specific physiologic data bears the price of reduced image resolution. In the case of adrenal imaging, the physiologic information is also often redundant, given that the anatomy and tissue characteristics have often been previously defined by CT and MR, and the biochemical issues by laboratory tests.

This chapter will make brief historical note of single photon agents previously used to study the adrenal gland, and devote itself to the remaining clinical applications of these agents today. These remaining applications owe their survival to the ability of single photon agents to target specific cellular characteristics while imaging the whole body in an acceptable time-frame and at an acceptable radiation burden.

Single photon agents have historically targeted both the adrenal cortex and medulla. The cortical imaging agents are largely of historic interest, given their limited anatomic resolution and redundancy to information provided by MR, CT, PET and laboratory studies. We will make brief note the cortical agents and then examine the medullary agents in greater detail.

M.A. Blake, G. Boland (eds.), *Adrenal Imaging*, DOI 10.1007/978-1-59745-560-2_10,
© 2009 Humana Press, a part of Springer Science+Business Media, LLC

Imaging of the Adrenal Cortex

Radionuclide techniques have also been used for adrenal cortical imaging, using investigational radiolabeled cholesterol derivatives. One agent, ^{131}I-iodo-methyl-19-norcholesterol, or NP-59, has been used in the evaluation of Cushing's syndrome [1]. Adrenal adenoma presents as unilateral adrenal uptake, while bilateral hyperplasia presents as bilateral, although possibly asymmetric, uptake. Adrenal carcinoma typically does not show increased uptake. Although this approach is a powerful use of radionuclide techniques, NP-59 has never been commercially available, and thus is of little practical clinical interest.

Imaging of the Adrenal Medulla

The primary single photon agents used to image the adrenal medulla are [131]I- or ^{123}I labeled metaiodobenzylguanidine (MIBG) and labeled somatostatin-receptor imaging (SRI) agents, the latter almost exclusively ^{111}In-octreotide.

Although the adrenal medulla is the primary source of physiologic catecholamine secretion, extramedullary paraganglia extend from the base of the skull to the lower pelvis. It is primarily in the detection of these extra-adrenal foci that the single-photon imaging agents have their use.

MIBG

Radionuclide techniques have proven useful in the detection and evaluation of adrenergic tumors, chiefly pheochromocytomas and extra adrenal paragangliomas. Because most pheochromocytomas are hormonally active, the excess catechol production typically allows a confident biochemical diagnosis to be made. Although virtually all adrenal tumors can be detected by abdominal CT and MRI, nuclear imaging using a radiolabeled norepinephrine analog, ^{123}I-meta-iodobenzylguanidine, or MIBG, may play an ancillary role in further characterizing uncertain findings, as well as in the evaluation of multifocal or metastatic disease. When presented with an adrenal mass that has CT or MRI characteristics suggesting pheochromocytoma, an abnormal MIBG study allows confident diagnosis because of the very high specificity of the agent in detecting adrenal medullary tissue present in pheochromocytoma or paraganglioma [1]. The presence of MIBG uptake in an adrenal mass confidently confirms the diagnosis of pheochromocytoma, which the absence of uptake makes the diagnosis unlikely.

In adults, about 90% of pheochromocytomas are located within the adrenal medulla [2], and these tumors are easily detected by CT. Most pheochromocytomas are benign, but about 10% show malignant characteristics, and may spread outside the adrenal gland [2]. In children, extra-adrenal tumors are much more common, representing up to 30% of tumors. Extra-adrenal tumors are most commonly located in the retroperitoneum, but may be found anywhere from the skull base to the pelvis. It is in these patients that nuclear imaging may be especially useful, as CT or MRI evaluation of the abdomen may miss small lesions. Thus, the MIBG scan may be useful to confirm the diagnosis of a suspected intra-adrenal pheochromocytoma, but is far more useful to evaluate for the presence of multifocal or extra-adrenal disease.

Radiolabeled MIBG was first introduced using an ^{131}I label in 1981 [3], and considerable experience was gained with this agent. More recently, an ^{123}I labeled version of the tracer has become widely available, providing markedly improved image quality and radiation dosimetry in comparison with the older, ^{131}I labeled version of the tracer [4]. The reported sensitivity of MIBG in the detection of phrochromocytoma is approximately 85% [5]. Some pheochromocytomas that are MIBG negative may show abnormal uptake of ^{18}F-FDG or ^{111}In-pentetreotide. The ultimate role of MIBG vis a vis FDG imaging has yet to be established. FDG PET examinations provide superior image quality, but lack the specificity shown by MIBG, as FDG imaging is abnormal in most adrenal malignancies. The role of FDG imaging is thus greater in the search for extra-adrenal disease than in the characterization of a known tumor.

The technical requirements for imaging with radiolabeled MIBG are more stringent than those needed in most nuclear imaging, requiring evaluation and interaction with the patient prior to dose administration. Any radioiodinated tracer will contain some unlabeled iodide, which localizes in the thyroid gland. To reduce unnecessary radiation exposure, it is standard practice to block thyroid uptake of radioiodine by administering a large dose of non-radioactive iodine prior to the study. Lugol's solution (a potassium iodide solution) is typically administered orally beginning a day or two before the study, and continuing for several days thereafter. Alternatively, some physicians pretreat with perchlorate to block thyroidal iodine uptake. This maneuver is less critical with the ^{123}I labeled agent than with the older ^{131}I agent, because of the much worse patient dosimetry with the latter. Nevertheless, it is an easy way to reduce patient absorbed radiation dose, and thus a prudent strategy.

It is also essential to ensure that patients are not taking any medications that might interfere with MIBG uptake by an adrenergic tumor. The list of medications that may block uptake is lengthy [4]. Common medications include calcium channel blockers, sympathomimetics (including ephedrine and pseudoephedrine), reserpine, cocaine, adrenergic blockers, and tricyclic antidepressants. If the patient is taking any of these medications, the drug must be withheld and the study postponed.

The standard adult radiopharmaceutical dosage is 370 MBq (10 mCi) of ^{123}I MIBG. The tracer is given as a slow intravenous injection, preferably via a peripheral vein rather than through a central line, in order to minimize the chance of patient reaction. Imaging is performed 24 h later, allowing time for uptake in tumor. If desired, earlier imaging at 2–4 h may be performed. This provides prompt information, but adds to patient inconvenience and rarely precludes the need for next-day imaging. Additional delayed imaging at 48 h is sometimes performed, but only adds diagnostic information in very selected cases. Both SPECT and planar imaging is performed, the latter using either whole body scanning or spot views. Because count rates are low, relatively long acquisition times of about 10 minutes are commonly used for spot images.

The normal radiopharmaceutical distribution depicts regions with rich sympathetic innervation, as well as the routes of excretion from the body. There is typically good definition of salivary glands and faint myocardial activity. There is more intense uptake in liver, and faint demonstration of the spleen. The bladder is typically visible, as is faint uptake in bowel. Lung uptake is commonly seen, although this is often greatest early after injection. In the absence of pharmacologic iodine pre-treatment, the thyroid would also be visible.

Normal adrenal glands may be faintly visible, usually better seen on SPECT images than on planar views (Fig. 10.1). Any more marked uptake or asymmetric appearance suggests an abnormality (Fig. 10.2). It is important to realize that a small fraction of pheochromocytomas may show little or no MIBG uptake (Fig. 10.3). Pheochomocytomas outside the adrenal gland are easily recognized by the presence of focally intense uptake (Fig. 10.4).

Somatostatin Receptor Imaging

Somatostatin receptors, of which there are five known subtypes, are glycoproteins located in the cell membrane of neuroendocrine-derived cells (including the pituitary, pancreas and thyroid), as well as in normal lymphocytes. Certain tumors, particularly those of neuro-endocrine origin, as well as lymphomas and activated lymphocytes over-express these receptors and this increased receptor density permits these cells to be targeted for imaging.

Clinical somatostatin receptor imaging is largely concerned with the evaluation of those neuroendocrine tumors with a high density of somatostatin receptors [6]. It is essentially a second-line agent in the specific context of the adrenal gland, best reserved for those cases where MIBG imaging fails to localize an abnormality but clinical suspicion of a catecholamine secreting lesion remains high. Although this may occur in a scenario where the primary tumor has undergone de-differentiation and become malignant, in general, somatostain receptors are found in the highest concentration in more well-differentiated tumors. Some reports do suggest an increased sensitivity of SRI for metastatic disease in dopamine secreting tumors when MIBG scanning is negative [7]. Even a complementary role with MIBG, however, would still leave SRI in a second tier position in adrenal imaging.

Although SRI is a secondary method in the particular context of the adrenal gland itself, it has much greater value in the search for additional sites of disease in the setting of potentially systemic processes. Increased concentrations of somatostatin receptors can be seen in pheochromoctyomas and paraganglionomas (both secretory and non-secretory) as well as neuroblastomas, among the

(a)

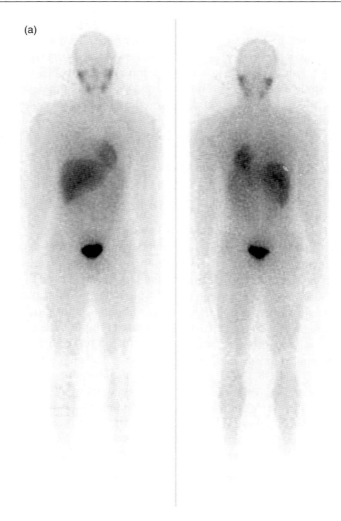

(b)

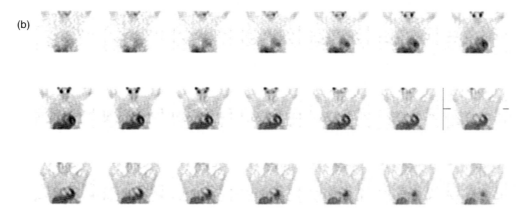

Fig. 10.1 (continued)

(c)

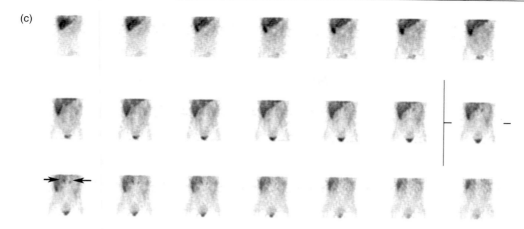

Fig. 10.1 **a** Anterior (*left*) and posterior (*right*) whole body images from a normal ^{123}I-MIBG scan. Note the salivary, myocardial, and liver uptake, as well as excretion via the bladder. **b** Coronal SPECT images of the chest better demonstrate the myocardial uptake. **c** Coronal SPECT images of the abdomen show faint uptake within both adrenal glands (*arrows*). Note bladder activity in the inferior pelvis

wide variety of tumor types over-expressing this receptor. SRI gains its clinical value primarily from its ability to detect metastastic disease in these somatostatin expressing tumor types.

There are many somatostatin analogues that have been labeled with radionuclides. The most common of these is Indium-111 DTPA pentetreotide. The somatostatin imaging agents have their greatest affinity

(a)

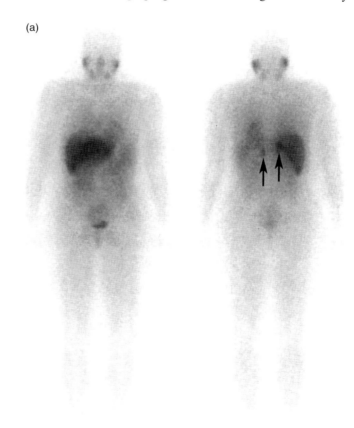

Fig. 10.2 (continued)

Fig. 10.2 a Anterior (*left*) and posterior (*right*) whole body images from a ^{123}I-MIBG scan in a patient with biochemical evidence of pheochromocytoma. Imaging with CT and MRI showed a 3-cm. right adrenal mass and slight thickening of the left adrenal. Both adrenals are unusually well seen (*arrows*), with clearly increased uptake on the right side. **b,c** Coronal and axial SPECT images of the abdomen better demonstrate that both adrenals show increased uptake (*arrows*), greater on the right side

(b)

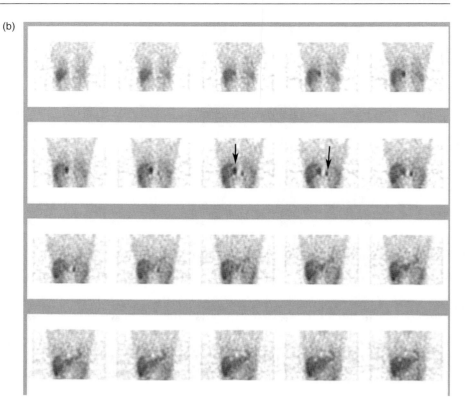

(c)

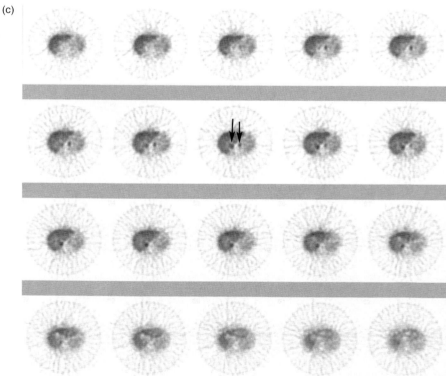

(a)

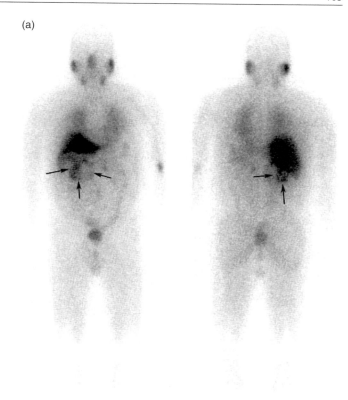

(b)

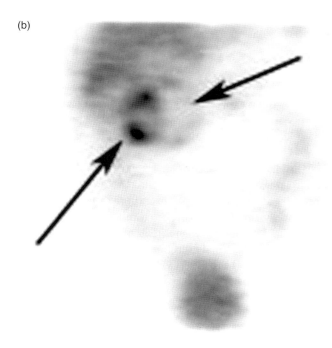

Fig. 10.3 (continued)

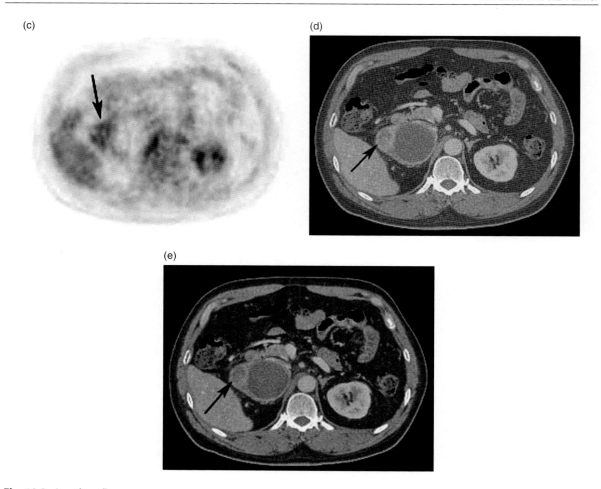

Fig. 10.3 (continued)

for the somatostatin receptor 2 subtype. As the adrenal medulla expresses type 2 somatostatin receptors, this provides the basis for uptake in the adrenal gland. Octreotide, an octapeptide analog of somatostatin, was the first agent to be used for imaging in clinical practice. Octreotide can also be labeled with ^{123}I-Tyr3 although this latter labeling method results in prominent gastrointestinal excretion rather than the primarily renal route of excretion seen with the DTPA label. As the abdomen is the primary region of concern, gastrointestinal excretion reduces diagnostic image quality, and thus the DTPA label is generally used for diagnostic purposes today. ^{111}In-DOTA-lanreotide has also proven successful, although showing somewhat less intense tracer accumulation in tumor foci [8]. The chelator DOTA (1,4,7,10-tetraazacyclododecane-N, N', N'', N'''-tetraacetic acid), however, permits labeling with a variety of metal ions so that tracers may be produced for therapeutic applications (using, for instance [90]Yr).

The technical procedure generally involves injecting at least 220 MBq of In-DTPA pentetreotide. The spleen and kidneys receive the highest radiation dose from this agent. Imaging is performed with a medium-energy parallel hole collimator (^{111}In photon energies are 172 keV and 245 keV) using a 20% window. Planar images are routinely obtained at 24 h after tracer injection, imaging for 10–15 min to acquire at least 500 K counts in the chest and abdomen, and if necessary additional 10–15-min images are acquired at 48 h. Images should also be obtained of the head and neck for

(f) (g) (h)

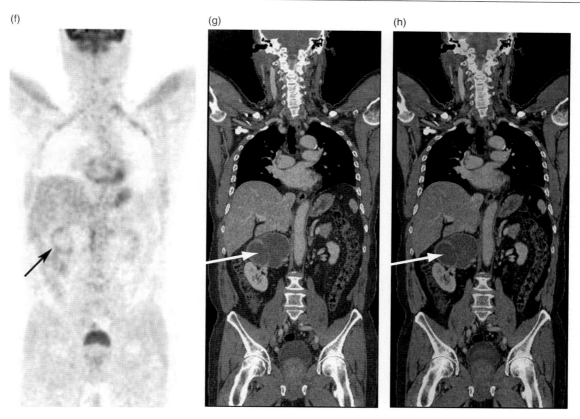

Fig. 10.3 **a** Anterior (*left*) and posterior (*right*) whole body images from a ^{123}I-MIBG scan in a patient with biochemical evidence of pheochromocytoma and a large, complex cystic right adrenal mass shown on CT and MRI demonstrate a faint zone of abnormal uptake in the region of the right adrenal gland (*arrow*). **b** Coronal SPECT imaging better defines a region of mixed increased and decreased uptake. Note the normal faint activity within colon. **c–e** Axial FDG PET scan (**c**) shows minor uptake in the solid component of the tumor (*arrow*), well demonstrated on axial CT (**d**) and PET/CT fusion overlay (**e**). **f–h** Coronal FDG (**f**), coronal CT image (**g**) and coronal PET/CT fusion overlay (**h**) demonstrate the extensive cystic nature of the tumor (*arrows*). At surgery, a 9 × 7.5 × 7 cm cystic and hemorrhagic pheochromocytoma was resected

about 300 K counts. SPECT imaging is necessary in the chest and abdomen. Some workers acquire an additional set of planar images at 4 h after injection, when there is less bowel activity, although these are usually not necessary since 24-h images have a higher lesion detection rate compared to those obtained at 4 h after injection [9]. In general, SPECT imaging is best obtained at 24 h even in the presence of intense bowel excretion, as this is often sufficient to document that the pattern of uptake conforms to the expected configuration of the bowel. Infrequently, when abdominal activity cannot be clearly attributed to normal bowel, or when excessive bowel excretion limits visibility of the abdomen, 48-h images may be useful. Oral laxatives help to reduce bowel uptake, and are usually given

immediately after tracer injection. Additional laxative treatment may be given after the 24-h images, should these show intense bowel excretion and 48-h images are then obtained. As Fig. 10.5a shows, occasionally bowel activity may be quite intense on 24-h images, even to the point of simulating a focus of disease. As Fig. 10.5b illustrates, the suspicious focus is absent on the 48-h planar images.

Tumor uptake of labeled somatostatin receptor analogues is reduced in the presence of higher plasma concentrations of unlabelled receptor agonists, so patients on octreotide therapy should have this withdrawn before the scan is obtained. The length of withdrawal will depend upon the type of therapy being administered. Immediate release preparations should be withdrawn 24 h before isotope

Fig. 10.4 Anterior (*left*) and posterior (*right*) whole body images from a ^{123}I-MIBG scan (**a**) show intense uptake in the midline lower abdomen (*arrows*), corresponding to a large retroperitoneal mass (*arrow*) shown on abdominal CT (**b**). The patient had initially presented with abdominal pain, although he had significant hypertension. At surgery, a 2.5-cm extra-adrenal pheochromocytoma was resected

(a)

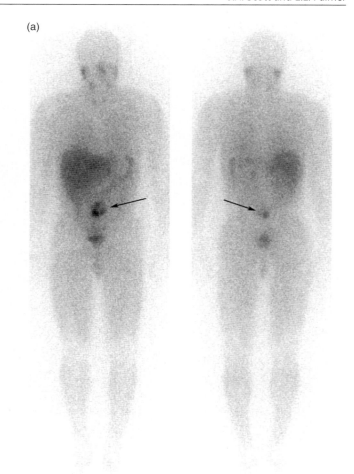

(b)

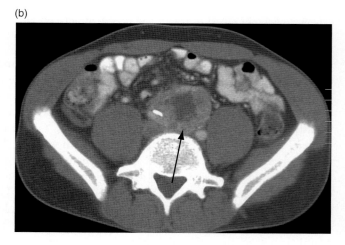

injection for the imaging procedure. If the patient is receiving a long-acting octreotide formulation, imaging should be performed immediately prior to the next scheduled dose administration of the long-acting agent. Although tumor foci can usually be identified even in those patients taking unlabeled octreotide, the degree of uptake will be reduced owing to competition with the unlabeled agent.

Fig. 10.5 **a** The normal pattern of ^{111}In-pentetreotide uptake includes activity in the liver, spleen, kidneys and bladder. Note the intense uptake on 24-h whole body images in the region of the mid ascending colon (*arrows*) in this patient being examined for a suspected paraganglionoma. **b** After laxative administration, repeat images of the abdomen at 48 h showed no evidence of abnormal uptake in this area, confirming that this focus had represented bowel excretion

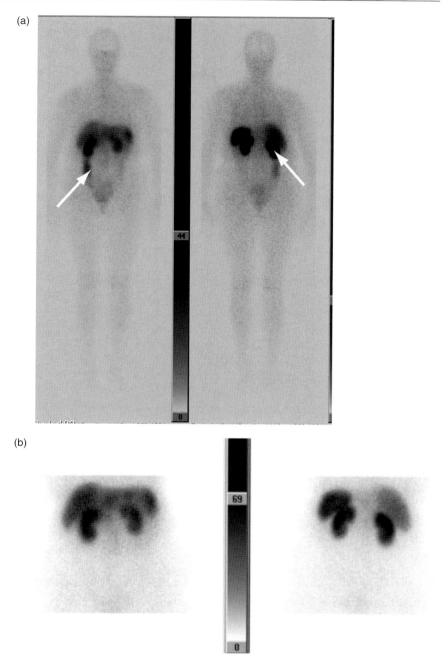

(a)

(b)

Familiarity with the normal pattern of uptake is critical for image interpretation. This normal pattern reflects both the normal distribution of somatostatin receptors as well as the route of tracer excretion. Uptake in structures due to normal expression of the somatostatin receptor includes the spleen, thyroid and pituitary. Uptake in the kidneys and urinary bladder represent the primary excretion path of octreotide. Activity in the gallbladder, liver and bowel represent a secondary hepatic excretion pathway. Some authors have noted faint uptake in breast tissue and in salivary glands [10]. Excretory accumulation in the urinary bladder, gallbladder and bowel occur to varying degrees, but can be quite prominent. It is interesting to note that the normal adrenal gland can be faintly seen on SPECT images on one or both sides in about 25% of adults using ^{111}In pentetreotide [11]. Scenarios giving rise to 'false positive' (in the sense of processes other than the tumor being sought expressing somatostatin receptors) have been described [12]. The degree of uptake in abnormal foci is often reported in qualitative terms by describing the intensity of uptake in the abnormality compared to uptake in the normal liver.

Recently, SPECT-CT imaging has been employed by fusing SPECT and CT data using internal or external markers, or by imaging with a dedicated SPECT-CT scanning device [13]. This may permit localization of suspected abnormalities to specific anatomic structures [14], although the success of the procedure is dependent on precise registration of the two image sets.

Somatostatin receptor imaging is somewhat limited in the adrenal region owing to the kidney being the primary excretory pathway for the agent. This lowers the ability of SRI to detect adrenal abnormalities as compared with MIBG. A large study showed a detection rate of 90% for ^{123}I-MIBG in detecting adrenal pheochromocytomas larger than 1 cm. with only a 25% detection rate for ^{111}In-pentetreotide [15]. Performance of SRI in the detection of pheochromoctyoma metastases is fortunately better than at the primary site, and is probably comparable to that of ^{123}I-MIBG. The overall accuracy for SRI and MIBG in neural crest tumors is thought to be similar by some authors [16]. An example of a pheochromocytoma is shown in Fig. 10.6, evident on both planar and SPECT images in a patient who had undergone previous resection of the contralateral adrenal. Figure 10.7 shows a ganglioneuroma in the sacral region, emphasizing the value of whole body imaging when there are concerns for extra-adrenal disease.

SRI has a diagnostic role in neuroblastoma and is capable of detecting many of the metastases in this tumor. The intensity of ^{111}In-pentetreotide uptake in these cases has prognostic value because high levels of somatostatin 2 expression correlate positively with survival [3, 17]. The sensitivity of SRI ranges from 55% to 70% across several studies of neuroblastoma, while that of MIBG is 83% to 94% [18]. These figures are somewhat difficult to interpret given the multitude of different imaging protocols used (for example SPECT vs planar images, ^{123}I vs ^{131}I MIBG), but they suggest that ^{111}In-pentetreotide is less sensitive than is ^{123}I-MIBG for neuroblastoma.

The specificity of SRI is limited by the occurrence of somatostatin receptors in many benign (often inflammatory) and malignant entities [19]. Malignant processes in which SRI scans are often abnormal include pheochromocytomas, paragangliomas, neuroblastomas, endocrine pancreatic tumors, medullary and other thyroid carcinomas, carcinoid tumors, small cell lung carcinoma, Merkel cell tumors, lymphomas, breast carcinoma, well-differentiated astrocytomas and melanomas. Benign processes that can show marked uptake include sarcoidosis (showing mediastinal, hilar, and parotid uptake), and Graves disease (with intense thyroid uptake) as well as other autoimmune and granulomatous diseases. This lack of specificity of SRI is one relative advantage for MIBG in the adrenal. On the other hand, medications interfere with SRI imaging less than with MIBG, making the procedure easier to perform on patients who must continue to take antihypertensive and other medications during the imaging process.

The sensitivity of SRI for benign pheochromocytoma and paraganglioma appears to be somewhat lower than MIBG scintigraphy and its use should probably be reserved for cases whether other imaging tests have failed to provide a definitive answer. A similar situation pertains in the case of neuroblastoma, for which MIBG is the preferred first line imaging agent. Somatostatin receptor imaging may be more useful to detect non-functioning paraganglionomas in extra-adrenal locations, such as the head and neck, where MIBG has proven less successful. When MIBG imaging is negative in a suspected pheochromocytoma, either FDG-PET imaging or SRI are appropriate [1].

Summary and Key Points

1. Single photon imaging plays an auxiliary role in the evaluation of adrenal masses.
2. ^{123}I-labeled MIBG is the most specific single photon agent for the detection of adrenergic tumors.
3. ^{111}In-pentetreotide is a less specific agent, binding to somatostatin receptors shared by a relatively broad range of malignant and benign processes. It thus has a secondary role to MIBG.
4. Single photon agents find their greatest application in the search for extra-adrenal sites of disease and when the primary imaging modalities have rendered indeterminate results.

Fig. 10.6 **a** This 56-year-old male with neurofibromatosis had a prior resection of the right adrenal for pheochromoctyoma and there was clinical concern for a pheochromoctyoma in the remaining adrenal given elevated urine metanephrine. ^{111}In-pentetreotide whole body images show a focus of abnormal accumulation in the area of the left adrenal (*arrow*). **b** CT shows an adrenal mass (*arrow*) which proved to be a pheochromoctyoma and adjacent ganglioneuroma, both tumors measuring between 2 and 3 cm

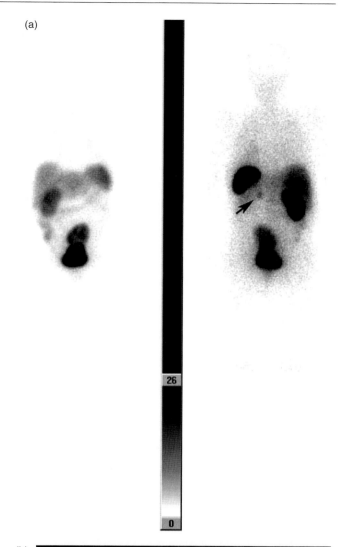

(a)

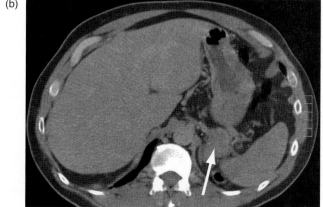

(b)

Fig. 10.7 A patient with a sacral paraganglionoma (*arrows*) is shown on whole body ^{111}In-pentetreotide images (**a**), SPECT of the pelvis (**b**) and CT (**c**). The advantages of single photon imaging largely derive from the ease of obtaining whole body images when there is clinical concern for multifocal disease

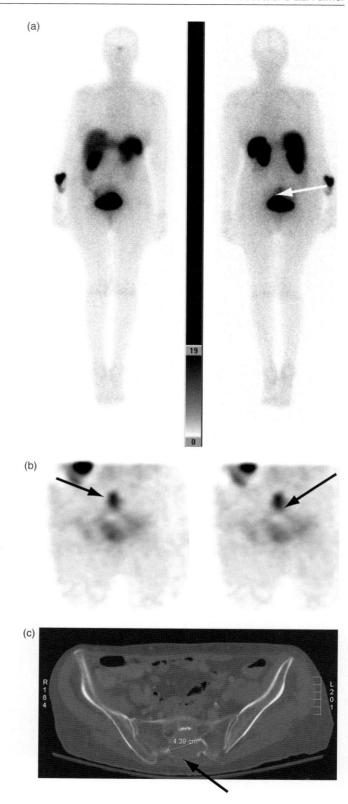

References

1. Avram AM, Fig LM, Gross MD (2006) Adrenal gland scintigraphy. Semin Nucl Med 36:212–227
2. Reisch N, Peczkowska M, Januszewicz A, Neumann H (2006) Pheochromocytoma: presentation, diagnosis and treatment. J Hypertension 24(12):2331–2339
3. Sisson JC, Frager MS, Valk TW et al. (1981) Scintigraphic localization of pheochromocytoma. N Engl J Med 305:12–17
4. McEwan AJ, Shapiro B, Sisson JC, Beierwaltes WH, Ackery DM (1985) Radio-iodobenzylguanidine for the scintigraphic location and therapy of adrenergic tumors. Semin Nucl Med 15:132–153
5. Shapiro B, Copp JE, Sisson JC, Eyre PL, Wallis J, Beierwaltes WH (1985) Iodine-131 metaiodobenzylguanidine for the locating of suspected pheochromocytoma: experience in 400 cases. J Nucl Med 26:576–585
6. van de Harst E, de Herder WW, Bruining HA et al. (2001) [^{123}I] metaiodobenzylguanidine and [^{111}In] octreotide uptake in benign and malignant pheochromocytomas. J Clin Endocrinol Metab 86:685–693
7. van Gelder T, Verhoeven GT, deJong P et al. (1995) Dopamine-producing paraganglionoma not visualized by iodine-123-MIBG scintigraphy. J Nucl Med 36:6320–6322
8. Virgiolini I, Traub T, Leimer M et al. (2000) New radiopharmaceuticals for receptor scintigraphy and radionuclide therapy. Q J Nucl Med 44:50–58
9. Jamar E, Fiasse R, Leners N et al. (1995) Somatostatin receptor imaging with indium-lll-pentetreotide in gastroenteropancreatic neuroendocrine tumors: safety, efficacy and impact on patient management. J Nucl Med 36:542–549
10. Krenning EP, Kwekkeboom DJ, Bakker WH et al. (1993) Somatostain receptor scintigraphy with [^{111}In-DTPA-D-Phe^1]- and [^{123}I-Tyr]-octreotide: the Rotterdam experience with more than 1000 patients. Eur J Nucl Med 20:716–731
11. Jacobsson H, Bremmer S, Larsson SA (2003) Visualisation of the normal adrenals at SPET examination with ^{111}In-pentetrotide. Eur J Nucl Med 30:1169–1172
12. Gibril F, Reynolds JC, Chen CC et al. (1999) Specificity of somatostatin receptor scintigraphy: a prospective study and effects of false positive localizations on management in patients with gastrinomas. J Nucl Med 40:539–553
13. Pfannenberg AC, Eschmann SM, Horger M et al. (2003) Benefit of anatomical-functional image fusion in the diagnostic work-up of neuroendocrine neoplasms. Eur J Nucl Med Mol Imag 30:835–843
14. Krausz Y, Israel O (2006) Single-photon emission computed tomography/computer tomography in endocrinology. Sem Nucl Med 36:267–274
15. Van der Harst E, de Herder WW, Bruining HA et al. (2001) [(123)I]Metalodobenzylguanidine and [(111)In]octreotide uptake in benign and malignant pheochromocytomas. J Clin Endocrinol Metab 86:685–693
16. Hoefnagel CA (1994) Metaiodobenzylguanidine and somatostatin in oncology: role in the management of neural crest tumors. Eur J Nucl Med 21:561–581
17. Orlando C, Raggi CC, Bagnoni L et al. (2001) Somatostatin receptor type 2 gene expression in neuroblastoma, measured by competitive RT-PCR, is related to patient survival and to somatostain receptor imaging by indium-111 pentetreotide. Med Pediat Oncol 36:224–226
18. Pashankar FD, O'Dorisio MS, Menda Y (2005) MIBG and somatostatin receptor analogs in children: Current concepts on diagnostic and therapeutic use. J Nucl Med 46:55S–61S
19. Hoefnagel CA (1997) Metaiodobenzylguanidine and somatostatin in oncology: role in the management of neural crest tumors. Eur J Nucl Med 38:60P

Contents

M.A. Blake (✉)
Division of Abdominal Imaging and Intervention,
Department of Radiology, Massachusetts General Hospital,
55 Fruit Street, Boston, MA 02114
E-mail: Mblake2@partners.org

Differentiation of Adrenal Lesions: The Need for Molecular Imaging

Since diagnostic imaging use has burgeoned in the last two decades, unsuspected adrenal gland lesions are now commonly found in clinical practice. They have been called "incidentalomas" when they are incidentally detected. The most important differential diagnosis of incidentalomas is between malignant and benign lesions. Some of the incidentalomas can be correctly diagnosed at computed tomography (CT) as benign adenomas due to high lipid content and therefore low attenuation values on unenhanced CT scans. However, in a large number of subjects, characterization of incidentalomas by unenhanced CT is not possible, and additional diagnostic work-up with contrast enhanced CT including a delayed acquisition of images post contrast injection or magnetic resonance imaging (MRI) is necessary. Still, up to one third of incidentalomas remain of unclear aetiology even after additional workup with MRI [1]. This illustrates the need for more accurate imaging techniques that reach beyond the morphologic level into the molecular characteristics of adrenal lesions. This is possible with positron emission tomography (PET) which visualizes the metabolic activity of tumors. In PET-CT, functional and morphologic information is synergistically combined in one exam. The radiotracer ^{18}F- fluoro-2-deoxy-D-glucose (FDG) is successfully used in differentiating benign from malignant adrenal lesions. Besides FDG, other radiopharmaceuticals specific for tumors arising from the adrenal cortex have been developed such as ^{11}C Metomidate (METO) or ^{18}F-fluoro-2-ethyl-desethyl-R-etomidate (FETO). Promising results have also been reported for ^{18}F-fluorodopamine (F-DA) and ^{18}F-dihydroxyphenylalanine (F-DOPA) in imaging of adrenal medullary tumors.

Principles of PET Imaging

Positron emission tomography (PET) and PET-CT have been shown to be very valuable in the differentiation of adrenal masses. In contrast to CT and MRI, PET is a functional and metabolic imaging modality. PET imaging is emission based, in that radiation is emitted from a tracer within the patient's body. Tracers or radiopharmaceuticals consist of a pharmaceutical/substrate that is labelled with a positron-emitting radionuclide. The most common radiopharmaceutical is ^{18}F-fluoro-2-deoxy-D-glucose (FDG), where the radionuclide ^{18}F labels the substrate deoxyglucose (DG) to create FDG. Tracers are injected intravenously and incorporated into the organ of interest through the metabolism of the pharmaceutical. For FDG, which is an analog of glucose, the metabolic process is glycolysis. Malignant lesions are known to be associated with enhanced glycolysis, and therefore accumulate FDG. FDG is transported into tumor cells by glucose membrane proteins (Glut-1 to Glut-5). Glut-1 in particular is expressed in many malignancies [2]. Intracellularly, the enzyme hexokinase phosphorylates FDG to FDG-6-phosphate. Unlike glucose, FDG-6-phosphate is not further

Table 11.1 Patient preparation for PET and PET-CT exams

1. Patient has to be non-pregnant and be fasting for 4–6 h prior to scan
2. No strenuous exercise for the patient within 24 h before study
3. Check blood glucose level (ideally between 120 and 150 mg/dL)
4. Metallic objects have to be removed
5. Protocol patient weight, height, injected tracer dose, and uptake time for SUV measurements
6. Patient should rest quietly on a cart during uptake time of tracer
7. Patient should void before scan

metabolized and remains in the incorporated cells because of its negative charge. Furthermore, the amount of FDG assimilation in malignant lesions has been associated with more aggressive tumors and the amount of viable cells [3]. In addition, PET permits semiquantitative analysis of tracer uptake through the calculation of standardized uptake values (SUVs). Since metabolic alterations in malignancies are present before morphologic changes, PET sometimes reveals diagnostic information at an earlier stage than CT or MRI. One of the most important advantages of PET imaging is that it is a whole-body imaging modality and a single exam identifies the overall extent of the cancer including lymph node, or distant organ metastases, and may even reveal unsuspected secondary malignancies. Careful patient preparation is essential for PET imaging since many confounding factors might interfere with tracer uptake and might have misleading consequences on the interpretation of findings. Table 11.1 summarizes the most important factors that have to be considered during patient preparation.

The Additional Value of PET-CT Over PET Alone

PET-CT is currently the fastest growing imaging modality in the world [4]. PET and CT are synergetic largely since PET offers high sensitivity and CT the necessary temporal and spatial resolution as well as other advantageous information. PET often detects the pathology, and CT helps to specify what is found and also contributes to the diagnostic power of the examination. In this multimodality imaging approach, CT and PET scans are obtained during a single imaging session in the same scanner. The PET and CT images are intrinsically spatially coregistered with no further need of labor-intensive and logistically challenging registration algorithms. Temporal misregistration effects due to patient or internal organ movements are minimized, since CT and PET images are obtained in close temporal proximity. PET-CT is a whole body imaging modality and can detect distant metastases and secondary tumors. FDG PET-CT has been shown to be very valuable in staging and therapy monitoring of most malignancies, including lung cancer, colorectal cancer, melanoma, lymphoma, and many more. However, for the characterization of prostate cancer, choline derivatives have been demonstrated to be superior to FDG. Besides the advantage of PET-CT in clinical diagnosis, the following technical advancements of combined PET-CT might explain why this new technology is so successful. In general, a PET camera detects the two gamma photons (each 511 keV) that emanate inside the body from the site of the positron-electron annihilation reaction close to the radionuclide. Since radiation from an annihilation reaction in the depth of the body is attenuated by tissue differently than radiation from an annihilation reaction at the body's surface, scans have to be corrected for attenuation in order to produce an image. This correction is done in PET standalone scanners by providing "attenuation maps" which are created in a germanium transmission scan from external radiation sources that rotate around the patient. This transmission scan is responsible for a significant portion of the duration of a complete PET exam. Fortunately, in combined PET-CT, the attenuation correction needed for PET can be obtained from the rapidly acquired CT component. This reduces examination time by about 30% compared to the conventional germanium transmission scan attenuation correction of PET standalone scanners. A PET-CT exam usually takes about 30 min or less. Therefore, PET-CT is not simply the addition of a PET to a CT scanner, rather, it benefits from the complementary synergism of both modalities at a diagnostic and a technical level [5]. Integrated PET-CT combines the best of its contributing modalities.

The Normal Adrenal Glands in FDG PET and PET-CT

Knowledge of the physiologic appearance of adrenal glands in FDG PET and PET-CT is necessary to correctly identify pathologic processes. Although adrenal glands are larger (size: about 4 mL; craniocaudal dimension: 2–3 cm) than the spatial resolution of PET (about 5 mm), and although they are rich in vascular supply and metabolically active, they are mostly not visible in PET alone. Differentiation of physiologic adrenal FDG uptake from normal background activity is usually not possible. Therefore, visualization of normal adrenal glands and quantification of their FDG uptake is not feasible with PET alone. Combined PET-CT examination, however, can assign the primarily nonspecific tracer uptake in FDG PET to the location of the adrenal glands visible in the coregistered CT component. In a study by Bagheri et al. [6] only 5% (2/40) of normal adrenal glands could be visualized with PET alone, whereas 68% (27/40) were identified with integrated PET-CT. In those adrenal glands which were detected in PET-CT, standardized uptake values (SUVs) of normal adrenal glands could be calculated. The average value of the maximum SUV and of the mean SUV was 0.90 ± 0.15 and 0.83 ± 0.17, respectively, for the right adrenal gland, and 1.10 ± 0.15 and 0.946 ± 0.15, respectively, for the left adrenal gland. In previous studies with CT, the left adrenal gland was found to be slightly larger than the right adrenal gland [7]. Thus, the higher SUV in the left adrenal gland compared to the right was suggested by Bagheri et al. to be related to its larger size and therefore less partial volume averaging. The maximum SUV of normal adrenal glands ranged from 0.95 to 2.46. Usually, adrenal FDG uptake is considered to be of malignant origin when intensity is higher than liver uptake. Considering that normal liver tissue has an average mean SUV between 1.5 and 2.0, physiologic adrenal uptake might in some cases be in the range of malignant lesions. Thus, the differential diagnosis of increased adrenal FDG uptake might not only include malignant or benign lesions, but also a normal adrenal gland. However, most normal adrenal glands have either FDG uptake less than normal liver tissue or are associated with uptake that is not different from background activity. This is in contrast to CT, where unenhanced soft tissue density of normal adrenals is similar to that of liver and where almost 100% of normal adrenals can be visualized [8]. Integrated PET-CT has the potential to combine information from both exams into one. Therefore, due to the exact anatomic information of integrated PET-CT it is now possible to perform SUV measurements in all normal and abnormal adrenal glands.

Differentiation of Adrenal Lesions – Benign vs Malignant

Unexpected adrenal masses (incidentalomas) in the general population are revealed in up to about 9% of autopsies [9] and about 5% of CT exams of the abdomen [10]. In healthy individuals, 80% of incidentally discovered adrenal masses are benign nonfunctioning adenomas [11]. The situation is more complex in subjects with known primary cancer, since adrenal metastases were observed in about 27% of autopsies in patients with carcinoma [12]. The most common malignancies associated with adrenal metastases are lung cancer, breast cancer, and melanoma. However, even in patients with primary malignant lesions, approximately 40%–57% of the incidentalomas are benign [12]. The accurate identification of metastases among incidentalomas in patients with primary carcinoma has major clinical importance since an isolated metastasis of the ipsilateral adrenal gland in a patient with resectable primary non small cell lung cancer is treated as localized disease. In these patients, resection of isolated adrenal metastases has been demonstrated to extend disease-free survival [13].

Differentiation of Adrenal Lesions with FDG PET – Results from Clinical Studies

Boland and colleagues [14] were the first to evaluate the feasibility of FDG-PET in adrenal imaging. In a prospective study with 24 adrenal lesions in patients with known cancer, all 14 adrenal metastases showed increased uptake relative to background activity (sensitivity and specificity 100%). Several further studies have followed: Erasmus et al. [15] studied 33 adrenal masses in 27 patients with lung cancer. PET findings were read as positive when FDG uptake was more intense in the adrenal lesions than in the background. The sensitivity for

detecting metastasis was 100%, and the specificity was 80%. Maurea et al. [16] investigated several benign adrenal masses, including seven adenomas, in comparison to malignant tumors. Only one benign lesion, a benign pheochromocytoma, showed increased uptake compared to background activity. For the detection of malignant adrenal lesions sensitivity was 100% and specificity was 93%. Subsequent investigators compared the activity of adrenal lesions in comparison to liver rather than background. In a study of 41 patients with 50 lesions (30 of whom had lung cancer), Yun et al. [17] found a sensitivity of 100% and a specificity of 94% when using lesion uptake more than or equal to liver uptake as the criterion of a positive result. Gupta et al. [18] evaluated 30 patients with lung cancer. Again, PET findings were read as positive when FDG uptake was higher than liver uptake. F-FDG PET showed abnormally increased uptake in 17 of 18 malignant lesions. In benign lesions, PET was true negative in 11 of 12 lesions. This resulted in a sensitivity of 94% and specificity of 92% in diagnosing metastases. Kumar et al. [19] evaluated PET in 113 adrenal masses detected by CT or MRI in 94 patients with lung cancer. Seventy-two lesions were malignant and 41 benign. Thirty-seven of the benign lesions were negative for ^{18}F-FDG uptake when compared with liver. A benign pheochromocytoma and three adenomas showed equal or greater uptake than liver. Sixty-seven of 72 malignant masses had uptake equal to or higher than liver. The overall sensitivity to differentiate between benign and malignant adrenal masses in patients with lung cancer was 93%, and specificity was 90%. Furthermore, positive predictive value was 94%, negative predictive value was 88%, and an accuracy was 92% for detecting metastasis in this study by Kumar et al.

Until this point, published studies have demonstrated a sensitivity and accuracy of more than 92% for PET. Following studies have evaluated the use of maximum or mean SUV measurements in the differentiation of benign and malignant adrenal disease. This quantitative method was compared with visual analysis. Furthermore performance of PET was compared with that of CT. Jana et al. [20] evaluated 50 benign and 30 metastatic adrenal lesions. PET was 93% sensitive and 96% specific for detecting metastases. A mean SUV threshold of

3.1 yielded a sensitivity of 95% and a specificity of 90%. Visual interpretation was as accurate as SUV calculation in this study by Jana et al. FDG-PET was most valuable in the 52.5% of cancer patients with inconclusive adrenal lesions on CT. In this group of lesions that were indeterminate in CT, PET was 88% sensitive and 96% specific. Two of the metastatic lesions fell into the category of indeterminate on CT, both of which were positive in PET.

Differentiation of Adrenal Lesions with FDG PET-CT – Results from Clinical Studies

By now there have been three studies evaluating incidentalomas with FDG PET-CT. Metser et al. [21] evaluated 100 adrenal adenomas (72 lipid rich, 29 lipid poor) and 75 non-adenomas. They found that a maximum SUV of 3.1 or more is useful for differentiating malignant from benign adrenal lesions. The sensitivity and specificity was 98.5% and 92% using this semiquantitative threshold. Figures 11.1 and 11.2 demonstrate two examples of adrenal metastases with intense uptake. However, interpretation should not solely be based on SUV measurements since this approach may produce false-negative findings in small (<1 cm) metastatic adrenal lesions or false positive results in FDG avid adenomas. The results by Metser et al. further improved when the SUV threshold was combined with attenuation analysis from unenhanced CT (<10 HU positive for adenoma; HU = Hounsfield Units) resulting in a sensitivity of 100% and specificity of 98%. In a study by Blake et al., 32 benign adrenal masses were compared with 9 non-adenomas compared in PET-CT. Of the 32 benign adrenal masses, 30 showed activity on visual analysis that was less than that of the liver (specificity: 94%). Sensitivity was 100% (12/12) for detecting adrenal malignant disease in this study by Blake et al. [22]. Similarly, Caoili et al. [23] recently demonstrated a sensitivity of 96% by identifying 45 of 47 adrenal metastases on combined PET-CT. Specificity was 100% (12/12) in their study. Table 11.2 summarizes studies that evaluated the performance of PET and PET-CT in the differentiation of adrenal lesions.

Adrenal Uptake Relative to Liver or Background Activity?

As shown in Table 11.2, the various studies on adrenal lesions have compared adrenal uptake either to background or to liver activity. Studies on PET alone exams reported that most of benign lesions including adenomas, presented with uptake equal to that of background [16, 17, 19]. In contrast to these studies on PET alone, Caoili et al. found a high percentage (87%) of adenomas with uptake higher than that of background in PET-CT examinations [23]. This may be explained by the use of PET-CT in the study by Caoili et al. which might more accurately assess uptake in an adrenal tumor and distinguish it from background intensity. Several investigations have demonstrated that when using liver activity as the threshold (rather than background activity) the accuracy of characterizing adrenal masses improved [17, 19, 22, 23]. In the study by Caoili et al., 87% (41 of 47) of adenomas had intensity higher than background, whereas only 11% (5 of 47) of adenomas had uptake higher than the liver. Eighteen adenomas and three non-adenomas demonstrated tracer activity equal to that of liver [23].

Lipid-poor Adenomas in FDG PET-CT

In the study by Metser et al. [21], FDG uptake was not significantly different between lipid-rich and lipid-poor adenomas. Sensitivity and specificity were 98.5% and 92% for differentiating lipid-poor adenomas and 98.5% and 93% for all adenomas. Identification of adenomas on unenhanced CT is dependent on the high lipid content of adenomas. Since about 30% of adenomas are low in lipid content and high in attenuation measurements (>10 HU), identification of such lipid-poor adenomas with CT alone is not possible. The PET component of integrated PET-CT might be complementary in these cases and provide the correct diagnosis by showing uptake less than liver. Contrast enhanced CT including a delayed acquisition of images post contrast injection ideally as part of the same PET/CT may provide further helpful diagnostic adrenal information. Occasionally MRI or adrenal biopsy may be necessary.

(a)

(b)

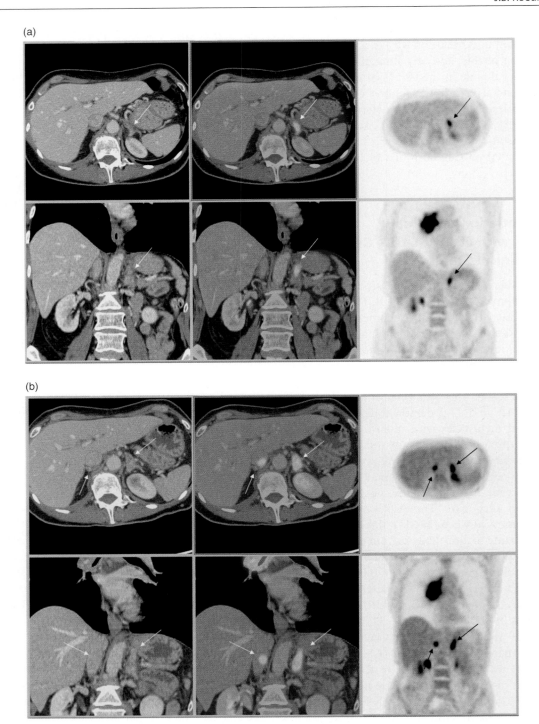

Fig. 11.1 A 70-year-old woman with lung cancer and metastatic disease to the right and left adrenal gland on PET/CT. **a** A first PET-CT scan for primary staging revealed intense FDG uptake in the left adrenal gland (SUVmax: 5.9) concordant with a mass seen on CT. **b** A follow-up scan 5 weeks later shows intense uptake both in the left (SUVmax: 8.4) and in the right (SUVmax: 6.1) adrenal gland. CT findings in the right adrenal gland are equivocal but subsequent imaging confirmed a metastasis. The *upper row* of selected images are axial views, the *lower row* are the corresponding coronal views. The *left* column shows the CT, the *right* column the PET component and the *middle* column the combined PET-CT

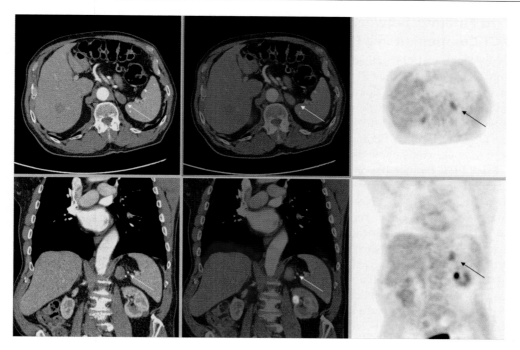

Fig. 11.2 Metastatic disease in a 72-year-old male with colon cancer. There is a 3.7-cm nodule in the left adrenal gland with intense FDG uptake (SUVmax: 5.3) consistent with metastatic disease. The *upper row* of selected images are axial views, the *lower row* are the corresponding coronal views. The *left* column shows the CT, the *right* column the PET component and the *middle* column the combined PET-CT

Table 11.2 Investigations on PET or PET-CT in the distinction of malignant from benign adrenal lesions

Study	Modality	Visual analysis	Sensitivity[a]	Specificity	Accuracy	SUV mean (range)
Boland et al. 1995 (14)	PET	>Background	100 (14/14)	100 (10/10)	100 (24/24)	7.4 (2.9–16.6) vs 0.8 (0.2–1.2)
Erasmus et al. 1997 (15)	PET	>Background	100 (23/23)	80 (8/10)	94 (31/33)	6.3 (3.2–14.4) vs 1.8 (0.93–3.70)
Maurea et al. 1999 (16)	PET	>Background	100 (13/13)	93 (13/14)	96 (26/27)	–
Yun et al. 2001 (17)	PET	≥Hepatic	100 (18/18)	94 (30/32)	96 (48/50)	–
Gupta et al. 2001(18)	PET	≥Hepatic	94 (11/12)	92 (17/18)	93 (28/30)	–
Kumar et al. 2004 (19)	PET	≥Hepatic	93 (67/72)	90 (37/41)	92 (104/113)	–
Jana et al. 2006 (20)	PET	>Hepatic	93 (28/30)	96 (48/50)	95 (76/80)	4.8 (2.1–13) vs 2.2 (1.2–3.3)
Metser et al. 2006 (21)	PET-CT	≥Hepatic	100 (68/68)	98 (105/107)	99 (173/175)	10.1 (1.1–26.2) vs 1.8 (0.3–6.4)
Blake et al. 2006 (22)	PET-CT	>Hepatic	100 (9/9)	94 (30/32)	95 (39/41)	SUV Ratio[b]: 4.0 (1.5–17.1) vs 0.7 (0.2–0.94)
Caoili et al. 2007 (23)	PET-CT	≥Hepatic	96 (45/47)	100 (12/12)	97 (57/59)	SUV Ratio[a]: 1.0±0.2 vs 2.1±1.1 (P = .006).

[a]In percent and absolute numbers in parenthesis
[b]SUV Ratio = Adrenal SUV/Liver SUV)

Discordant Findings Between the PET and the CT Component in a PET-CT Exam

In the study by Caoili et al. [23] 17 lipid-rich adenomas (<10 HU on unenhanced CT) had SUV uptake equal to that of the liver and three lipid-rich adenomas demonstrated activity greater than liver. Using adrenal uptake equal or greater than liver uptake as the criterion for a PET positive finding, 20 cases in the study by Caoili et al. would show discordant results between CT and PET. It might be concluded that if an adrenal gland lesion shows intensity equal to or slightly higher than that of the liver on FDG PET, the scan should be read as indeterminate. Only if a lesion shows FDG uptake less than that of the liver, or uptake that is significantly higher than the liver (more than twice that of the liver) the study can be interpreted with high confidence. If attenuation values on unenhanced CT are also indeterminate, then additional imaging should be performed for further characterization of the lesion. There have been no other studies besides that of Caoili et al. that reported about discordant findings in PET-CT meaning increased FDG activity in the PET component and an attenuation value <10 HU on the CT part. In the study by Blake et al. [22] both false-positive PET interpretations also had an attenuation value measured at nonenhanced CT of more than 10 HU. Thus, the PET and the CT component were essentially concordant in all cases in this study [22]. It is yet unclear which component of PET-CT should be relied upon when there are discordant results.

Absolute or Relative SUV Measurements of Adrenal Lesions?

Blake et al. and other groups (Table 11.2) demonstrated that there was a significant difference in SUVs between benign and malignant adrenal masses. Metser et al. [21] reported promising results in detecting malignant adrenal disease with a sensitivity of 98.5% and a specificity of 92% by using a SUV threshold of 3.1. However, in the study by Blake et al. SUV ratios (adrenal lesion SUV/liver SUV) have been shown to be more accurate in differentiating benign lesions from metastases than absolute SUVs. This is partially consistent with the investigation by Caoili et al. [23] who found significant differences only in SUV ratios (adrenal/liver) but not in absolute SUVs between adenomas and metastases to the adrenals. SUV measurement is dependent on a number of factors, such as an accurate recording of dose, duration of time tracer uptake time, and patient body weight. Other parameters such as tumor size, noise, image resolution, region of interest, serum glucose levels, type of reconstruction used, and renal function have also been reported to alter the measured SUV [24–26]. Some of these factors are difficult to quantify and are not accounted for in current SUV calculations potentially causing misleading SUVs. SUV ratios (tumor SUV/reference tissue SUV) would "normalize" many of these factors. Considering this, SUV ratios might be preferred over absolute SUV measurements. However, further studies are warranted to determine whether absolute or relative values should be used for characterizing adrenal lesions.

The Additional Value of PET-CT Over PET Alone in Adrenal Gland Imaging

FDG PET–CT is better able to differentiate benign from malignant adrenal lesions than is FDG PET alone. With PET-CT the characterization of adrenal lesions combines the diagnostic value of CT and PET in a single exam. This advantage applies to both visual and quantitative evaluation of adrenal lesions. The complementary advantage of quantitative results was demonstrated by the study of Metser et al. where the combination of a SUV threshold of 3.1 with a CT attenuation value of <10 HU resulted in a sensitivity of 100% and specificity of 98% for characterizing adrenal lesions [21]. In this study of 175 adrenal lesions, PET alone (maximum SUV, 3.1) achieved a sensitivity, specificity, and accuracy of 99% (67 of 68 nodules), 92% (98 of 107), and 94% (165 of 175), respectively, compared to integrated PET-CT with values of 100% (68 of 68 nodules), 98% (105 of 107), and 99% (173 of 175), respectively. Furthermore, specificity was significantly higher for PET-CT compared to PET alone [21]. Furthermore, in this study, even the small adrenal lesions detected on the CT component were correctly diagnosed on the PET part by evaluating tracer uptake. This might be explained by the precise fusion capabilities of PET-CT with the ability to identify adrenal lesions that would not accurately be localized on PET alone. Besides that, PET-CT has the previously discussed advantages including the possibility of SUV measurements in lesions with low FDG uptake and shorter examination time by using CT for attenuation correction. Furthermore, if contrast enhanced CT including a delayed acquisition of images post contrast injection is incorporated as part of the PET/CT examination this may provide additional diagnostic adrenal information.

False Negatives in FDG PET and PET-CT

In metastastic adrenal lesions FDG uptake depends on size, differentiation, and the primary tumor of the metastasis. PET scanners have spatial resolution of about 5 mm. Therefore, in small metastases (<10 mm) uptake is lower than in larger lesions due to partial volume averaging. Uptake in lesions smaller than 10 mm is mostly less than in normal liver tissue [19]. These small metastatic lesions might also be missed due to the absence of sufficient tumor cells with increased glycolysis. Hemorrhage and necrosis are also known to cause false negative results in FDG-PET [17, 20, 21]. Kumar et al. found five false-negative lesions in their study on adrenal lesions: one necrotic metastasis, one metastasis with central hemorrhage, and three small metastatic

lesions [19]. Furthermore, metastases from primary carcinomas that are non-FDG avid have been found to be false negative in PET including carcinoid (neuroendocrine tumors), and pulmonary carcinoma of the bronchioloalveolar type [15, 17, 20].

False Positives in FDG PET and PET-CT

FDG accumulates not only in malignant tumor cells but also in activated inflammatory cells such as granulocytes and macrophages which can be mistaken for malignancy in patients with proven or suspected cancer. In general, both acute and chronic infections (36–40) including sarcoidosis, tuberculosis [27], and autoimmune disease such as Grave's disease [28] might be associated with increased FDG uptake. Moreover, the ^{18}F-FDG uptake can be enhanced by postoperative healing scars and postradiation therapy. Approximately, 5% of adrenal pathologies interpreted as positive in PET are false-positive for malignancy. This is secondary to inflammatory lesions, adrenal endothelial cysts, adrenal adenomas and periadrenal pathology (Fig. 11.3). There is no

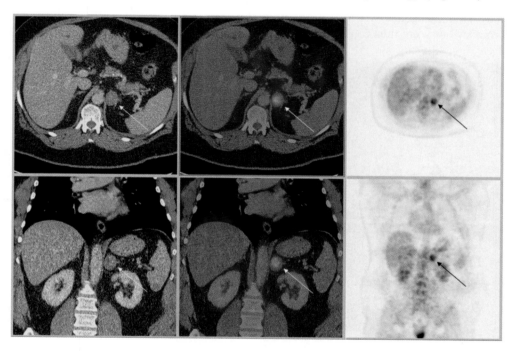

Fig. 11.3 Erroneous PET false positive finding for metastatic disease to the adrenal in a 53-year-old female with esophageal carcinoma periadrenal lymphadenopathy. The left adrenal gland region demonstrates marked tracer uptake (SUVmax: 5.6) on PET. A lymph node medial to and displacing a normal adrenal gland is seen on CT which was the cause of FDG uptake. The correct diagnosis of metastatic periadrenal lymph node was made with PET/CT. The *upper row* of selected images are axial views, the *lower row* are the corresponding coronal views. The *left* column shows the CT, the *right* column the PET component and the *middle* column the combined PET-CT

proven explanation why some adenomas demonstrate high FDG uptake, and simulate malignant disease. It has been assumed, however, that the functional state of an adenoma determines the intensity of tracer uptake, with increased uptake in functionally active adrenal masses [29]. In Figs. 11.4 and 11.5 two examples of FDG avid adenomas are presented. Yun et al. [17] has reported variable FDG uptake in adenomas, resulting in false positive findings. Furthermore, adrenal cortical hyperplasia without chronic inflammatory cell infiltration might also mimic metastases, because it has been associated with increased FDG uptake. Furthermore, FDG PET cannot differentiate between malignant lesions e.g. between metastases, adrenocortical carcinoma, malignant pheochromocytoma, and lymphoma (Figs. 11.6 and 11.7), each of which might present with increased FDG uptake [30]. Pheochromocytoma, whether benign or malignant, might accumulate FDG. It was reported, however, that among malignant pheochromocytomas the percentage with increased uptake is higher than among benign pheochromocytomas [17]. In addition, even pathologically benign pheochromocytomas may have malignant systemic effects and all pheochromocytomas are thus considered surgical lesions. Last but not least, false positive findings might occur in false adrenal masses that actually arise from a nearby organ such as the liver, kidney, or stomach [31, 32]. Brown fat deposition with increased FDG uptake in the retroperitoneum and periadrenal fat might also mimic a primary adrenal mass (Fig. 11.8). Although sceptics complain about the lack of specificity of FDG, its accumulation in tissue is still more specific than the accumulation of extracellular fluid agents, such as most iodinated contrast agents and gadolinium chelates used for contrast enhancement in CT and MRI.

Why PET/PET-CT When There is Already CT, MRI and Biopsy?

It is desirable to evaluate adrenal lesions non-invasively in order to avoid unnecessary complications associated with adrenal biopsy. Adrenal biopsy was reported to have a complication rate of 8.4%–11.3% [33]. Besides that, biopsy does not always provide the final diagnosis considering that it has a failure rate of 14%–50% from the first attempt. This is secondary to either non-diagnostic pathology findings or the failure to

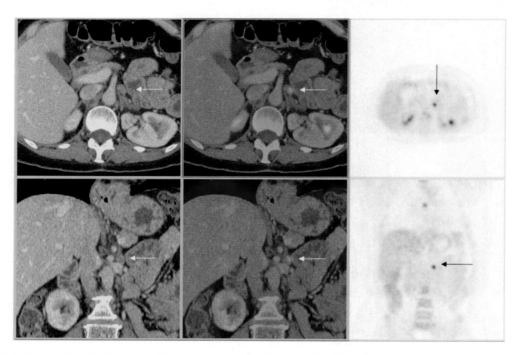

Fig. 11.4 A 51-year-old male with primary leiomyosarcoma and highly FDG avid adenoma. Intense FDG uptake (SUVmax: 9.2) was incidentally found in the left adrenal gland correlating with a mass seen in the concurrent CT. This finding was highly suspicious for metastatic disease. However, biopsy revealed benign adenoma. Image quality of the CT component is degraded by increased noise due to obesity of the patient. The *upper row* of selected images are axial views, the *lower row* are the corresponding coronal views. The *left* column shows the CT, the *right* column the PET component and the *middle* column the combined PET-CT

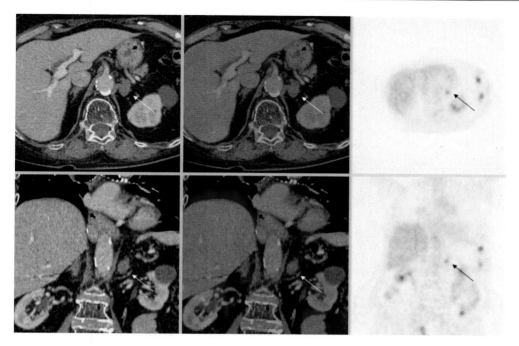

Fig. 11.5 An 83-year-old male with lung cancer and "hot adenoma". Moderate FDG uptake (SUVmax: 3.3) was found and metastatic disease was suspected in this patient with a history of lung cancer. However, on CT the nodule remained stable in size on follow-up exams and surgery finally revealed benign adenoma. The *upper row* of selected images are axial views, the *lower row* are the corresponding coronal views. The *left* column shows the CT, the *right* column the PET component and the *middle* column the combined PET-CT

obtain adequate tissue [34]. Moreover, there is a potential risk of dissemination of malignant cells in invasive procedures. The current imaging modalities besides PET and PET-CT used for the differentiation of incidentalomas include CT and MRI. The diagnosis of adrenal lesions with CT and MR is based on the high lipid content of adrenal adenomas. Several studies showed that adenomas have lower attenuation values compared to non-adenomas [35–37]. It was demonstrated that lower HU correlate with the concentration of intracellular lipid content [38]. Boland found that a threshold attenuation value of 10 HU on unenhanced CT provides the optimal sensitivity (71%) and specificity (98%) for the diagnosis of adrenal adenoma [36]. Despite the high specificity of this method about 30% of adenomas are lipid poor and associated with attenuation values that fall in the range of malignant lesions such as metastases. Besides CT, chemical shift MRI is valuable in the distinction of adrenal adenomas and metastases. In high lipid tissues chemical shift MR imaging shows a decrease

in the signal intensity [39]. It should be considered, however, that adrenal cortical carcinomas or metastases from hepatoma, renal cell carcinoma, or liposarcoma could give the same lipid signal loss seen in adenomas. Furthermore, failure rate for diagnosis with MRI is high (13%–17%) in lipid-poor adenomas [40] and signal intensity of benign and malignant lesions might show considerable overlap with adrenal MRI imaging [41].

Suggested Diagnostic and Therapeutic Approach for Adrenal Lesions

The diagnostic approach to the correct diagnosis of adrenal lesions begins with standard biochemical evaluation to rule out pheochromocytoma, Cushing syndrome, and primary hyperaldosteronism. However, adrenal lesions do not usually cause adrenal hyperfunction because they are either nonhypersecreting or secrete inactive products. Although both the PET and CT components expose the patient to a not insignificant radiation dose, FDG-PET-CT might still be the most

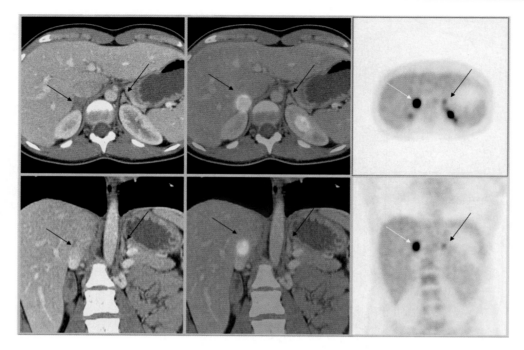

Fig. 11.6 A 23-year-old female with bilateral lymphomatous involvement of the adrenals. Hypermetabolic activity (SUVmax: 17.4) involving the right adrenal gland with underlying mass on the CT scan was consistent with lymphoma. The moderate FDG uptake (SUVmax: 3.2) in the left adrenal gland without a definite finding in the CT component was also found to be lymphoma. This example illustrates that metabolic imaging with PET-CT can detect malignant disease earlier than CT alone. However, the CT component is necessary for the exact localisation of the abnormal uptake. The *upper row* of selected images are axial views, the *lower row* are the corresponding coronal views. The *left* column shows the CT, the *right* column the PET component and the *middle* column the combined PET-CT

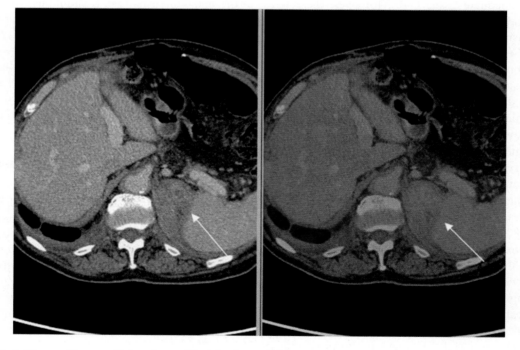

Fig. 11.7 A 79-year-old man with lymphoma. The left adrenal gland showed moderate to intense FDG uptake (SUVmax: 3.6) in the left adrenal mass (*arrow*) with a grossly conserved adreniform shape consistent with known history of lymphoma

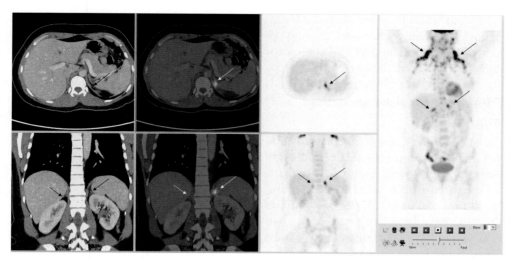

Fig. 11.8 A 36-year-old female with periadrenal brown fat deposition. Bilateral supraclavicular foci of brown fat with increased uptake (*neck arrows*). Similarly, enhanced uptake is seen bilaterally in the periadrenal fat (*suprarenal arrows*) with no uptake in the adrenal glands. Brown adipose tissue accumulates FDG since it is associated with increased glycolysis. Brown fat is usually not visible in adults, but might become apparent after exposure to cold temperatures. It is especially seen in the supraclavicular area, may extend into the retroperitoneum surrounding the kidneys, adrenals and the aorta. The CT component in the presented case helps to allocate the increased uptake to the periadrenal fat tissue. The *upper row* of selected images are axial views, the *lower row* are the corresponding coronal views. The *left* column shows the CT, the *right* column the PET component and the *middle* column the combined PET-CT

appropriate imaging modality for oncology patients with adrenal lesions since it combines CT attenuation data and PET FDG uptake information. PET-CT has better accuracy than CT or chemical shift MRI. FDG PET and PET-CT have demonstrated very good diagnostic performance in differentiating adrenal lesions with sensitivities of 93%–100%, and accuracies of 92%–100% [14, 16, 20, 22, 23] (see also Table 11.2). Furthermore, PET-CT allows the evaluation of primary lesions as well as metastases in one exam. PET was shown to reveal 19%–34% additional metastatic foci compared with conventional imaging methods [14, 15, 42]. In case of discordant findings between the components of PET-CT the patient should undergo further evaluation. Delayed contrast enhanced CT for washout analysis again might be integrated in a PET-CT protocol if previous findings are inconclusive. Furthermore, chemical shift MR with decreased signal intensity might be performed to determine the final diagnosis. Fine-needle aspiration biopsy can be reserved for cases where previously performed clinical and imaging results remain

indeterminate. Hormone secreting adrenal lesions as well as non functional lesions that appear malignant on imaging exams have to be surgically removed. Any adrenal lesions greater than 4 cm are also generally resected. The stability of non-hypersecreting adrenal lesions suggestive of benign entity should be confirmed on regular imaging and endocrinological follow-ups [43].

Identification of Adrenocortical Lesions

Primary Adrenocortical Tumors

Primary adrenocortial tumors include adrenocortical carcinoma (ACC) and adenomas. Although ACCs account for only 0.05%–0.2% of all cancers and although the estimated annual incidence in the United States is only about 1–2 per million, the reported prevalence of ACCs among incidentalomas is significant at about 4.1% [44]. These cases may be surgically resected at an early stage with improved prognosis [45]. On average, patients are about 45 years old when they are diagnosed with ACC. Prognosis is usually poor and etiology of ACC is unknown, but smoking and oral contraceptives are suggested to be risk factors [46].

FDG PET Imaging for Adrenocortical Carcinoma

First results of FDG PET in adrenocortical carcinomas (ACC) came from non-specific studies on adrenal lesions where a small number of patients had ACC. Increased FDG uptake was demonstrated in all of these ACCs [45–47]. Specific studies focusing on ACC have been performed after that: Becherer et al. [48] found a sensitivity of 100% and a specificity of 95% in identifying ACC in 10 patients. FDG was able to detect multiple lesions that were negative in other modalities. Leboulleux et al. [49] recently evaluated the role of FDG PET-CT with a non contrast enhanced CT component compared to a standalone i.v. contrast enhanced CT in the evaluation of metastatic disease in 22 patients with ACC and a total of 269 lesions. Sensitivities for the detection of metastatic lesions were found to be 90% and 93% for PET-CT and 88% and 82% for CT, respectively. Eighteen percent of the metastatic lesions were seen only in the PET-CT and 7% only in the contrast enhanced CT. PET-CT was especially valuable for the diagnosis of local recurrence. Five of 13 (38%) of the local recurrences were detected with PET-CT, but not with CT. The investigation of Mackie et al. [50] suggested that most ACC accumulate and retain FDG with the exception of very small tumors. Similar to the result of Leboulleux et al. they found FDG PET to detect local relapse of disease more reliably than morphologic imaging modalities.

Principals of METO PET Imaging

As described previously, FDG PET is used to differentiate benign from malignant masses. FDG is not specific for adrenal malignant lesions, and cannot distinguish between ACC and metastases or other malignancies. Radiotracers have been developed for PET that accumulate specifically in primary adrenocortical lesions (benign or malignant). Radiolabelled enzyme inhibitors can be used for specifically visualizing the adrenal cortex and its tumors. Etomidate and Metomidate (METO) labelled with ^{11}C were developed as PET tracers with the aim of identifying primary adrenocortical lesions. Etomidate is a potent inhibitor of 11b-hydroxylase, (enzyme of the cytochrome P45011B family, CYP11B) which is essential for the biosynthis of cortisol and aldosterone by the adrenal cortex [51]. For clinical applications, however, ^{11}C-metomidate was selected because of its better synthetic characteristics [52]. The major advantages of PET compared to conventional scintigraphy (e.g. with radiocholesterol) are rapid completion of the imaging, within 1 h, and a resolution and sensitivity better than those of adrenal scintigraphy.

METO PET Imaging: Results from Clinical Studies

The first results with ^{11}C METO were demonstrated by Bergstrom et al. in rhesus monkeys with a very high uptake and excellent visualisation of the adrenal glands [52]. In a following investigation by the same group on 15 patients with incidentalomas, this tracer showed very high uptake in all adrenocortical adenomas, whereas other 'masses' were negative [53]. In a study by Khan et al. [1] all 11 viable ACCs were visualised by METO PET. Two more lesions were revealed with METO PET than were seen on CT. In an investigation by Minn et al. [54], endocrinological analysis, METO and FDG PET were performed on 21 patients. High uptake of ^{11}C-metomidate was demonstrated in adrenocortical tumors and normal adrenal glands. The highest accumulation of ^{11}C-metomidate was seen in adrenocortical carcinoma (SUV = 28.0), followed by active adenomas (median SUV = 12.7), nonsecretory adenomas (median SUV = 12.2), and non-cortical tumors (median SUV = 5.7). METO PET was clearly superior to FDG PET for depicting adrenal lesions if they were adenomas. In a recent study by Hennings et al. [55], 73 patients were evaluated METO PET. Sensitivity was 89% and specificity was 96% for METO PET for the identification of tumors with adrenocortical origin. Non-adrenal masses, pheochromocytomas and adrenal metastases did not show increased METO uptake.

First Experiences with FETO PET

As described above, the results with METO- PET have been promising for adrenocortical lesions.

However, the use of METO is limited due to its short half-life (20 min). An analog of METO labelled with ^{18}F-fluoro-2-ethyl-desethyl-R-etomidate (FETO) has been developed which has longer half life and makes longer imaging protocols possible. First results in rats demonstrated that FETO accumulates almost solely in the adrenal glands and no significant accumulation was demonstrated in any other organs [56]. Wadsack et al. recently published the first experiences with this tracer in ten healthy volunteers [57]. As in the previous animal studies, strong uptake of FETO was seen in the adrenal glands of the study participants. The low uptake in structures close to the adrenals such as the liver and stomach make delineation of adrenal uptake more accurate in FETO than in METO.

Imaging of Adrenocortical Tumors: Conclusions

METO PET can distinguish adrenal metastases from adrenocortical tumors (adenomas, ACC). However, METO PET usually cannot discriminate adrenocortical cancers from adenomas. Newly developed FETO might improve performance of METO by combining its long half-life of ^{18}F with high 11β-hydroxylase and therefore provide adrenal selectivity. For patients presenting with adrenal masses and a history or strong suggestion of neoplastic disease, FDG PET is still the study of choice because whole-body imaging may reveal other additional metastatic cancer foci in addition to adrenal metastasis [17]. However, supporters of METO-PET argue that METO PET performed as the first imaging modality in patients with lesions would split patients into two groups with high specificity. METO-positive lesions encompass the adrenocortical tumors including adrenocortical adenomas, hyperplasias and ACC, whereas the METO-negative lesions consist of all other adrenal tumors. In cases of negative METO-PET, metastasis is a likely diagnosis, and a FDG-PET study could be performed to search for the primary tumor.

Identification of Medullary Lesions (Pheochromocytomas)

Pheochromocytomas are benign or malignant chromaffin cell tumors that produce catecholamines [1]. About 1% of all patients with hypertension are found to have a pheochromocytoma. Since these tumors are curable with surgical resection, identification and precise localization is clinically important [58].

PET for Pheochromocytoma Imaging

Functional (molecular imaging) methods are useful in diagnosing pheochromocytoma. Conventional scintigraphy with ^{131}I-MIBG yields very good specificity (95%–100%) but relatively low sensitivity (approximately 77%) [59, 60] in detection of pheochromocytomas. Sensitivity has been shown to be higher for ^{123}I-MIBG (MIBG) reaching up to 90%. However, availability of ^{123}I-MIBG scintigraphy has been limited to only some academic centers in the United States [61]. MIBG scanning necessitates withdrawal of drugs before the examination, and a delay of 48 h between MIBG injection and scanning because of the slow clearance of radioactivity from normal organs. Furthermore, limited spatial resolution, relatively high radiation exposure, and false negative results when tumors are smaller than 2.0 cm or associated with necrosis or hemorrhage are further disadvantages of MIBG [58]. Most of these disadvantages do not apply for PET imaging. Using FDG PET Shulkin et al. localized pheochromocytomas in 15 of 17 patients with malignant pheochromocytomas compared to 7 out of 12 patients with benign pheochromocytomas. Malignant lesions in general showed more intense uptake. In addition, the first PET tracer specific for the sympathetic nervous system has been developed: ^{11}C-hydroxyephedrine (HED) accumulates in organs with sympathetic innervation because it is a catecholamine analog. In a first series, Shulkin et al. [62] identified pheochromocytomas in 9 of 10 patients with HED-PET. PET scanning localized more lesions, with better spatial resolution and a faster scan time than ^{131}I MIBG. In a study by Trampal et al. [63] evaluating 13 pheochromocytomas, all but one were identified with HED-PET. In the remaining seven patients without pheochromocytoma HED-PET did not show increased uptake. Sensitivity, specificity, positive predictive value, negative predictive value, and accuracy for HED PET were 92%, 100%, 100%, 87.5%, and 95%, respectively for the detection of pheochromocytoma. Mann et al. [64] included eight patients with pheochromocytoma in their study. HED-PET was 100% sensitive in sites of confirmed disease, whereas in four out of eight patients with pheochromocytoma MIBG missed one or more sites of disease. Other tracers have been used for evaluating pheochromocytomas. Two reports indicate that ^{18}F-fluorodopamine (F-DA) is valuable for identification of primary and metastatic pheochromocytoma [65, 66]. These studies have demonstrated that F-DA is a highly specific radiopharmaceutical for depicting adrenal and extra-adrenal pheochromocytoma [67]. In detail, Pacak et al. demonstrated a high positive and negative predictive value of PET scanning for pheochromocytoma with F-DA. In their study of 28 patients, pheochromocytoma could be detected in all patients. In a study by Ilias et al. [65] on patients with metastatic pheochromocytoma, more metastatic foci were identified with F-DA-PET than with MIBG scintigraphy. While F-DA-PET was positive in all lesions, MIBG scintigraphy was false negative in 7 out of 16 lesions. Furthermore, ^{18}F dihydroxyphenylalanine (F-DOPA), a precursor of dopamine, has been found to be valuable in PET imaging of pheochromocytomas with a high sensitivity and specificity [68]. In a series of 14 patients, Hoegerle et al. demonstrated that this novel radiotracer F-DOPA had a higher sensitivity (100%) than ^{123}I MIBG (71%) in the depiction of pheochromocytoma. Another catecholamine analog is ^{18}F fluorobenzylguanidine that so far has only been tested in dogs with pheochromocytomas. High PET uptake was demonstrated in all tumors [69].

Conclusions for Pheochromocytoma Imaging: PET Compared to MIBG

HED PET, DA PET and DOPA PET may provide several potential advantages to conventional MIBG scintigraphy. Tomographic imaging has higher spatial resolution compared to the planar imaging of MIBG. Since scans can be performed immediately or within a few hours of injection, patient throughput is significantly higher with PET. PET technique also provides quantification of tracer uptake by calculating SUVs. The shorter half-life of ^{11}C in HED (20 min) allows injection of larger doses with

lower radiation exposure compared to MIBG. This results in better quality of the images [53]. However, the short half-life of ^{11}C necessitates on-site production of the radiopharmaceutical and makes it difficult to perform whole-body examinations in the evaluation of metastatic disease. These disadvantages do not exist for the F-DA and F-DOPA since both are labelled with ^{18}F and therefore have longer half-lives (110 min) than HED. In contrast to MIBG, the PET based tracers have no adverse effect on the thyroid and do not require thyroid blocking. It is expected that PET and PET-CT will replace the conventional planar scintigraphic imaging.

Key Points

1. PET-CT combines functional information from the PET component with primarily morphologic information from the CT part. PET-CT is the fast growing imaging modality worldwide. Almost all newly bought PET systems are PET-CT scanners.
2. PET imaging with ^{18}F-FDG is based on the enhanced glucose metabolism in malignant cells.
3. PET-CT with FDG is currently the imaging modality of choice for most malignant lesions, including adrenal tumors especially in the evaluation for metastatic disease.
4. PET-CT with FDG yielded sensitivity of 96%–100%, specificity of 94%–100% and accuracy of 95%–100% in the differentiation of malignant vs benign adrenal lesions.
5. An adrenal lesion can be interpreted with high confidence as malignant when FDG uptake is significantly higher than liver uptake and when attenuation values in unenhanced CT are >10 HU.
6. A maximum SUV value >3.1 is suggestive for adrenal malignancy. However, SUV ratios (relative to liver uptake) might be more accurate than absolute numbers.
7. False negative FDG uptake might be seen in small, necrotic, and hemorrhagic lesions, and in metastases from non FDG avid primary tumors.
8. False positive FDG uptake might be seen in inflammatory lesions, adrenal endothelial cysts, and functioning adrenal adenomas.

9. FDG uptake is non-specific and differentiation among malignant lesions including metastases, adrenocortical carcinoma, lymphoma and pheochromocytoma is not possible.

10. In cases of discordant findings between the PET and CT component, delayed contrast enhanced CT for washout – analysis might be incorporated in the PET-CT protocol, or chemical shift MRI might be subsequently performed to indicate the correct diagnosis.

11. PET-CT is progressively replacing much conventional scintigraphic imaging. Instead of radiocholesterol, adrenal cortex lesions are identified with ^{18}F-FDG, METO (11C-Metomidate) or FETO (^{18}F-fluoro-2-ethyl-desethyl-R-etomidate) PET-CT. These radiotracers can distinguish primary adrenal cortex tumors (adenomas and adrenocortical carcinoma) from other adrenal lesions (including metastases and pheochromocytoma). Further studies are warranted to evaluate their value in clinical practice.

12. ^{123}I-MIBG, PET-CT with FDG, F-DA (^{18}F-fluorodopa) or F-DOPA (^{18}F dihydroxyphenylalanine) have all been advocated by different investigators as helpful in the diagnosis of pheochromocytomas.

References

1. Khan TS, Sundin A, Juhlin C, Langstrom B, Bergstrom M, Eriksson B (2003) 11C-Metomidate PET imaging of adrenocortical cancer. Eur J Nucl Med Mol Imaging 30(3):403–410

2. Brown RS, Leung JY, Fisher SJ, Frey KA, Ethier SP, Wahl RL (1996) Intratumoral distribution of tritiated-FDG in breast carcinoma: correlation between Glut-1 expression and FDG uptake. J Nucl Med 37(6): 1042–1047

3. Higashi K, Clavo AC, Wahl RL (1993) Does FDG uptake measure proliferative activity of human cancer cells? In vitro comparison with DNA flow cytometry and tritiated thymidine uptake. J Nucl Med 34(3):414–419

4. Von Schulthess GK, Steinert HC, Hany TF (2006) Integrated PET/CT: current applications and future directions. Radiology 238(2):405–422

5. Cohade C, Wahl RL (2003) Applications of positron emission tomography/computed tomography image fusion in clinical positron emission tomography – clinical use, interpretation methods, diagnostic improvements. Semin Nucl Med 33(3):228–237

6. Bagheri B, Maurer AH, Cone L, Doss M, Adler L (2004) Characterization of the normal adrenal gland with 18F-FDG PET/CT. J Nucl Med 45(8):1340–1343

7. Karstaedt N, Sagel SS, Stanley RJ, Melson GL, Levitt RG (1978) Computed tomography of the adrenal gland. Radiology 129(3):723–730

8. Abrams HL, Siegelman SS, Adams DF, Sanders R, Finberg HJ, Hessel SJ, McNeil BJ (1982) Computed tomography versus ultrasound of the adrenal gland: a prospective study. Radiology 143(1):121–128

9. Hedeland H, Ostberg G, Hokfelt B (1968) On the prevalence of adrenocortical adenomas in an autopsy material in relation to hypertension and diabetes. Acta Med Scand 184(3):211–214

10. Korobkin M, Francis IR, Kloos RT, Dunnick NR (1996) The incidental adrenal mass. Radiol Clin North Am 34(5):1037–1054

11. Paulsen SD, Nghiem HV, Korobkin M, Caoili EM, Higgins EJ (2004) Changing role of imaging-guided percutaneous biopsy of adrenal masses: evaluation of 50 adrenal biopsies. AJR Am J Roentgenol 182(4):1033–1037

12. Dunnick NR, Korobkin M (2002) Imaging of adrenal incidentalomas: current status. AJR Am J Roentgenol 179(3):559–568

13. Kocijancic I, Vidmar K, Zwitter M, Snoj M (2003) The significance of adrenal metastases from lung carcinoma. Eur J Surg Oncol 29(1):87–88

14. Boland GW, Goldberg MA, Lee MJ, Mayo-Smith WW, Dixon J, McNicholas MM, Mueller PR (1995) Indeterminate adrenal mass in patients with cancer: evaluation at PET with 2-[F-18]-fluoro-2-deoxy-D-glucose. Radiology 194(1):131–134

15. Erasmus JJ, Patz EF Jr, McAdams HP, Murray JG, Herndon J, Coleman RE, Goodman PC (1997) Evaluation of adrenal masses in patients with bronchogenic carcinoma using 18F-fluorodeoxyglucose positron emission tomography. AJR Am J Roentgenol 168(5):1357–1360

16. Maurea S, Mainolfi C, Bazzicalupo L, Panico MR, Imparato C, Alfano B, Ziviello M, Salvatore M (1999) Imaging of adrenal tumors using FDG PET: comparison of benign and malignant lesions. AJR Am J Roentgenol 173(1):25–29

17. Yun M, Kim W, Alnafisi N, Lacorte L, Jang S, Alavi A (2001) 18F-FDG PET in characterizing adrenal lesions detected on CT or MRI. J Nucl Med 42(12):1795–1799

18. Gupta NC, Graeber GM, Tamim WJ, Rogers JS, Irisari L, Bishop HA (2001) Clinical utility of PET-FDG imaging in differentiation of benign from malignant adrenal masses in lung cancer. Clin Lung Cancer 3(1):59–64

19. Kumar R, Xiu Y, Yu JQ, Takalkar A, El Haddad G, Potenta S, Kung J, Zhuang H, Alavi A (2004) 18F-FDG PET in evaluation of adrenal lesions in patients with lung cancer. J Nucl Med 45(12):2058–2062

20. Jana S, Zhang T, Milstein DM, Isasi CR, Blaufox MD (2006) FDG-PET and CT characterization of adrenal lesions in cancer patients. Eur J Nucl Med Mol Imaging 33(1):29–35

21. Metser U, Miller E, Lerman H, Lievshitz G, Avital S, Even-Sapir E (2006) 18F-FDG PET/CT in the evaluation of adrenal masses. J Nucl Med 47(1):32–37

22. Blake MA, Slattery JM, Kalra MK, Halpern EF, Fischman AJ, Mueller PR, Boland GW (2006) Adrenal lesions: characterization with fused PET/CT image in

patients with proved or suspected malignancy – initial experience. Radiology 238(3):970–977

23. Caoili EM, Korobkin M, Brown RK, Mackie G, Shulkin BL (2007) Differentiating adrenal adenomas from nonadenomas using (18)F-FDG PET/CT quantitative and qualitative evaluation. Acad Radiol 14(4):468–475

24. Jaskowiak CJ, Bianco JA, Perlman SB, Fine JP (2005) Influence of reconstruction iterations on 18F-FDG PET/CT standardized uptake values. J Nucl Med 46(3):424–428

25. Stahl A, Ott K, Schwaiger M, Weber WA (2004) Comparison of different SUV-based methods for monitoring cytotoxic therapy with FDG PET. Eur J Nucl Med Mol Imaging 31(11):1471–1478

26. Zasadny KR, Wahl RL (1993) Standardized uptake values of normal tissues at PET with 2-[fluorine-18]-fluoro-2-deoxy-D-glucose: variations with body weight and a method for correction. Radiology 189(3): 847–850

27. Bakheet SM, Powe J, Ezzat A, Rostom A (1998) F-18-FDG uptake in tuberculosis. Clin Nucl Med 23(11): 739–742

28. Boerner AR, Voth E, Theissen P, Wienhard K, Wagner R, Schicha H (1998) Glucose metabolism of the thyroid in Graves' Disease measured by F-18-fluoro-deoxyglucose positron emission tomography. Thyroid 8(9):765–772

29. Shimizu A, Oriuchi N, Tsushima Y, Higuchi T, Aoki J, Endo K (2003) High [18F] 2-fluoro-2-deoxy-D-glucose (FDG) uptake of adrenocortical adenoma showing subclinical Cushing's Syndrome. Ann Nucl Med 17(5):403–406

30. Shulkin BL, Thompson NW, Shapiro B, Francis IR, Sisson JC (1999) Pheochromocytomas: imaging with 2-[fluorine-18]fluoro-2-deoxy-D-glucose PET. Radiology 212(1):35–41

31. Barzon L, Boscaro M (2000) Diagnosis and management of adrenal incidentalomas. J Urol 163(2):398–407

32. Bertherat J, Mosnier-Pudar H, Bertagna X (2002) Adrenal incidentalomas. Curr Opin Oncol 14(1):58–63

33. Mody MK, Kazerooni EA, Korobkin M (1995) Percutaneous CT-guided biopsy of adrenal masses: immediate and delayed complications. J Comput Assist Tomogr 19(3):434–439

34. Silverman SG, Mueller PR, Pinkney LP, Koenker RM, Seltzer SE (1993) Predictive value of image-guided adrenal biopsy: analysis of results of 101 biopsies. Radiology 187(3):715–718

35. Korobkin M, Brodeur FJ, Yutzy GG, Francis IR, Quint LE, Dunnick NR, Kazerooni EA (1996) Differentiation of adrenal adenomas from nonadenomas using CT attenuation values. AJR Am J Roentgenol 166(3):531–536

36. Boland GW, Lee MJ, Gazelle GS, Halpern EF, McNicholas MM, Mueller PR (1998) Characterization of adrenal masses using unenhanced CT: an analysis of the CT literature. AJR Am J Roentgenol 171(1): 201–204

37. Lee MJ, Hahn PF, Papanicolaou N, Egglin TK, Saini S, Mueller PR, Simeone JF (1991) Benign and malignant adrenal masses: CT distinction with attenuation coefficients, size, and observer analysis. Radiology 179(2):415–418

38. Korobkin M, Brodeur FJ, Francis IR, Quint LE, Dunnick NR, Goodsitt M (1996) Delayed enhanced CT for differentiation of benign from malignant adrenal masses. Radiology 200(3):737–742

39. Mitchell DG, Crovello M, Matteucci T, Petersen RO, Miettinen MM (1992) Benign adrenocortical masses: diagnosis with chemical shift MR imaging. Radiology 185(2):345–351

40. Outwater EK, Siegelman ES, Huang AB, Birnbaum BA (1996) Adrenal masses: correlation between CT attenuation value and chemical shift ratio at MR imaging with in-phase and opposed-phase sequences. Radiology 200(3):749–752

41. Tsushima Y, Ishizaka H, Matsumoto M (1993) Adrenal masses: differentiation with chemical shift, fast low-angle shot MR imaging. Radiology 186(3):705–709

42. MacManus MP, Hicks RJ, Matthews JP, Hogg A, McKenzie AF, Wirth A, Ware RE, Ball DL (2001) High rate of detection of unsuspected distant metastases by pet in apparent stage III non-small-cell lung cancer: implications for radical radiation therapy. Int J Radiat Oncol Biol Phys 50(2):287–293

43. Alves A, Scatton O, Dousset B (2002) Diagnostic and therapeutic strategy for an incidental finding of an adrenal mass [in French]. J Chir (Paris) 139(4):205–213

44. Siren JE, Haapiainen RK, Huikuri KT, Sivula AH (1993) Incidentalomas of the adrenal gland: 36 operated patients and review of literature. World J Surg 17(5):634–639

45. Wooten MD, King DK (1993) Adrenal cortical cCarcinoma. Epidemiology and treatment with Mitotane and a review of the piterature. Cancer 72(11):3145–3155

46. Wajchenberg BL, Albergaria Pereira MA, Medonca BB, Latronico AC, Campos Carneiro P, Alves VA, Zerbini MC, Liberman B, Carlos Gomes G, Kirschner MA (2000) Adrenocortical carcinoma: clinical and laboratory observations. Cancer 88(4):711–736

47. Zettinig G, Mitterhauser M, Wadsak W, Becherer A, Pirich C, Vierhapper H, Niederle B, Dudczak R, Kletter K (2004) Positron emission tomography imaging of adrenal masses: (18)F-fluorodeoxyglucose and the 11beta-hydroxylase tracer (11)C-metomidate. Eur J Nucl Med Mol Imaging 31(9):1224–1230

48. Becherer A, Vierhapper H, Potzi C, Karanikas G, Kurtaran A, Schmaljohann J, Staudenherz A, Dudczak R, Kletter K (2001) FDG-PET in adrenocortical carcinoma. Cancer Biother Radiopharm 16(4):289–295

49. Leboulleux S, Dromain C, Bonniaud G, Auperin A, Caillou B, Lumbroso J, Sigal R, Baudin E, Schlumberger M (2006) Diagnostic and prognostic value of 18-fluorodeoxyglucose positron emission yomography in adrenocortical carcinoma: a prospective comparison with computed tomography. J Clin Endocrinol Metab 91(3):920–925

50. Mackie GC, Shulkin BL, Ribeiro RC, Worden FP, Gauger PG, Mody RJ, Connolly LP, Kunter G, Rodriguez-Galindo C, Wallis JW, Hurwitz CA, Schteingart DE (2006) Use of [18F]fluorodeoxyglucose positron emission tomography in evaluating locally

recurrent and metastatic adrenocortical carcinoma. J Clin Endocrinol Metab 91(7):2665–2671

51. Weber MM, Lang J, Abedinpour F, Zeilberger K, Adelmann B, Engelhardt D (1993) Different inhibitory effect of etomidate and ketoconazole on the human adrenal steroid biosynthesis. Clin Investig 71(11):933–938

52. Bergstrom M, Bonasera TA, Lu L, Bergstrom E, Backlin C, Juhlin C, Langstrom B (1998) In vitro and in vivo primate evaluation of carbon-11-etomidate and carbon-11-metomidate as potential tracers for PET imaging of the adrenal cortex and its tumors. J Nucl Med 39(6):982–989

53. Bergstrom M, Juhlin C, Bonasera TA, Sundin A, Rastad J, Akerstrom G, Langstrom B (2000) PET imaging of adrenal cortical tumors with the 11beta-hydroxylase tracer 11C-metomidate. J Nucl Med 41(2):275–282

54. Minn H, Salonen A, Friberg J, Roivainen A, Viljanen T, Langsjo J, Salmi J, Valimaki M, Nagren K, Nuutila P (2004) Imaging of adrenal incidentalomas with PET using (11)C-metomidate and (18)F-FDG. J Nucl Med 45(6):972–979

55. Hennings J, Lindhe O, Bergstrom M, Langstrom B, Sundin A, Hellman P (2006) [11C]Metomidate positron emission tomography of adrenocortical tumors in correlation with histopathological findings. J Clin Endocrinol Metab 91(4):1410–1414

56. Mitterhauser M, Wadsak W, Wabnegger L, Sieghart W, Viernstein H, Kletter K, Dudczak R (2003) In vivo and in vitro evaluation of [18F]FETO with respect to the adrenocortical and GABAergic system in rats. Eur J Nucl Med Mol Imaging 30(10):1398–1401

57. Wadsak W, Mitterhauser M, Rendl G, Schuetz M, Mien LK, Ettlinger DE, Dudczak R, Kletter K, Karanikas G (2006) [18F]FETO for adrenocortical PET imaging: a pilot study in healthy volunteers. Eur J Nucl Med Mol Imaging 33(6):669–672

58. Moreira SG Jr, Pow-Sang JM (2002) Evaluation and management of adrenal masses. Cancer Control 9(4):326–334

59. Fujita A, Hyodoh H, Kawamura Y, Kanegae K, Furuse M, Kanazawa K (2000) Use of fusion images of I-131 metaiodobenzylguanidine, SPECT, and magnetic resonance studies to identify a malignant pheochromocytoma. Clin Nucl Med 25(6):440–442

60. Sisson JC, Shulkin BL (1999) Nuclear medicine imaging of pheochromocytoma and neuroblastoma. Q J Nucl Med 43(3):217–223

61. Eisenhofer G, Pacak K, Goldstein DS, Chen C, Shulkin B (2000) 123I-MIBG scintigraphy of catecholamine systems: impediments to applications in clinical medicine. Eur J Nucl Med 27(5):611–612

62. Shulkin BL, Wieland DM, Schwaiger M, Thompson NW, Francis IR, Haka MS, Rosenspire KC, Shapiro B, Sisson JC, Kuhl DE (1992) PET scanning with hydroxyephedrine: an approach to the localization of pheochromocytoma. J Nucl Med 33(6):1125–1131

63. Trampal C, Engler H, Juhlin C, Bergstrom M, Langstrom B (2004) Pheochromocytomas: detection with 11C hydroxyephedrine PET. Radiology 230(2):423–428

64. Mann GN, Link JM, Pham P, Pickett CA, Byrd DR, Kinahan PE, Krohn KA, Mankoff DA (2006) [11C]Metahydroxyephedrine and [18F]fluorodeoxyglucose positron emission tomography improve clinical decision making in suspected pheochromocytoma. Ann Surg Oncol 13(2):187–197

65. Ilias I, Yu J, Carrasquillo JA, Chen CC, Eisenhofer G, Whatley M, McElroy B, Pacak K (2003) Superiority of 6-[18F]-fluorodopamine positron emission tomography versus [131I]-metaiodobenzylguanidine scintigraphy in the localization of metastatic pheochromocytoma. J Clin Endocrinol Metab 88(9):4083–4087

66. Pacak K, Eisenhofer G, Carrasquillo JA, Chen CC, Whatley M, Goldstein DS (2002) Diagnostic localization of pheochromocytoma: the coming of age of positron emission tomography. Ann N Y Acad Sci 970:170–176

67. Pacak K, Eisenhofer G, Carrasquillo JA, Chen CC, Li ST, Goldstein D (2001) S. 6-[18F]Fluorodopamine positron emission tomographic (PET) scanning for diagnostic localization of pheochromocytoma. Hypertension 38(1):6–8

68. Hoegerle S, Nitzsche E, Altehoefer C, Ghanem N, Manz T, Brink I, Reincke M, Moser E, Neumann HP (2002) Pheochromocytomas: detection with 18F DOPA whole body PET – initial results. Radiology 222(2):507–512

69. Berry CR, DeGrado TR, Nutter F, Garg PK, Breitschwerdt EB, Spaulding K, Concannon KD, Zalutsky MR, Coleman RE (2002) Imaging of pheochromocytoma in 2 dogs using P-[18F] fluorobenzylguanidine. Vet Radiol Ultrasound 43(2):183–186

Adrenal Trauma and Intervention

12

Brian C. Lucey

Contents

Introduction

From an interventional perspective, there is not a wide range of interventional procedures performed on the adrenal glands. The vast majority of adrenal procedures are percutaneous biopsies of an adrenal mass. Other procedures occasionally performed include radiofrequency ablation of an adrenal mass and adrenal vein sampling. Retrograde venous ablation for treatment of endocrine abnormalities has fallen out of favor as it results in only temporary reduction in adrenal function while causing significant long standing pain with questions concerning the safety of the procedure. Chemoembolization of adrenal cortical carcinoma has been reported in a few patients with inoperable disease [1]. Adrenal abscesses and cysts are infrequently encountered yet may be drained percutaneously safely in a manner identical to abscess or cyst elsewhere in the abdomen. Percutaneous ablation for functioning adenomas with acetic acid and ethanol has also been reported in small series [2, 3].

Percutaneous Adrenal Biopsy
Indications

The indication for percutaneous biopsy of the adrenal gland is to characterize definitively an adrenal mass identified on prior imaging. Traditionally, unsuspected adrenal masses are reported to be present in 5%–8.7% of patients [4, 5]. With the dramatic increase in cross sectional imaging over the past few years, this figure is likely to increase. A vast majority of these masses are benign, even in patients

B.C. Lucey (✉)
Department of Radiology, VA Healthcare System,
1400 VFW Parkway, West Roxbury, MA 02132
E-mail: brian.lucey@bmc.org

M.A. Blake, G. Boland (eds.), *Adrenal Imaging*, DOI 10.1007/978-1-59745-560-2_12,
© 2009 Humana Press, a part of Springer Science+Business Media, LLC

with a known primary malignancy. The traditional indication for adrenal mass biopsy is to characterize an adrenal mass seen on imaging in a patient that may or may not have a primary malignancy. One study of adrenal biopsies performed in the decade spanning the mid 1980 s to the mid-1990 s [6] found that 53% of patients undergoing adrenal mass biopsy for suspected metastatic disease had malignancy in the gland. These results were mirrored by other groups [6–9]. This means that almost half (40%–57%) of adrenal biopsies were essentially unnecessary. Advances in both CT and MR imaging permit definitive characterization of a great number of these incidentally discovered adrenal masses. Given the increasing ability of imaging to characterize adrenal masses, the role of percutaneous biopsy has changed. Currently, biopsy is restricted to two indications. Most frequently, it is performed to confirm the already suspected diagnosis of metastatic disease to the adrenal gland prior to initiating therapy. Less commonly, biopsy is performed to provide a definitive diagnosis on the rare occasion when imaging cannot provide a definitive diagnosis. This is reflected in work performed from 1998 to 2002 [10] which showed that almost 80% of adrenal mass biopsies performed during this period showed malignancy. In 12% of cases, benign adrenal adenoma was found that was unsuspected following imaging prior to biopsy. Further advances in adrenal mass characterization with the introduction of absolute percentage washout [11, 12] will likely drive this number down further.

Patient Preparation and Care

Prior to performing the biopsy, the patient's coagulation status needs to be checked. This includes the INR, APTT and platelet count. An INR of less than 1.3 is advisable particularly as this is usually a non urgent procedure most frequently performed as an out patient. An APTT of less than 50 is ideal and a platelet count over 50,000 platelets per mL is required. An elevated INR may be corrected with fresh frozen plasma if required and platelets may be given to patients with a platelet count <50,000 platelets per mL. For patients on coumadin, it is advisable to cease the coumadin for 5 days prior to the procedure

and repeat the INR on the morning of the procedure. Ideally, non steroidal anti inflammatory drugs are stopped 5–7 days prior to the procedure. This includes clopidogrel, an anti platelet agent.

As with all procedures, written informed consent is required prior to performing the biopsy. This includes an open discussion with the patient including the risks, benefits and alternatives to the procedure.

For patient comfort, conscious sedation may be given at the start of the procedure. This is usually given intravenously in the form of midazolam (2–6 mg and fentanyl 50–200 µg). The patient's heart rate, respiratory rate and oxygen saturation need to be continually monitored during the procedure. Once the procedure is over, the patient is then returned to an observation unit where vital signs are monitored every 15 min for up to 2 h following the procedure. If all vital signs are stable and the patient is asymptomatic at this stage, the patient is permitted to go home. If conscious sedation has been used, the patient is not permitted to drive home and should be accompanied.

Biopsy Technique

Due to the relatively deep location of the adrenal glands within the retroperitoneum, most adrenal mass biopsies are performed using CT guidance. Occasionally, when the mass is large, usually of the order of 4 cm or larger, the procedure may be performed using sonographic guidance. When using sonography, a more anterior approach is often employed frequently using a trans hepatic route. A relatively low frequency probe is required, of the order of 2–5 MHz and a curved array transducer is usually used. Before attempting sonographic guidance to perform the biopsy, it is important to ensure that the mass is clearly identified on a preliminary sonographic examination. Once the mass has been identified, the overlying skin is cleaned, prepared and draped in a sterile manner. Local anesthetic, usually as lidocaine 1%–2%, 10 mL is given subcutaneously at the skin entry site. A small, 4–5-mm dermatotomy is made and the biopsy needle introduced using direct sonographic guidance. A coaxial technique is preferred as this permits multiple aspirations and core biopsies to be obtained without requiring multiple punctures of the adrenal gland. A 17 gauge coaxial needle with an 18 gauge biopsy gun is best. Once the coaxial needle has been guided into the mass, the position should be confirmed and documented with an image showing the echogenic needle tip within the adrenal mass. Once the needle tip location is confirmed, the inner stylet can be removed and 22 gauge aspirations obtained through the coaxial needle. These may be spread onto sterile slides and examined on site by a cytologist if available. Following this, 18 gauge core biopsies may be obtained and the specimens placed into formalin. Should adrenal involvement by lymphoma be suspected, samples should be sent for flow cytometry. Once adequate samples have been obtained, the stylet is placed back into the coaxial needle and the entire coaxial system is withdrawn. A small bandage may then be placed over the puncture site.

Most adrenal mass biopsies are performed using CT guidance. For this, the patient is placed onto the CT table in the lateral decubitus position with the side of interest closest to the CT table (Fig. 12.1). This is done to decrease the expansion of the dependent lung and thus help to create a window into the retroperitoneum that does not traverse the lung parenchyma. A marking grid is placed over the patient's back at the estimated site of skin entry. A preliminary CT scan through the area of interest is acquired using thin slices of the order of 1–3 mm. A slice for optimal access is selected and the patient moved to that specific table position. The laser light on the CT scanner is then used to triangulate the skin entry site. On

the image selected for the needle entry site, a line is drawn from the skin site to the mass and the angle and distance is recorded. Once this is done, the overlying skin is cleaned, prepared and draped as for a sonographic procedure. Again, a minor dermatotomy is performed. A 17 gauge coaxial needle is then guided into the mass and the needle position confirmed with a CT image. The needle is repositioned as required based on the CT image acquired and further images obtained until the needle position is confirmed within the mass. Once this is achieved, the biopsy may proceed as described for a sonographic procedure. A post procedure CT scan through the area is advised following removal of the coaxial needle to ensure that no immediate complications are present. Post procedure care is as described for a sonographic procedure.

There are several variations on the CT technique that may be used if required. For adrenal masses that lie superiorly, in order to safely access the mass without traversing lung parenchyma, an angled gantry approach may be employed. Most CT scanners will permit angulation of up to 20–24°. This may help to create a safe route that did not exist with true axial imaging. This technique does introduce an extra angle to be considered when guiding the coaxial needle but is easily accomplished by trained interventional radiologists.

An alternative technique that may occasionally be useful is the use of saline to create a window for biopsy. This involves guiding a 22 gauge needle between the pleura and diaphragm using CT

(a)

(b)

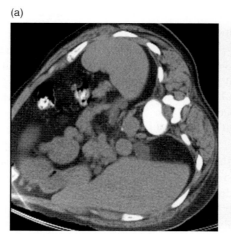 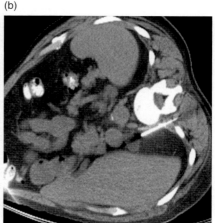

Fig. 12.1 **a** CT image of a 53-year-old male patient with a right sided adrenal mass in the right lateral decubitus position. **b** The biopsy needle in situ

guidance and through this needle, a small volume of saline in the order of 5–20 mL, is slowly injected. This displaces the pleura laterally sufficiently that may permit an access route that extends from the skin, through the saline and into the adrenal mass without needing to traverse the lung parenchyma.

Results

The acceptable success rate threshold for adrenal biopsy as set out by the Quality Improvement Guidelines for Image-guided Percutaneous Biopsy in Adults is 80%. Reported accuracy rates are generally between 85% and 93% [6] with sensitivity and specificity of 81% and 99% respectively and are almost always in excess of the figures suggested by the guidelines. More recent results for adrenal biopsy report diagnostic accuracy of 96% with 48 of 50 masses providing a definitive answer [10]. In contrast to this, the reported success rate for fine needle aspiration of the adrenal using endoscopic ultrasound is 88% although EUS is almost universally restricted to biopsy of the left adrenal gland [13].

Complications

The complications related to percutaneous adrenal mass biopsy are similar to those encountered with most biopsy procedures in the abdomen. Infection at the skin entry site is always a possibility but its occurrence is vanishingly rare. The major potential complication is bleeding. This has been reported to occur in up to 5%–10% of cases although transfusion is rarely required. Inadvertent puncture of the lung may occur despite all the aforementioned precautions and the post procedure CT scan should be assessed for this possibility particularly for adrenal masses that are located superiorly. Damage to adjacent organs is uncommon yet may occur and the organs involved depend upon the side of the adrenal that is being biopsied. On the right, this includes the liver, right kidney and colon. On the left, this includes the left kidney, pancreas and colon. The overall major complication rate for adrenal biopsy is similar to that of biopsy in other abdominal organs and is reported at approximately 2% [6].

Percutaneous Adrenal Radiofrequency Ablation

Percutaneous radiofrequency ablation (RFA) of the adrenal gland has been performed relatively infrequently when compared to the liver, kidney and lung. Given the dramatic increase in the total number of RFA procedures over the past 5 years or so, and given the excellent patient tolerance for the procedure, it is almost inevitable that RFA of the adrenal gland will increase in popularity. There are two distinct patient populations in whom RFA of the adrenal gland has been performed. These are primary adrenal cortical tumors and adrenal metastatic disease with a primary malignancy elsewhere. Indication for RFA is usually restricted to patients that are unfit for surgical resection or who refuse surgical intervention. Ideally, adrenal metastases that are treated with RFA should be the only site of metastatic disease.

Patient Preparation and Care

Patient preparation for adrenal RFA is similar to that for adrenal biopsy. Coagulation status needs to be assessed and corrected where appropriate. Informed consent is required with a complete discussion of the potential complications. Conscious sedation is required for RFA although general anesthesia may be preferred by some interventionists. The procedure may be performed as an outpatient as with biopsy although some operators may prefer to observe the patient overnight. Immediate post procedural care is similar to that for adrenal biopsy.

RFA Technique

Prior to performing the procedure, grounding pads need to be placed on the thighs of the patient. These conduct the electrical current away from the patient and prevent the current remaining in the patient.

The localization of the mass and positioning of the RFA probe into the adrenal mass is identical to that for adrenal biopsy. Once the position is confirmed by an image, if a multi tined deployable probe is used, the tines are deployed as directed by the manufacturer of the specific probe. Once the tines are deployed or once the probe is in position for non deployable probes, the ablation may commence. Depending upon the probe manufacturer used, the length of the ablation varies and is terminated either by time, temperature or impedance. One or more treatments may be performed until the ablated zone is larger than the original mass. At this stage, the probe is removed and a post procedure CT image should be obtained to assess for any immediate complications. A successful ablation is defined as the absence of contrast enhancement in the target mass following intravenous contrast administration.

Results

In a small series of 13 patients that underwent adrenal mass RFA, 11 of 13 adrenal masses were successfully ablated as defined by the absence of contrast enhancement at follow up CT imaging with a mean follow up of 11 months [14]. Two patients had residual disease with one patient developing progression of disease. Most patients, however, developed metastatic disease elsewhere on follow up imaging. A second study with 8 patients with 15 adrenal masses had a mean follow up of 10 months [15]. Of the masses, 53% were successfully treated as defined by absence of contrast enhancement on follow up CT; 20% showed interval growth indicating incomplete treatment or recurrent tumor and 27% showed no change in size on follow up imaging although two of these four masses showed some contrast enhancement. This study found that ablation was more successful in tumors of less than 5 cm in size.

Complications

Complications related to adrenal RFA may be divided into two discrete groups. Those related to probe placement and those related to thermal treatment. The first group is similar to adrenal biopsy and includes infection, bleeding and pneumothorax. The latter group includes skin burns at the grounding pad sites in addition to thermal injury to structures adjacent to the adrenal mass. Although the potential for significant complication is always present, the real incidence of major complications is low and lies in the 2%–5% range for RFA in the liver and kidney. There is very little data on complications specific to adrenal RFA although no major complications were reported by the largest reported series to date [14].

Miscellaneous Adrenal Procedures

There are a variety of rarely performed interventional procedures related to the adrenal gland (Fig. 12.2). One of these involves the percutaneous ablation of functioning adrenal adenomas using acetic acid [2]. Surgical resection is considered to be the treatment of choice for functioning adenomas; however, there are infrequently encountered cases where patients are either unfit for surgery or refuse surgical intervention for one reason or another. A similar compound (ethanol) has been used successfully to percutaneously ablate hepatocellular carcinoma, parathyroid adenoma and functioning thyroid nodules. Acetic acid has approximately three times the potency of ethanol. Ideally, small adrenal adenomas are the best candidates for percutaneous ablation with masses of the order of 1.5–3.5 cm as these are also rarely malignant. Larger masses may not be completely ablated easily. The patient preparation and technique for the procedure is similar to adrenal biopsy. Under CT guidance, a 19 gauge coaxial needle is guided into the mass. Through this a 22 gauge needle is advanced into the center of the mass. A 50% acetic acid solution is then slowly injected into the center of the mass. A total of 5–12 mL of the 50% solution is usually required with the volume used calculated by the formula $4/3(\pi + 0.5) r^3$ where 'r' is the radius of the mass. The addition of the 0.5 in the formula allows for some cell death at the periphery of the mass. This has been reported to result in excellent biochemical result with patients laboratory values normal at over one year follow up. Injection of ethanol has also been reported as successful for the treatment of small functioning adrenal adenomas [3].

Adrenal cysts are infrequently encountered lesions that seldom manifest clinically. True endothelial cysts account for almost half of adrenal cysts and pseudocysts account for most of the remainder. Pseudocysts usually result from cystic involution of prior adrenal hematoma. Hydatid cysts of the adrenal are extremely uncommon. Adrenal cysts become symptomatic either through compressive symptoms due to large size or less commonly, super infection of the cyst. The cyst may be drained percutaneously either under sonographic or CT guidance [16]. The patient preparation and technique is again similar to adrenal

(a)   (b)   (c)

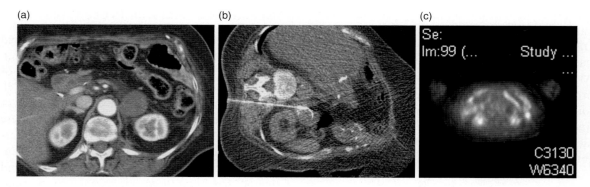

Fig. 12.2 A 68-year-old woman with cystic adrenal metastasis from ampullary carcinoma underwent deployable microwave with trio antenna from Vivant Medical. There is complete macroscopic necrosis on CT and 6-month follow-up PET. Images courtesy of Damian Dupuy, Rhode Island

biopsy. Once the cyst has been accessed, the contents are aspirated until the cyst is completely drained. Recurrent cysts may be sclerosed using alcohol if required. Percutaneous aspiration and or sclerosis of an adrenal cyst obviate the necessity for surgical excision with all the accompanying possible morbidity and mortality.

Adrenal Vein Sampling

Indications

The principal indication for performing adrenal venous sampling is in the investigation of hyperaldosteronism. The purpose is to differentiate between unilateral and bilateral hormone production. Occasionally adrenal venous sampling is performed in patients with biochemical evidence of pheochromocytoma when no adrenal mass is identified on imaging (Fig. 12.3). The prevalence of primary aldosteronism in hypertensive patients has been reported at between 5% and 10% of all hypertensive patients [17, 18]. In many cases of hyperaldosteronism, either bilateral adrenal hyperplasia or an adrenal mass may be identified on CT or MR imaging although cross sectional imaging is an unreliable screening test for hyperaldosteronism and patients with symptoms suggesting adrenocortical excess production should undergo adrenal vein sampling. An aldostreone to renin ratio is a useful screening test for primary aldosteronism as the levels of the individual hormones may lie within normal limits but an elevated ratio is strongly suggestive of the diagnosis. The difficulty with using CT or MR to make the diagnosis is that many tumors resulting in

aldosteronism are extremely small and may be missed on imaging. In addition, the presence of an adrenal mass is not necessarily indicative that the mass is the underlying cause. One study showed that CT was not contributory in 68% of patients with primary hyperaldosteronism [19].

Patient Preparation and Care

As with all interventional procedures, written informed consent is required. Coagulation status needs to be checked and corrected where necessary. Conscious sedation is given as detailed above.

The value of CT for adrenal vein sampling lies in the planning. This allows identification of the adrenal veins pre procedure in many cases. The right adrenal vein may be identified in approximately 50% of patients and its position relative to other structures may be noted. This aids in locating the vein during the procedure.

Technique

With the patient sedated, a peripheral line is required to draw samples for peripheral cortisol and aldosterone levels. A femoral vein puncture is used to gain access to the venous system. Sonographic guidance may be used if required. Once access is obtained, a guide wire is placed into the IVC and the puncture needle removed. A 5 French catheter is then threaded over the guide wire and into the IVC. The catheter then needs to be manipulated into the adrenal veins. This must be performed carefully as the veins are small. The position is then

(a)

(b)

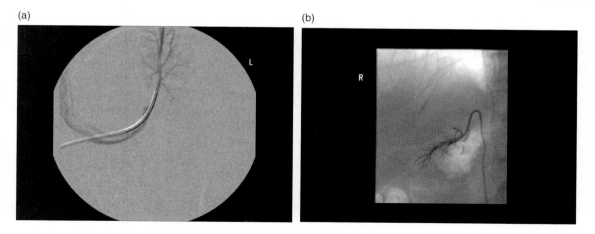

Fig. 12.3 Left and right adrenal venogram during adrenal vein sampling in a 46-year-old female patient with hypertension

confirmed with an injection of a small volume (2–4 mL) of contrast. The contrast injection should be performed gently so as not to rupture the delicate veins. To engage the right adrenal vein, the catheter should be placed at the level identified on the prior CT scan. The catheter is then rotated to the posterior wall of the IVC as the right adrenal vein always arises on the posterior wall. In searching for the adrenal vein, the catheter may initially engage a number of different vessels such as the phrenic vessels or accessory hepatic vessels. The catheter should not be placed too deeply into the vein to avoid missing venous drainage from a potential tumor. If the vein cannot be successfully canulated, an acceptable alternative may be to place the catheter tip in the mid posterior wall of the IVC a few millimeters above the suspected level of the vein based on the CT image.

With the catheter in position, the samples are obtained. 5–6 mL of blood is aspirated using a 10-mL syringe. Gentle suction is required so as not to allow the vein to collapse around the catheter tip. It is important to ensure that no iodinated contrast is collected in the sample. At least two samples should be obtained from the right adrenal vein.

Once the samples have been obtained from the right vein, the catheter is withdrawn to the level of the left renal vein and advanced into the left renal vein. The left adrenal vein usually arises from the superior surface of the renal vein approximately 3 cm from the origin of the renal vein from the IVC. As with the right vein, care must be taken with both catheter placement and contrast injection. As a last resort, if the left adrenal vein cannot be canulated, the catheter may be placed in the left renal vein just proximal to the expected orifice of the adrenal vein. Again, at least two samples are obtained from the left adrenal vein. Peripheral samples are obtained simultaneously for each adrenal vein sample taken.

Results

The reported success rate for adrenal vein sampling in experienced hands is 97% for left-sided samples and 96.6% for right-sided samples [20]. Success is defined as successful canulation of the veins with an adequate hormone gradient and with results influencing clinical management. The cortisol level from the adrenal vein sample should be significantly higher than the simultaneously obtained peripheral sample. A ratio greater than 3:1 for adrenal to peripheral cortisol level is diagnostic [21] although ratios between 2 and 3 to 1 often provide sufficient clinical information. When there is hyperfunction of the adrenal gland, the aldosterone to cortisol ratio is higher in the adrenal vein sample than the peripheral sample whereas normal glands tend to have a ratio that is similar to the peripheral value. In patients with a unilateral adrenal adenoma, the contralateral gland has decreased aldosterone production.

Complications

The overall reported complication rate for adrenal vein sampling is 4% [22] although others have reported higher figures in the 5%–10% range [23].

The most serious complication is adrenal vein rupture with hemorrhage both into the adrenal gland and in the retroperitoneum. It is believed to occur more commonly in patients with Conn and Cushings syndromes and also more commonly on the right [23]. Other potential complications that are infrequently encountered include adrenal infarction, adrenal vein thrombosis, hypertensive crisis and adrenal insufficiency although the exact incidence of these complications is not well known. Features suggestive of adrenal hemorrhage are prolonged pain after contrast injection often accompanied by fever that both persist for up to 48 h. As formal adrenal venography is performed with decreasing frequency and very small and gentle injections are required for venous sampling, the complication rate for adrenal vein canulation is decreasing. In one large series of over 800 adrenal vein samplings, only one adrenal hemorrhage was encountered resulting in a complication rate of less than 0.2% [20].

Conclusions

Adrenal intervention does not have a large volume in busy interventional radiology departments when compared to other organs or body systems; however, trends in adrenal intervention have changed radically over the years. Adrenal venography has been replaced by cross sectional imaging but adrenal vein sampling remains a useful diagnostic tool in the evaluation of aldosteronism. The indications for adrenal biopsy have changed dramatically with improved CT and MR imaging. This has resulted in few adrenal biopsies being performed for benign disease and indeed adrenal mass biopsy is most frequently performed to confirm already suspected malignancy. Radiofrequency ablation of the adrenal gland is a growth area that has yet to hit its peak and although remains somewhat in its infancy, will undoubtedly grow significantly over the coming years.

Adrenal Trauma

Introduction

The adrenal glands are infrequently involved following blunt abdominal trauma. Although the incidence of adrenal injury has been reported at 28% on autopsy in patients sustaining severe abdominal trauma [24], the incidence on CT imaging is closer to 2% [25]. Other authors have identified adrenal injury in 0.8% of trauma patients and 1.9% of trauma patients that undergo CT imaging [26]. The right adrenal gland is far more frequently involved than the left gland by a ratio between 3 and 4 to 1. Isolated adrenal injury is exceedingly rare and is frequently associated with laceration to the liver, spleen or kidney, fractures of the ribs, spine, pelvis or extremities and often accompany head injuries. The mortality in patients sustaining adrenal trauma is reported to be over twice that of patients sustaining blunt trauma without adrenal injury [26]. The relatively low incidence of adrenal injury is not surprising given that the glands are small and well protected in the retroperitoneum surrounded by fat. Mechanism of injury is postulated as direct compression between the spine and the other abdominal organs such as the liver. This could account for the greater incidence in right sided adrenal injury given the relatively smaller space available for the right adrenal gland and the size of the adjacent liver.

Imaging Characteristics

CT is the imaging modality of choice in the initial evaluation of patients sustaining blunt abdominal trauma provided that the patient is hemodynamically stable. Pan scanning is routine and this involves imaging the brain, cervical spine, chest, abdomen and pelvis in one imaging acquisition. Additional CT angiography may also be performed if vascular injury is suspected. Images are acquired using 1.25–2.5 mm slice collimation following the administration of 100 mL of 350 mg/mL iodinated contrast injected intravenously at 2.5–3.5 mL/s. Oral contrast is not routinely required for blunt trauma patients. Adrenal injury is usually identified as a discrete round or oval mass representing hematoma within a limb or body of the gland. Occasionally, the hematoma may lie between the two limbs and the mass splays the limbs around the hematoma. Adrenal hematoma has an average Hounsfield Unit (HU) value of 50–80 HU or so. Uniform diffuse enlargement of the gland with preservation of the adreniform shape may also be seen. In these cases, the margins of the gland are irregular with haziness in the surrounding fat (Fig. 12.4). Bilateral

Fig. 12.4 CT image of a 38-year-old male following blunt abdominal trauma. There is enlargement of the right adrenal gland (*arrow*) with haziness in the periadrenal fat representing blood. Note the left upper pole renal injury

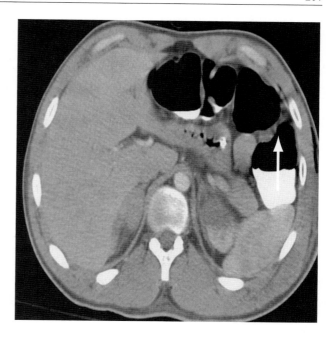

injury may be seen on occasion with similar features seen in both adrenal glands. Blood may extend into the fat surrounding the adrenal gland and this appears as soft tissue stranding infiltrating the peri-adrenal fat. Blood may also collect in the anterior or posterior para renal space and occasionally adrenal hemorrhage may result in thickening of the ipsilateral diaphragmatic crus.

When an adrenal hematoma is identified on CT, it is important to differentiate this entity from an incidental adrenal mass unrelated to the recent trauma. A majority of incidental adrenal masses are non functioning adenomas and approximately 70% of these are lipid rich adenomas that measure less than 10 HU on non contrast CT. The difficulty lies in that a vast majority of trauma CT scans are performed with intravenous contrast and hence non-contrast HU are not available. One option is to obtain delayed images at 10 min and calculate the percentage wash out of contrast from the mass. In the absence of other injuries, an isolated mass in the adrenal gland is almost certainly an adrenal incidentaloma. When other injuries are present and delayed images are either not obtained or are not useful, follow up imaging may help to differentiate these entities. Follow up CT scans will show varying degrees of resolution if the mass is a hematoma.

Hematomas that presented as round or oval masses will show gradual decrease in both size and attenuation. Patients with diffuse enlargement of the adrenal gland will also show evidence of decreased enlargement with time. Adrenal adenomas will not change on short term interval follow up. One caveat to consider, despite the fact that it is extremely rare, is the possibility of hemorrhage into an existing tumor. To this end, unless the appearances are characteristic of traumatic injury, follow up imaging is required to exclude an underlying mass. Fortunately, almost all patients sustaining significant trauma with multiple organ injury will get follow up imaging routinely.

Adrenal injury is for the most part of little clinical significance. Adrenal function is seldom affected following adrenal trauma and may only occur if bilateral adrenal injury is present. A large right sided adrenal hematoma may result in compression of the IVC leading to symptoms of venous congestion and potentially long term IVC thrombosis. One potential concern in patients sustaining adrenal hemorrhage is the possibility of delayed recurrent hemorrhage if the patient is placed on anticoagulation. This may be required if the patient sustains significant concomitant orthopedic injuries.

One feature of imaging that is peculiar to the adrenal gland in patients who have sustained abdominal trauma is the intense enhancement of the adrenal glands following the administration of intravenous contrast. This is thought to result from profound hypotension with extensive blood loss although the exact mechanism is disputed. This sign is often seen along with a collapsed IVC and the so called 'shock bowel' appearance of intense mucosal enhancement of the small bowel following severe blood loss.

Conclusion

The prevalence of adrenal injury following trauma in patients undergoing CT scan is approximately 2%. The frequency of detecting adrenal injury increases with increasing severity of trauma. Adrenal injuries are almost always associated with injuries elsewhere and patients with adrenal injury have a higher mortality. If an adrenal injury is identified, a search should be made for further injuries. In addition, if an isolated adrenal mass is seen on a trauma scan, a pre existing adrenal mass is more likely. Adrenal injuries are easily recognized on CT as a hyperdense mass particularly when associated with surrounding periadrenal stranding.

References

1. Regge D, Balma E, Lasciarrea P, Martina C,Serrallonga M, Gandini G (1995) Interventional radiology of the adrenal glands. Minerva Endocrinol 20(1):15–26
2. Liang HL, Pan HB, Huang JS, Wu TD, Chang CT, Liang HL, Yang TL, Yang F (1999) Small functional adrenal cortical adenoma: treatment with CT-guided percutaneous acetic acid injection–report of three cases. Radiology 213:612–615
3. Rossi R, Savastano S, Tommaselli AP, Valentino R, Iaccarino V, Tauchmanova L, Luciano A, Gigante M, Lombardi G (1995) Percutaneous computed tomography-guided ethanol injection in aldosterone-producing adrenocortical adenoma. Eur J Endocrinol 132:302–305
4. Korobkin M, Francis IR, Kloos RT, Dunnick NR (1996) The incidental adrenal mass. Radiol Clin North Am 34:1037–1054
5. Kenney PJ, Lee KT (1998) The adrenals. Computed body tomography with MRI correlation, vol. 2, 3rd edn. Lippincott-Raven, Philadelphia, PA, p 1190
6. Welch TJ, Sheedy PF II, Stephens DH, Johnson CM, Swensen SJ (1994) Percutaneous adrenal biopsy: review of a 10 year experience. Radiology 193:341
7. Silverman SG, Mueller PR, Pinkney LP, Koenker RM, Seltzer SE (1993) Predictive value of image-guided adrenal biopsy: analysis of results of 101 biopsies. Radiology 187:715–718

8. Mody MK, Kazerooni EA, Korobkin M (1995) Percutaneous CT-guided biopsy of adrenal masses: immediate and delayed complications. J Comput Assist Tomogr 19:434–439
9. Bernardino ME, Walther MM, Phillips VM, Graham SD Jr, Sewell CW, Gedgaudas-McClees K, Baumgartner BR, Torres WE, Erwin BC (1985) CT-guided adrenal biopsy: accuracy, safety, and indications. AJR Am J Roentgenol 144:67–69
10. Paulsen SD, Nghiem HV, Korobkin M, Caoili EM, Higgins EJ (2004) Changing role of imaging-guided percutaneous biopsy of adrenal masses: evaluation of 50 adrenal biopsies. AJR Am J Roentgenol 182(4):1033–1037
11. Caoili EM, Korobkin M, Francis IR, Cohan RH, Platt JF, Dunnick NR, Raghupathi KI (2002) Adrenal masses: characterization with combined unenhanced and delayed enhanced CT. Radiology 222(3):629–633
12. Blake MA, Kalra MK, Sweeney AT, Lucey BC, Maher MM, Sahani DV, Halpern EF, Mueller PR, Hahn PF, Boland GW (2006) Distinguishing benign from malignant adrenal masses: multi-detector row CT protocol with 10-minute delay. Radiology 238(2):578–585
13. Stelow EB, Debol SM, Stanley MW, Mallery S, Lai R, Bardales RH (2005) Sampling of the adrenal glands by endoscopic ultrasound-guided fine-needle aspiration. Diagn Cytopathol 33(1):26–30
14. Mayo-Smith WW, Dupuy DE (2004) Adrenal neoplasms: CT-guided radiofrequency ablation–preliminary results. Radiology 231(1):225–230
15. Wood BJ, Abraham J, Hvizda JL, Alexander HR, Fojo T (2003) Radiofrequency ablation of adrenal tumors and adrenocortical carcinoma metastases. Cancer 197(3):554–560
16. Tung GA, Pfister RC, Papanicolaou N, Yoder IC (1989) Adrenal cysts: imaging and percutaneous aspiration. Radiology 173(1):107–110
17. Gordon RD (1994) Mineralocorticoid hypertension. Lancet 344:240–243
18. Calhoun DA, Nishizaka MK, Zaman MA, Thakkar RB, Weissmann N (2002) Hyperaldosteronism among black and white subjects with resistant hypertension. Hypertension 40:892–896
19. Magill SB, Raff H, Shaker JL, Brickner RC, Knechtges TE, Kehoe ME, Findling JW (2001) Comparison of adrenal vein sampling and computed tomography in the differentiation of primary aldosteronism. J Clin Endocrinol Metab 86:1066–1071
20. Daunt N (2005) Adrenal vein sampling: how to make it quick, easy, and successful. RadioGraphics 25:S143–S158
21. Stowasser M, Gordon RD, Rutherford JC, Nikwan NZ, Daunt N, Slater GJ (2001) Diagnosis and management of primary aldosteronism. J Renin Angiotensin Aldosterone Syst 2:156–169
22. Bookstein JJ (1983) The roles of angiography in adrenal disease. In: Abram's angiography, 3rd edn. Little, Brown, Boston, Mass, pp 1395–1424
23. Walters NA, Thomson KR (1993) Urogenital venography. In: Rifkin MD, Thomson K, Rickards D, Jones S (eds) Practical interventional uroradiology. Edward Arnold, Edinburgh, Scotland, chap 11
24. Sevitt S (1955) Post-traumatic adrenal apoplexy. J Clin Pathol 8:185–194

25. Burks DW, Mirvis SE, Shanmuganathan K (1992) Acute adrenal injury after blunt abdominal trauma: CT findings. AJR Am J Roentgenol 158(3):503–507

26. Rana AI, Kenney PJ, Lockhart ME, McGwin G Jr, Morgan DE, Windham ST III, Smith JK (2004) Adrenal gland hematomas in trauma patients. Radiology 230(3):669–675

13

Evolving Functional and Advanced Image Analysis Techniques for Adrenal Lesion Characterization

Nagaraj Setty Holalkere and Michael A. Blake

Contents

N.S. Holalkere (✉)
Department of Radiology, Boston Medical Center,
820 Harrison Ave, FGH Building, 3rd floor, Boston,
MA 02118
E-mail: Nagaraj.Holalkere@bmc.org

Introduction

Recent advances in imaging techniques and the widespread use of high-resolution thin slice CT imaging has led to an increased detection of adrenal lesions as has been discussed in earlier chapters [1, 2]. It is again essential to characterize all adrenal lesions in patients with known cancer elsewhere in the body because many tumors particularly lung cancer have a propensity to metastasize into the adrenal glands [3]. However, the majority of adrenal lesions are still benign cortical adenomas and only 26%−36% of adrenal lesions in patients with a known cancer are metastatic [4, 5]. Nonetheless, it is critical to differentiate benign from malignant lesions because the presence of metastasis might contraindicate a curative surgery or radiotherapy and may have significant impact on life expectancy [6]. Conventional imaging techniques with measurement of Hounsfield units on non enhanced CT, washout characteristics on CT and drop in signal intensity on out-of-phase chemical shift MR imaging help to characterize the majority of the adrenal lesions again as discussed in detail in Chaps. 9 and 10. However, still a sizable percent of adrenal lesions require either biopsy or surgery or interval follow-up to determine the type of lesion. Recent advances in image acquisition and post processing techniques on both CT and MR are helping to expand the research tools available for adrenal imaging. In this chapter, the evolving concepts and principles of advanced image analysis that can be utilized for adrenal lesion characterization such as dual energy

M.A. Blake, G. Boland (eds.), *Adrenal Imaging*, DOI 10.1007/978-1-59745-560-2_13,
© 2009 Humana Press, a part of Springer Science+Business Media, LLC

CT and histogram analysis as well as functional techniques such as diffusion weighted imaging, MR spectroscopy and perfusion imaging will be discussed.

Advanced Image Analysis Techniques
Dual Energy CT

Similar to CT densitometry performed on non-enhanced CT scans to identify microscopic fat in adrenal lesions to differentiate adenomatous from non-adenomatous lesions, dual energy CT can also be performed to detect fat in adrenal lesions. This technique is a well-established in determination of bone mineral density and has been used for differentiating fatty liver from low density masses in the liver [7, 8].

Basic Principle

Dual energy CT is based on the principle that differences in X-ray attenuation diminishes with increasing energy of X-rays used. When low-density substance such as fat increases, the CT attenuation values at different energy levels tend to decrease, and the CT attenuation values at low-energy levels decrease more than those at high-energy levels [9].

We can take advantage of this phenomenon to quantify fat in the adrenal glands by measuring the difference in CT attenuation acquired at 140 and 80 kVp. If the difference of attenuation between the two kVp images is >6 HU then it is suggestive of fat containing lesions such as adenomas or myelolipomas:

$$\text{If HU 140 kVp} - \text{HU 80 kVp} \geq 6\text{, then fat is present.}$$

There are no published data utilizing this technique for adrenal lesion characterization; however, a recent abstract presented by Li et al. have shown a mean change in attenuation values between 140 kVp and 80 kVp of 11.2 ± 2.3 HU for adenoma as compared to 1.7 ± 0.6 HU for normal adrenal gland and 3.4 ± 0.6 HU for malignant masses with an average change in attenuation value significantly higher for adenoma compared to the other group ($p < 0.001$) [10] (Fig. 13.1). The technique is relatively simple and can be performed on any scanner using routine software available on picture archiving and communication systems (PACS) for analysis. The main limitations of this technique are that there is minimal increase in radiation dose as compared to standard non-enhanced CT and images at 80 kVp have

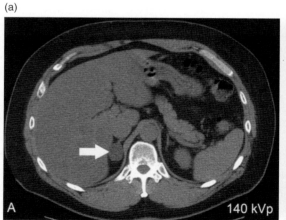
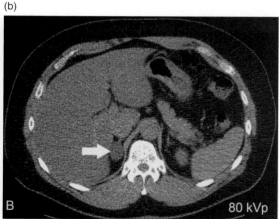

Fig. 13.1 Axial CT sections of the right upper abdomen in a 55-year-old male using dual energy CT, i.e. 140 kVp (**a**) and 80 kVp (**b**) demonstrate a right adrenal nodule that has a mean attenuation of 12 HU on 140 kVp and 4 HU on 80 kVp images with a difference of 8 HU consistent with lipid containing adrenal adenoma

increased noise that results in a wide standard deviation of estimated attenuation values. In addition, it is also important to note that the region of interest (ROI) for measurement of attenuation should again be within the lesion since inclusion of peripheral fat results in false positive results for fat. Further studies are essential in understanding its role in characterization of adrenal lesions including lipid poor adenomas in comparison to other well-established imaging techniques.

Histogram Analysis

As was discussed in detail in Chap. 9, adrenal adenomas often contain intracytoplasmic lipid in the adrenal cortex unlike metastases and thus demonstrate low attenuation at unenhanced CT. The region of interest based 10 HU threshold mean attenuation measurement for differentiating adenomas from indeterminate lesions on unenhanced CT has a sensitivity of only 71% with specificity of 98% for diagnosis of adrenal adenoma [11] likely due to the presence of lipid poor adenomas. Further, with contrast enhancement, there is too much overlap between adrenal adenomas and non-adenomas partly due to the heterogeneous tissue composition in adrenal adenomas and partly due to enhancement and overall increase in mean attenuation even though lipid tissue is present in adenomas. Thus an alternative method of identification of lipid and thus adenoma on unenhanced and contrast enhanced CT is to perform histogram or pixelogram analysis, where the density in each pixel can be measured that helps to characterize the lesion more accurately.

Basic Principle

The histogram is a graphical plot of pixel attenuation (CT numbers) along the x-axis vs the frequency of pixels at each attenuation value along the y-axis. Thus it allows estimation of distribution of tissue attenuation in a mass rather than calculation of an overall mean attenuation in a ROI. It also allows the measurement of mean attenuation, number of pixels, and range of pixel attenuation for all pixels in the ROI placed carefully within the boundaries of the lesion. ROI can be placed on either a single axial section or on all the sections of the adrenal lesion by manually or by using computer software that generates semi automatic segmentation of lesions to obtain a volumetric data. The percentages of negative pixels are calculated from the total number of pixels and the number of negative pixels in each ROI.

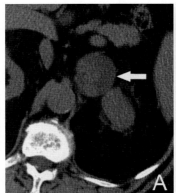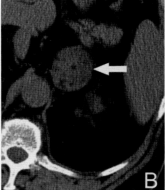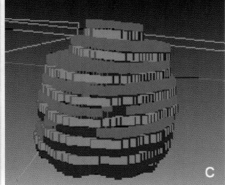

Fig. 13.2 Axial CT sections of left adrenal lesion at lower (**a**) and upper (**b**) level of the lesion demonstrate varying consistency of the lesion with minimal heterogeneity at the lower level (**b**). Single slice histogram from each of these slices may give different results and hence a volume histogram analysis performed by computing pixel wise HU values for entire tumor volume (**c**). Here, the volume histogram was more uniform and demonstrated 32% of pixels with <0 HU which was consistent with a feature of adenoma

Table 13.1 Results from various studies on Histogram analysis

Study	Comment[a]	Sensitivity	Specificity
Bae et al. [12]	Both NECT and CECT with −ve pixel	–	100%
Remer et al. [13] Pathologically proven adrenal masses	NECT with >10% −ve pixel	77%	88%
	CECT with >10% −ve pixel	12%	99%
Jhaveri et al. [14] Histogram vs Chemical shift (CSI) MRI	>10% −ve pixel	46%	100%
	>20% signal drop on CSI	71%	100%

[a]NECT = Non-enhanced CT and CECT = Contrast enhanced CT

A value of 10% negative pixels or pixels with ≤0 HU is used for detection of significant fat and thus adenoma using histogram analysis (Fig. 13.2). The results of various published studies on histogram analysis are discussed in Table 13.1 [12–14]. In our experience from 72 biopsy proven indeterminate adrenal lesions, the volumetric histogram analysis demonstrates a higher specificity of 93.3% as compared to 80% for single slice analysis.

Functional Imaging Techniques

Nuclear Medicine

FDG-PET and PET/CT provide metabolic information with radiotracers such as ^{18}F fluorodeoxyglucose and can help to differentiate benign and malignant lesions. Malignant lesions display intense FDG uptake greater than that of liver due to increased glucose metabolism. The other conventional metabolic studies such as adrenal scintigraphy

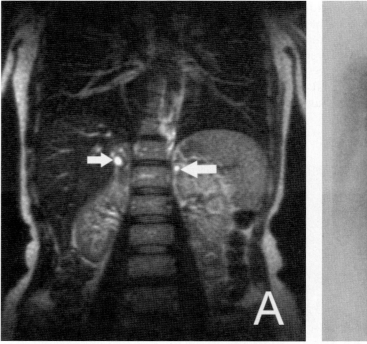
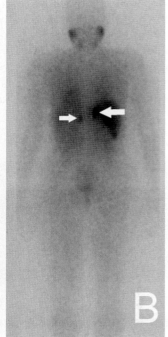

Fig. 13.3 Bilateral hyperintense focus in the adrenal glands on T2W coronal section MRI in a 32-year-old (**a**) that demonstrates an avid meta-iodo-benzyl-guanidine (MIBG) uptake on adrenal scintigraphy (**b**) representing bilateral pheochromocytoma

using ^{131}I-6-beta-iodomethyl-19-norcholesterol or 6-methyl-^{75}Se-methyl-19-norcholesterol meta-iodobenzyl-guanidine (MIBG), marked with ^{131}I or ^{123}I provide adrenal cortical and medullary function respectively (Fig. 13.3). The comprehensive role of these nuclear metabolic imaging methods for adrenal imaging is discussed in Chaps. 11 and 12.

Diffusion-weighted MR Imaging (DWI)

Diffusion is thermally induced motion of water molecules in biologic tissues, called Brownian motion. Water molecules are in constant motion, and the rate of movement or diffusion depends on the kinetic energy of the molecules and is temperature dependent. In biological tissues, diffusion is not truly random because tissue has structure. Changes in cell membranes, vascular structures and viscosity of the media can limit or restrict the amount of diffusion. Also, chemical interactions of water and macromolecules affect diffusion properties. DWI was primarily used in brain imaging but with the advent of the echo-planar MR imaging technique, DWI of the abdomen has become possible with fast imaging times, which minimize the effect of gross physiologic motion from respiration and cardiac movement.

Basic Principle

DWI can provide an insight into water composition within a tumor. Benign tumors tend to have proportionate increase of cells as well as intercellular space whereas malignant tumors usually have a disproportionate increase of cells (mitotic activity) as compared to interstitial tissue as well as disrupted cell membranes. These properties of malignancies result in selective restriction of diffusion of water molecules that may provide strong evidence for malignancy in an adrenal lesion (Fig. 13.4). On the other hand, the lack of restricted diffusion may correlate with a benign or borderline neoplastic tumor (Fig. 13.5). This information if validated would have significant implications on the management of patients with adrenal lesions. For example a benign appearing adrenal lesion on DWI exam would be managed conservatively whereas a malignant result would guide appropriate treatment.

Technique

To obtain diffusion-weighted images, a pair of strong gradient pulses is added to the pulse sequence. The first pulse dephases the spins, and the second pulse rephases the spins if no net movement occurs. If net movement of spins occurs between the gradient pulses, signal attenuation occurs. The degree of attenuation depends on the magnitude of molecular translation or diffusion of water molecule that and can be related through the following equation:

$$S/S_0 = e^{-\gamma^2 G^2 \delta^2 (\Delta - \delta/3)D} = e^{-bD}$$

where S_0 is the signal intensity without the diffusion weighting, S is the signal with the gradient, γ is the gyromagnetic ratio, G is the strength of the gradient pulse, δ is the duration of the pulse, Δ is the time between the two pulses, b is the diffusion sensitizing factor and D is the diffusion constant. The amount of diffusion weighting is determined by the strength of the diffusion gradients, the duration of the gradients, and the time between the gradient pulses. Therefore, the use of high field gradient systems with faster and more sensitive sequences makes diffusion weighting more feasible [15–17].

Diffusion imaging is performed optimally on a high-field (1.5 T or above) systems using either conventional spin-echo or stimulated echo, fast spin-echo, gradient-echo (e.g., steady-state free precession), echo planar imaging (EPI), and line

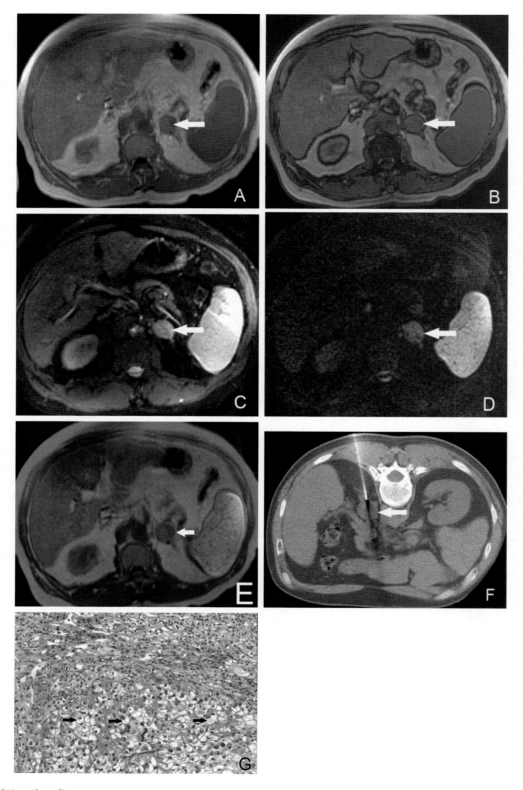

Fig. 13.4 (continued)

Fig. 13.4 MRI, DWI and histopathology images in a 52-year-old man with a history of renal cell cancer demonstrates an adrenal lesion on left side (*arrow*). On chemical shift MRI in in-phase (**a**) and out-of-phase (**b**) there was no fat and DWI with b = 50 (**c**) and b = 500 (**d**) demonstrate a hyperintense lesion suggesting restricted diffusion and malignant lesion. The lesion was less hyperintense on DWI with b = 1000 and when it was fused with the corresponding T1 weighted image (**e**) the signal intensity can be localized to the adrenal gland. Tissue sample was obtained using CT guided biopsy (**f**) and histopathology (**g**) demonstrated clear cells (*small arrows*) from renal cell cancer. The DWI findings thus correlated with the histopathological features of metastasis

scan diffusion imaging [18]. Each of these techniques has its advantages and limitations [18, 19]. DWI of the adrenal gland can be performed using either breath-hold or non-breath-hold imaging sequences. The diffusion data can be presented as signal intensity or as an image map of the apparent diffusion coefficient (ADC). Calculation of the ADC requires two or more acquisitions with different diffusion weightings. A low ADC corresponds to high signal intensity (restricted diffusion), and a high ADC to low signal intensity on diffusion-weighted images. Breath-hold imaging allows a target volume to be rapidly assessed. The images retain good anatomic detail and are usually not degraded by respiratory motion or volume averaging. Small lesions may be better perceived and the quantification of ADC

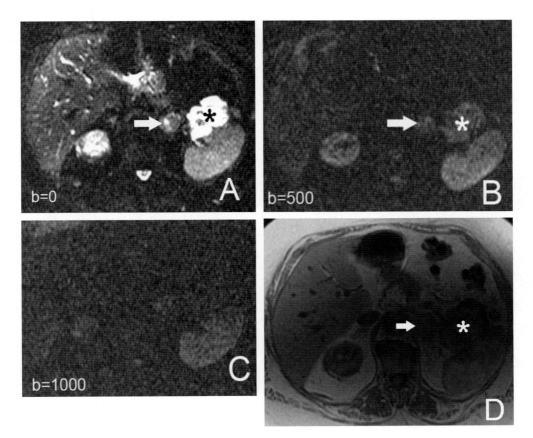

Fig. 13.5 DWI demonstrated a lesion in left adrenal gland (*arrow*) and a large mass in the tail of the pancreas (*). Signal intensity of adrenal lesion on DWI was iso to hypo intense and dropped as the b value increased from 0 (**a**) to 500 (**b**) and to 1000 (**c**) suggesting lack of restricted diffusion. Fused imaged (**d**) helped to localize the signal intensity of DWI to the adrenal gland. Subject underwent surgery and both the adrenal and pancreatic lesions were benign and correlated with DWI features of benignity

is theoretically more accurate than with a non-breath-hold technique. Authors prefer to use breath-hold single-shot spin-echo EPI with parameters of TE = minimum, TR = 3000, NEX = 1, thickness/skip = 5/0 mm, b value = 0, 250 and 500 s/mm², matrix = 128 × 128, combined with parallel imaging (e.g., sensitivity encoding) and fat suppression for adrenal imaging due to the advantages discussed before [20–22]. The image acquisition time at each breath-hold is 12–20 s. Earlier published studies on DWI of upper abdomen and liver imaging have also suggested similar parameters [16, 18]. The disadvantages of breath-hold imaging include a limited number of b-value images that can be acquired over the duration of a breath-hold, poorer signal-to-noise ratio compared with multiple averaging methods, and greater sensitivity to pulsatile and susceptibility artifacts.

To date there are no published studies on the utility of DWI and ADC maps in characterization of adrenal lesions. However, Uhl et al. have demonstrated restricted diffusion in 7/7 (100%) neuroblastoma cases including two in adrenal glands [23]. Based on this and our initial experience, we believe that the DWI and ADC maps will increase the accuracy of detection of malignancy in the adrenal gland. The main advantages of DWI are no associated radiation and no requirement for intravenous contrast administration. At present the main limitations of DWI remain technique related and it is hoped that this can be optimized in the near future for routine clinical application.

MR Spectroscopy (MRS)

MR spectroscopy has been shown to be useful in quantification of liver fat in the abdomen and thus may prove to be useful in identifying fat in benign adrenal lesions. In vivo nuclear magnetic resonance spectroscopy (MRS) is growing rapidly as a result of the development of effective MR instrumentation and increasing availability of whole-body MR imaging systems for diagnostic radiology. Many clinical MR systems now have state-of-the-art in vivo MRS capabilities, allowing the systematic use of MRS in many

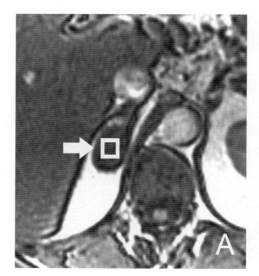
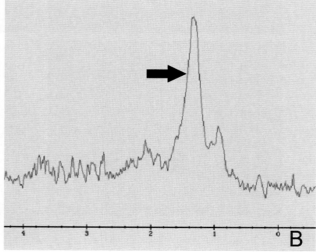

Fig. 13.6 Single voxel proton MR spectroscopy obtained by defining a voxel (**a**) from adrenal nodule demonstrates the spectrum (**b**) with a raised lipid peak at 1.3 ppm consistent with adrenal adenoma

areas of medicine. It is a non-invasive technique, which allows the study of cellular biochemistry and metabolism. It is a diverse research tool, widely used by biochemists to investigate pathophysiological processes in vitro and more recently, by physicians to determine disease abnormalities in vivo [24–27].

Basic Principle

Absolute quantization of metabolite concentrations offers a number of advantages for the evaluation of in vivo MR spectroscopic data. The presence of a lipid peak at 1.3 ppm on the MR spectra in an adrenal lesion could confidently characterize adrenal lesions into a benign category (Fig. 13.6). Quantification of choline-containing compounds (Cho) at 3–3.3 ppm is also of great interest because such compounds have shown to be increased in malignancy [28]. Researchers are actively investigating adrenal lesion characterization as a practical application of MR spectroscopy.

Technique

MRS provides information about the normal chemical composition of a tissue and thus can detect changes in chemical composition, which may occur in disease processes [29]. High levels of homogeneity of the main magnetic field are a prerequisite to resolve different chemical species in tissues, which can be achieved by shimming the magnetic field in the region of interest to the resonance of water. Water is the dominant peak in hydrogen spectroscopy. The intensity of all metabolites is scaled relative to that of water when an analog-to-digital conversion is performed. The most common technique used to suppress the water peak is by Chemical Shift Selective Imaging Sequence (CHESS). This technique uses a frequency-selective 90° pulse to excite the water signal selectively , which is followed by a spoiler gradient to dephase the resulting magnetization. These gradients may be repeated several times in different directions to increase its effectiveness [30].

Diagnostically resolvable hydrogen MR spectra may be obtained using routinely used clinical instruments (1.5 T or greater) and surface coils. However, the new generation of 3-T clinical scanners offer better signal to noise ratio and spectral resolution. A basic step in spectroscopy is the localization of the region of interest in all three spatial dimensions, thus generating the volume of interest. This can be performed using two methods [31]:

1. Single-voxel spectroscopy (SVS)
2. Chemical-shift imaging (CSI)

SVS is more useful for adrenal lesion evaluation for the following reasons: it provides metabolic information from a small volume of tissue, water suppression is more effective and the acquisition time is shorter with less susceptibility to motion, quantum effects, and diffusion [32].

Point Resolved Spectroscopy (PRESS) is the most commonly used SVS technique. It uses longer echo times and therefore allows visualization of metabolites with longer relaxation times that is optimal for adrenal imaging. Acquisition parameters of TR (repetition time) = 2000–3000 ms, TE (echo time) = 20–30 m, spectral width = 1000–2500 Hz spectral width and data points of 1000–2000 with 16–32 acquisitions are commonly used. A voxel of 8–30 cm^3 is used for data acquisition by avoiding adjacent fat places and restricting the edge of voxel to a position more than 5 mm from the inner margin of the adrenal lesion. This will help to prevent the spectrum from being contaminated by strong signals originating from the fat, which can mask resonance from adrenal adenoma fat. Signals can be acquired either during quiet regular respiration without respiratory interruption by respiratory gating or during breath hold. If a breath-hold technique is employed, the acquisition is split into 2 or 3 parts and a compression belt is used to reduce respiratory motion [26].

In vivo single voxel proton MRS is a non-invasive technique for evaluating the various biochemical processes [26, 27, 30, 33]. Currently, clinical applications of adrenal proton MRS are limited. However, a study by Johnsen et al. on

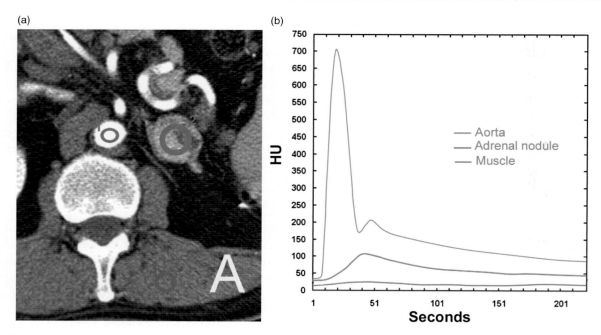

Fig. 13.7 CT Perfusion source image (**a**) illustrating selection of the arterial (*1*) and regions-of-interest (ROIs) left adrenal nodule (*2*), needed to construct the representative time attenuation curves (TACs). TACs (**b**) of aorta (*1*) and adrenal nodule (*2*) depicts highest peak enhancement in aortic TAC as compared to adrenal nodule

adrenal neuroblastoma following treatment with NSAIDs demonstrated depletion of choline on MRS [28]. Thus, MRS has the potential to emerge as a promising tool in adrenal imaging with the continuing advances in MR scanners and post processing techniques.

Perfusion Imaging

Perfusion imaging has been well established for brain tumors and has also been proven to be valuable in other abdominal tumors such as HCC and rectal cancers [34–36]. Similar to these tumors, malignant adrenal tumors are likely to demonstrate higher permeability surface due to the presence of disorganized neovasculature and increased blood flow in contrast to benign adenomatous lesions where vascular organization is preserved [37]. Thus, CT or MR perfusion (dynamic or functional) imaging may also prove useful in further characterization of indeterminate adrenal lesions.

Basic Principle

The determination of tissue perfusion using CT or MR is based on the relationships between the arterial, tissue and potentially the venous enhancement after the introduction of a bolus of contrast material. Malignant tumors tend to have disorganized and highly permeable blood vessels with resulting early enhancement and washout of contrast on CT and MRI. This phenomenon is utilized and quantification of perfusion performed by measuring tumor blood flow, blood volume and permeability surface or k-trans on CT or MR perfusion imaging [37–39]. Dynamic rapid repeated CT or MRI scans acquired at the same location of the tumor after contrast administration is used for estimation of these perfusion parameters. A change in attenuation or signal intensity due to contrast material is directly proportional to the concentration of the contrast material and plotting of attenuation or signal intensity with time gives time-attenuation curves (TAC) or time-signal intensity curve (TSC) on CT or MRI respectively [38] (Fig. 13.7). Initially, a non-contrast enhanced images are acquired

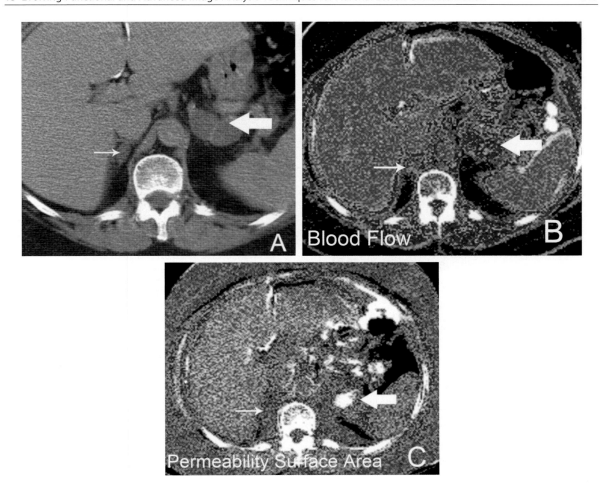

Fig. 13.8 Axial CT scan (**a**) in a patient with lung cancer demonstrates the normal right adrenal (*thin arrow*) and metastasis (*thick arrow*) in the left adrenal gland. Dynamic CT perfusion (parameters of gantry rotation time of 1 s, kVp 100, mA 240, acquisition in 4i axial mode, 5 mm reconstructed slice thickness, 6 s delay following injection of 50 cc contrast media at 5 cc/s and scanned continuously in breath hold for 25 s, and then followed by intermittent scanning once every 12 s for a total duration of 150 s) with blood flow map (**b**) depicts a higher blood flow (*mixture of blue and red color*) in the metastasis compared to normal right gland (*blue and green color*). On absolute quantification the difference was 40%. Permeability surface area product map (**c**) also depicts a higher (*red and bright yellow*) value for metastasis as compared to normal right gland (*green color*). On absolute quantification the difference was 55%

and are subtracted from the contrast-enhanced images to obtain time enhancement data. Also, use of regions of interest allows the generation of organ, regional or pixel time enhancement curves. Later, TAC or TSC curves are used to generate perfusion values using different post processing techniques. The key differences between CT (Fig. 13.8) and MR perfusion (Fig. 13.9) are summarized in Table 13.2 [40].

Currently, both CT and MRI perfusion imaging are being evaluated for various organs in the body and their application in adrenal lesion evaluation has not yet been explored much. However from our experience with a few selected patients, perfusion imaging is another potential tool for adrenal lesion characterization but will need to be studied further before it can be adopted for clinical applications.

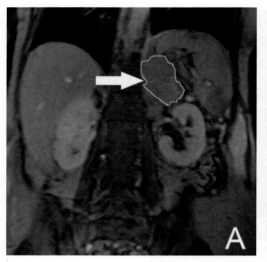
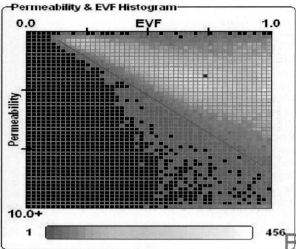

Fig. 13.9 MR perfusion (parameters of coronal VIBE sequence, TR/TE = 5/1.5 ms, flip angle = 15°, matrix = 192 × 123, delay of 10 s following 0.2 mmol/kg of gadolinium injection and scanned intermittently for every 14 s in breath hold for 5 min with 14 s between breath hold) with region of interest placed for adrenal metastasis in a 62-year-old male with hepatocellular cancer (**a**) and mapping of pixel wise k trans (permeability) vs extra vascular fraction (**b**) demonstrate a mean k trans value of 2.5 (*red line*) suggestive of high permeability and a feature of malignant lesion

Table 13.2 Differences between CT and MRI perfusion imaging

Parameter	CT perfusion	MR perfusion
Contrast enhancement	Linear	Exponential (some times unpredictable)
Models for analysis	Simple	Relatively complex
Temporal resolution <1 s	Possible	Not possible
Respiration, motion, co-registration issues	Common	More common
Scanning parameters	Few	Many
Variability between vendors	Less frequent	Frequent
Area covered for imaging	Up to 4 cm (64 MDCT)	Unlimited
Kinetic parameters measured	Blood flow, blood volume, mean transit time, permeability	Transfer constants, leakage space, blood volume and flow

Conclusion and Summary

In summary, CT and MR remain the primary imaging modalities for characterization of adrenal lesions. Recently developed techniques of dual energy CT and histogram analysis may offer additional information. The value of PET and PET/CT has already been proven and other new functional imaging techniques such as perfusion; diffusion-weighted imaging and MR spectroscopy may play an important role in lesion characterization in the near future. These exciting techniques may soon to be routinely available and could potentially further obviate the need for adrenal biopsies that are performed in indeterminate cases. The final goal of adrenal imaging is to achieve accurate characterization of all adrenal lesions in order to optimize patient care.

References

1. Sahdev A, Reznek RH (2004) Imaging evaluation of the non-functioning indeterminate adrenal mass. Trends Endocrinol Metab 15(6):271–276
2. Dunnick NR, Korobkin M, Francis I (1996) Adrenal radiology: distinguishing benign from malignant adrenal masses. AJR Am J Roentgenol 167(4):861–867
3. Lam KY, Lo CY (2002) Metastatic tumours of the adrenal glands: a 30-year experience in a teaching hospital. Clin Endocrinol (Oxf) 56(1):95–101

4. Oliver TW Jr, Bernardino ME, Miller JI, Mansour K, Greene D, Davis WA (1984) Isolated adrenal masses in nonsmall-cell bronchogenic carcinoma. Radiology 153(1): 217–218

5. Katz RL, Patel S, Mackay B, Zornoza J (1984) Fine needle aspiration cytology of the adrenal gland. Acta Cytol 28(3):269–282

6. Mitchell IC, Nwariaku FE (2007) Adrenal masses in the cancer patient: surveillance or excision. Oncologist 12(2):168–174

7. Wang B, Gao Z, Zou Q, Li L (2003) Quantitative diagnosis of fatty liver with dual-energy CT. An experimental study in rabbits. Acta Radiol 44(1):92–97

8. Raptopoulos V, Karellas A, Bernstein J, Reale FR, Constantinou C, Zawacki JK (1991) Value of dual-energy CT in differentiating focal fatty infiltration of the liver from low-density masses. AJR Am J Roentgenol 157(4):721–725

9. Cann CE, Gamsu G, Birnberg FA, Webb WR (1982) Quantification of calcium in solitary pulmonary nodules using single- and dual-energy CT. Radiology 145(2):493–496

10. Li J, Udayasankar UK, Kalra MK, Small WC (2007) Genitourinary (renal and adrenal gland imaging). Adrenal mass: differentiation by attenuation characteristics using dual-energy MDCT. AJR Am J Roentgenol 188(Suppl 5):A59-62

11. Boland GW, Lee MJ, Gazelle GS, Halpern EF, McNicholas MM, Mueller PR (1998) Characterization of adrenal masses using unenhanced CT: an analysis of the CT literature. AJR Am J Roentgenol 171(1):201–204

12. Bae KT, Fuangtharnthip P, Prasad SR, Joe BN, Heiken JP (2003) Adrenal masses: CT characterization with histogram analysis method. Radiology 228(3):735–742

13. Remer EM, Motta-Ramirez GA, Shepardson LB, Hamrahian AH, Herts BR (2006) CT histogram analysis in pathologically proven adrenal masses. AJR Am J Roentgenol 187(1):191196

14. Jhaveri KS, Wong F, Ghai S, Haider MA (2006) Comparison of CT histogram analysis and chemical shift MRI in the characterization of indeterminate adrenal nodules. AJR Am J Roentgenol 187(5):1303–1308

15. Mori S, Barker PB (1999) Diffusion magnetic resonance imaging: its principle and applications. Anat Rec 257(3): 102–109

16. Naganawa S, Kawai H, Fukatsu H et al. (2005) Diffusion-weighted imaging of the liver: technical challenges and prospects for the future. Magn Reson Med Sci 4(4):175–186

17. Luypaert R, Boujraf S, Sourbron S, Osteaux M (2001) Diffusion and perfusion MRI: basic physics. Eur J Radiol 38(1):19–27

18. Koh DM, Collins DJ (2007) Diffusion-weighted MRI in the body: applications and challenges in oncology. AJR Am J Roentgenol 188(6):1622–1635

19. Bammer R (2003) Basic principles of diffusion-weighted imaging. Eur J Radiol 45(3):169–184

20. Squillaci E, Manenti G, Di Stefano F, Miano R, Strigari L, Simonetti G (2004) Diffusion-weighted MR imaging in the evaluation of renal tumours. J Exp Clin Cancer Res 23(1):39–45

21. Yamashita Y, Tang Y, Takahashi M (1998) Ultrafast MR imaging of the abdomen: echo planar imaging and diffusion-weighted imaging. J Magn Reson Imaging 8(2):367–374

22. Park SW, Lee JH, Ehara S et al. (2004) Single shot fast spin echo diffusion-weighted MR imaging of the spine; Is it useful in differentiating malignant metastatic tumor infiltration from benign fracture edema? Clin Imaging 28(2):102–108

23. Uhl M, Altehoefer C, Kontny U, Il'yasov K, Buchert M, Langer M (2002) MRI-diffusion imaging of neuroblastomas: first results and correlation to histology. Eur Radiol 12(9):2335–2338

24. Chang JS, Taouli B, Salibi N, Hecht EM, Chin DG, Lee VS (2006) Opposed-phase MRI for fat quantification in fat-water phantoms with 1 H MR spectroscopy to resolve ambiguity of fat or water dominance. AJR Am J Roentgenol 187(1):W103–106

25. Longo R, Ricci C, Masutti F et al. (1993) Fatty infiltration of the liver. Quantification by 1 H localized magnetic resonance spectroscopy and comparison with computed tomography. Invest Radiol 28(4):297–302

26. Szczepaniak LS, Nurenberg P, Leonard D et al. (2005) Magnetic resonance spectroscopy to measure hepatic triglyceride content: prevalence of hepatic steatosis in the general population. Am J Physiol Endocrinol Metab 288(2):E462–468

27. Thomas EL, Hamilton G, Patel N et al. (2005) Hepatic triglyceride content and its relation to body adiposity: a magnetic resonance imaging and proton magnetic resonance spectroscopy study. Gut 54(1):122–127

28. Johnsen JI, Lindskog M, Ponthan F et al. (2005) NSAIDs in neuroblastoma therapy. Cancer Lett 28(1/2): 195–201

29. Castillo M, Kwock L, Mukherji SK (1996) Clinical applications of proton MR spectroscopy. AJNR Am J Neuroradiol 17(1):1–15

30. Cousins JP (1995) Clinical MR spectroscopy: fundamentals, current applications, and future potential. AJR Am J Roentgenol 164(6):1337–1347

31. Frahm J, Bruhn H, Gyngell ML, Merboldt KD, Hanicke W, Sauter R (1989) Localized high-resolution proton NMR spectroscopy using stimulated echoes: initial applications to human brain in vivo. Magn Reson Med 9(1):79–93

32. Hsu YY, Chang C, Chang CN, Chu NS, Lim KE, Hsu JC (1999) Proton MR spectroscopy in patients with complex partial seizures: single-voxel spectroscopy versus chemical-shift imaging. AJNR Am J Neuroradiol 20(4):643–651

33. Kim DY, Kim KB, Kim OD, Kim JK (1998) Localized in vivo proton spectroscopy of renal cell carcinoma in human kidney. J Korean Med Sci 13(1):49–53

34. Guan S, Zhao WD, Zhou KR, Peng WJ, Tang F, Mao J (2007) Assessment of hemodynamics in precancerous lesion of hepatocellular carcinoma: evaluation with MR perfusion. World J Gastroenterol 13(8):1182–1186

35. Sahani DV, Holalkere NS, Mueller PR, Zhu AX (2007) Advanced hepatocellular carcinoma: CT perfusion of liver and tumor tissue–initial experience. Radiology 243(3):736–743

36. Lankester KJ, Taylor JN, Stirling JJ et al. (2007) Dynamic MRI for imaging tumor microvasculature: comparison of susceptibility and relaxivity techniques in pelvic tumors. J Magn Reson Imaging 25(4):796–805

37. Miller JC, Pien HH, Sahani D, Sorensen AG, Thrall JH (2005) Imaging angiogenesis: applications and potential for drug development. J Natl Cancer Inst 97(3):172–187

38. Goh V, Padhani AR (2006) Imaging tumor angiogenesis: functional assessment using MDCT or MRI? Abdom Imaging 31(2):194–199

39. Miles KA, Griffiths MR (2003) Perfusion CT: a worthwhile enhancement? Br J Radiol 76(904):220–231

40. Jeswani T, Padhani AR (2005) Imaging tumour angiogenesis. Cancer Imaging 5:131–138

Index